Inside you'll find:

- **SHAREABLE PLATES:** Invite your friends to share Roasted Eggplant with Tahini & Walnuts.

- **SPREADS & DIPS:** Make them a lifestyle with Baba Ghanoush and Garlic Feta Dip.

- **SALADS:** Hearty faves like Spicy Tuna Salad and Mediterranean Chicken Salad won't leave you hungry.

- **MAINS:** You'll crave the main event with Lamb Koftas with Cucumber Dill Yogurt Sauce, Ricotta-Stuffed Eggplant Rolls, and Spicy Walnut Jumbo Scallops.

- **PASTA & RICE:** Pasta Carbonara and "Marry Me" Chicken Pasta will soothe your soul.

- **POWER BOWLS:** Arash's viral Salmon Power Bowl and Korean Beef Bowl will crush your macros and your hunger.

- **SAUCES & SALSAS:** Chili Lime Everything Sauce, Zhoug, Chermoula, and Spicy Yum Yum Sauce are absolute game-changers that elevate the most basic plate of protein and veggies into a whole new dimension.

- **DESSERTS:** Satisfy your sweet tooth minus the carbs with Lemon Ricotta Crepes and Baklava Pancakes.

shred happens

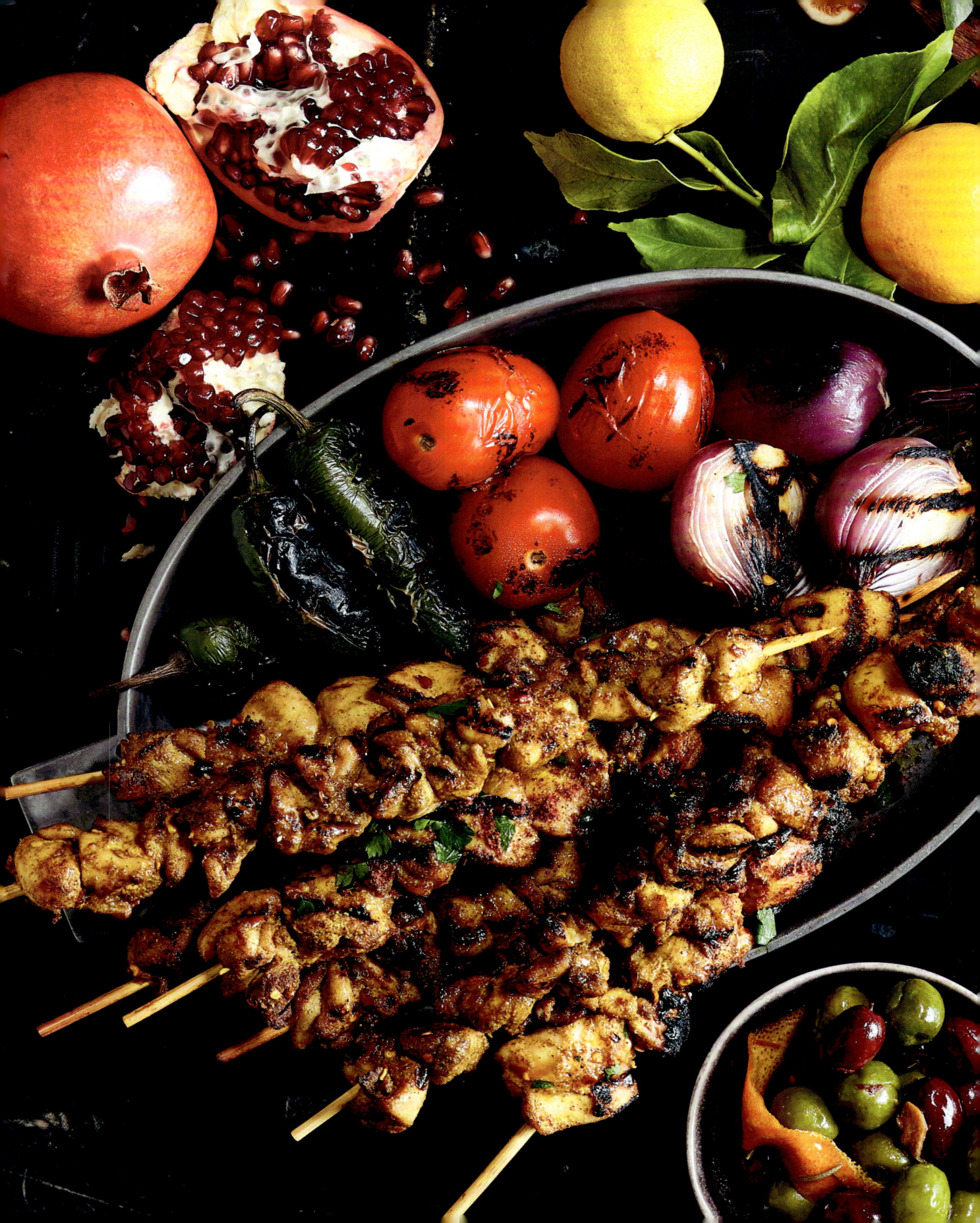

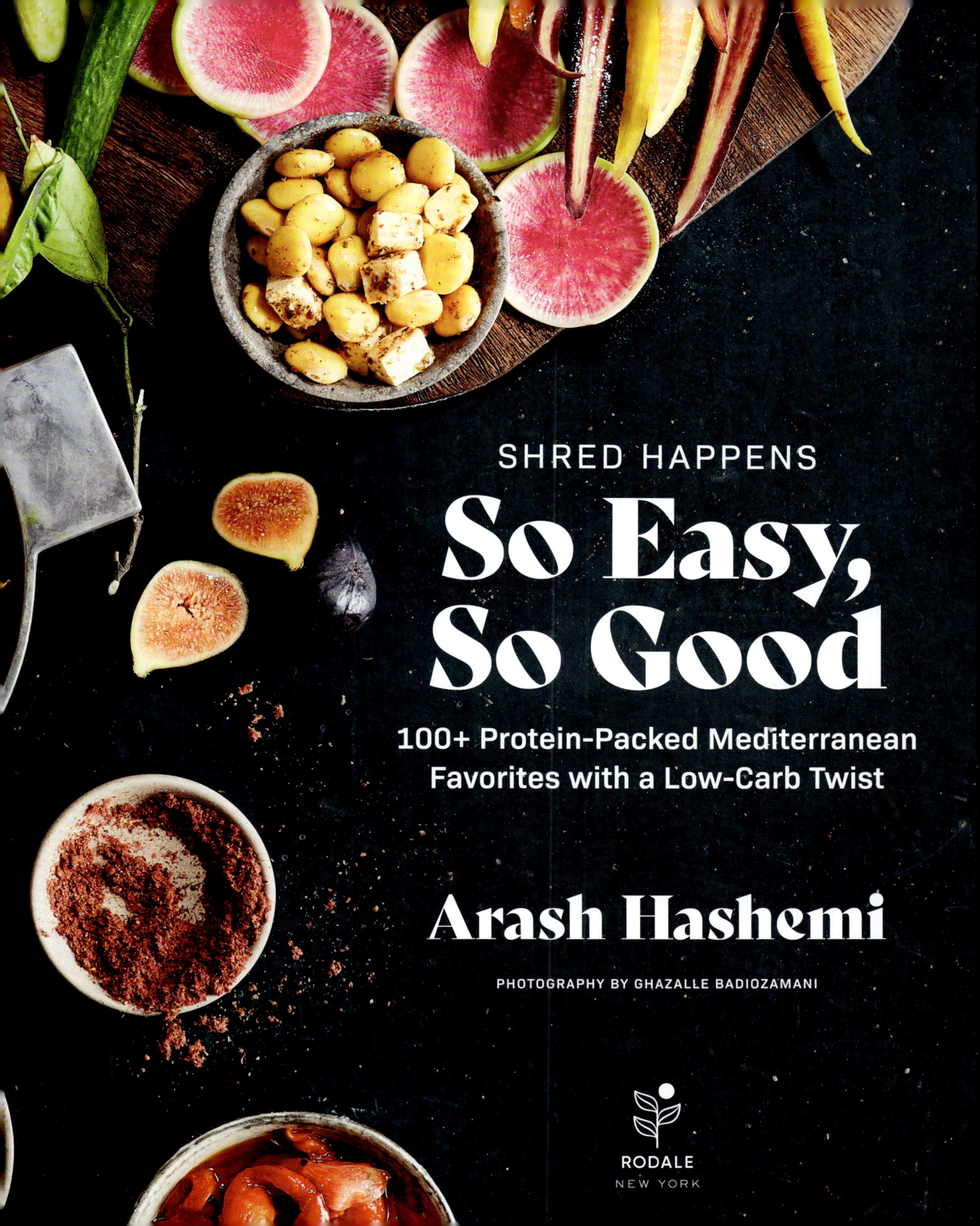

SHRED HAPPENS

So Easy, So Good

100+ Protein-Packed Mediterranean Favorites with a Low-Carb Twist

Arash Hashemi

PHOTOGRAPHY BY GHAZALLE BADIOZAMANI

RODALE

NEW YORK

Published in the United States by Rodale Books, an imprint of Random House, a division of Penguin Random House LLC, New York.

RODALE and the Plant colophon are registered trademarks of Penguin Random House LLC.

Library of Congress Cataloging-in-Publication Data
Names: Hashemi, Arash, author.
Title: Shred happens / Arash Hashemi.
Description: First edition. | New York, NY: Rodale, [2025] | Includes index.
Identifiers: LCCN 2024034020 (print) | LCCN 2024034021 (ebook) |
ISBN 9780593796535 (hardcover) | ISBN 9780593796542 (ebook)
Subjects: LCSH: Cooking.
Classification: LCC TX714 .H3824 2025 (print) | LCC TX714 (ebook) | DDC 641.5—dc23/eng/20240813
LC record available at https://lccn.loc.gov/2024034020
LC ebook record available at https://lccn.loc.gov/2024034021

Printed in China

RodaleBooks.com | RandomHouseBooks.com

9 8 7 6 5 4 3 2

First Edition

Book design by Jan Derevjanik

Photography by Ghazalle Badiozamani
Food styling by Barrett Washburne
Prop styling by Paige Hicks

To Madalina:

The best part of my day and the secret ingredient in my success.
This book is full of recipes, but none of them taste quite right without you.

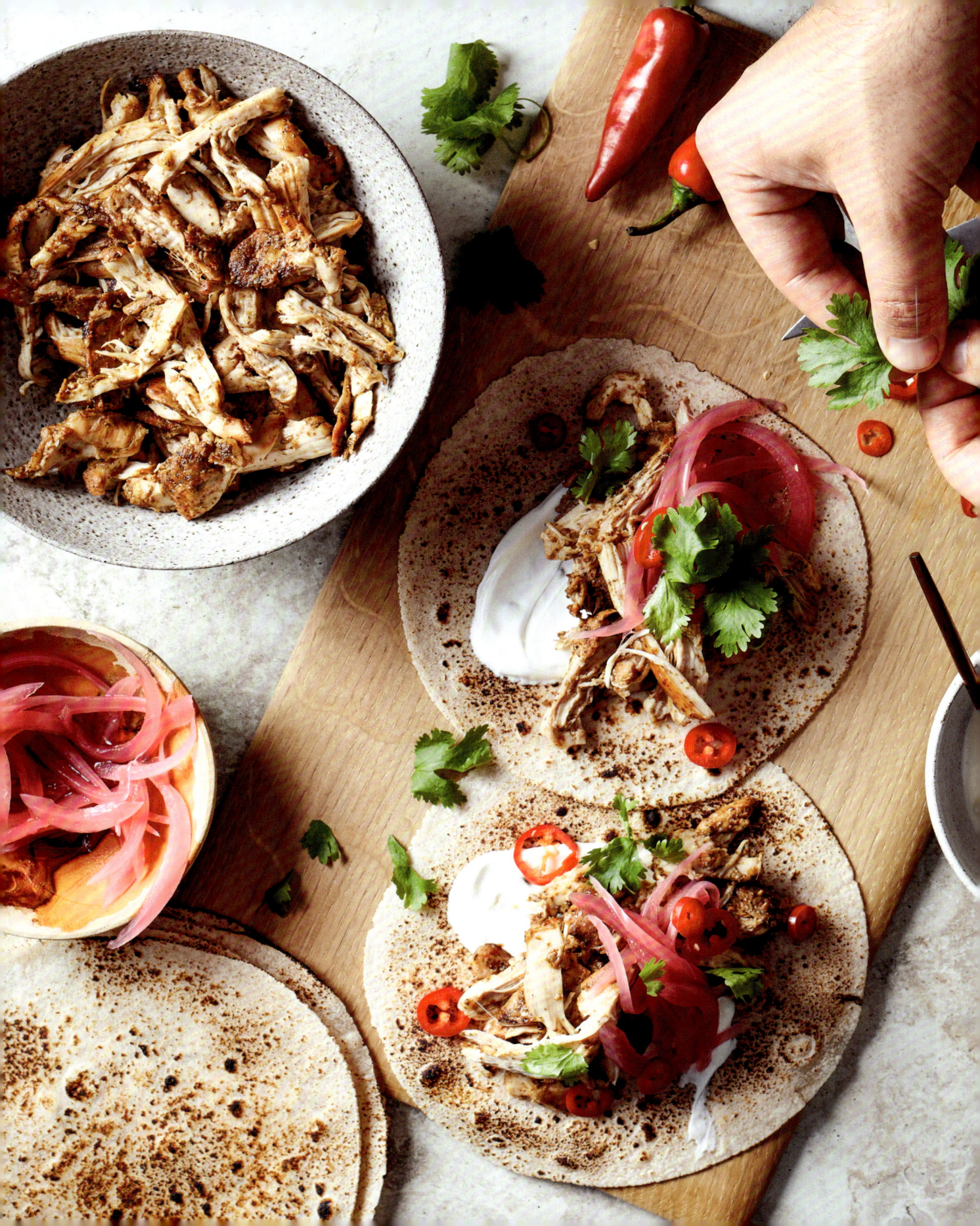

Contents

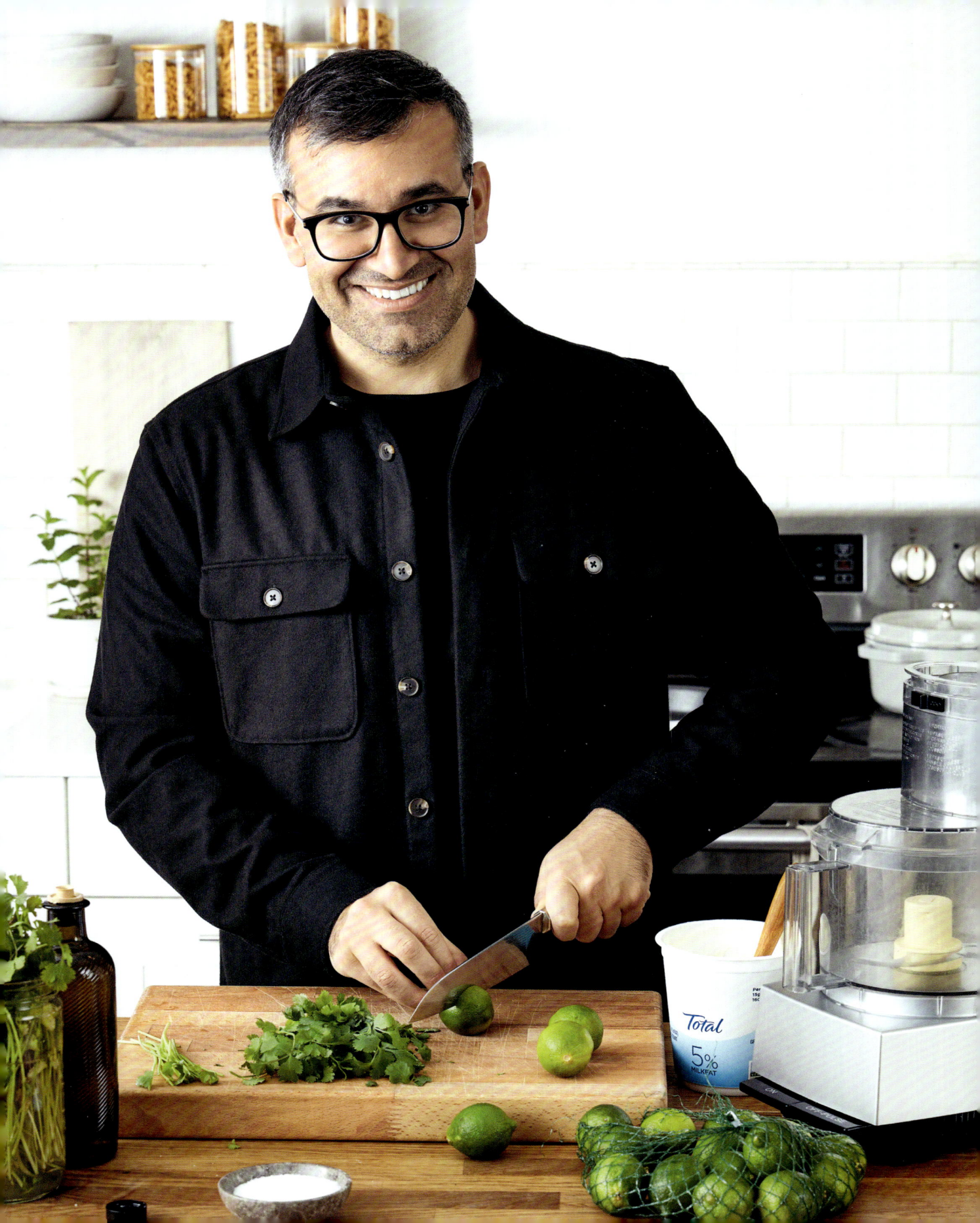

Introduction

HOW I GOT TO BE MORE THAN 330 POUNDS

I never thought I'd be writing this book.

I'm just a regular guy with a long record of failing at every diet imaginable. You name it, I've tried it. And trust me, there were plenty growing up in the 1990s and 2000s. From the big names like WeightWatchers, Jenny Craig, the Atkins diet, and the South Beach Diet, to the realm of the unconventional, with diets like the cabbage soup diet, the egg diet, and a myriad of other fad diets. Instead of weight loss, they ultimately led to me have a horrible relationship with food. What they did lead to was overeating, emotional eating, and binges.

I had all the books, magazines, and subscriptions you can think of, yet continued to get bigger and bigger.

For years (read: decades) I chased the miracle solution to lose weight, get healthy, and take control over my relationship with food. I aimed to lose x amount of weight by y date. By this birthday, by this summer, by this school year, by this wedding, by this party, by this family gathering.

It never happened.

By the time I was twenty years old, I weighed more than 330 pounds and was completely miserable. So much so that I stopped stepping on the scale. I just didn't want to know anymore. I was uncomfortable in my own skin, had to continue buying bigger clothes, and felt trapped in my own head and body.

I wasn't completely sedentary throughout all this either. During practically all this time, I did work out a bit. I had gym memberships and even personal trainers. But I learned very quickly you cannot

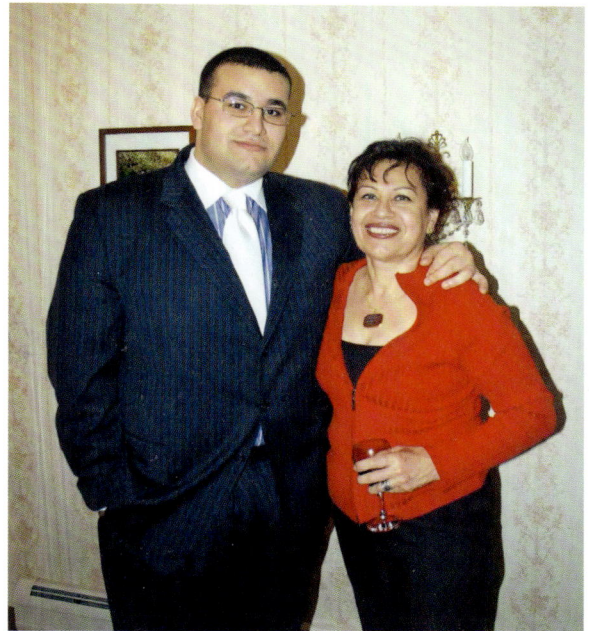

With my mom; at this point, I weighed more than 320 pounds and wore a size 56 men's suit.

outrun a poor diet, no matter how fast you run. I would undo an hour of effort in a few bites.

The problem wasn't my activity level. My biggest impediment to health was my relationship with food.

While my friends could enjoy eating a scoop or two of ice cream or a single meal from the drive-through, I needed more. One fast-food meal was never satisfying on its own. A scoop of ice cream would turn into the whole carton. I needed to eat until I was uncomfortably full.

For as long as I could remember, I had been chronically overeating, while concurrently hoping, wishing, and "aiming" to lose weight. I would sometimes manage to "do well" for a few days, only to bounce back and go the opposite direction.

Years of constant failure in this endeavor impacted my confidence and how I showed up in life. I was ashamed. Beyond the physical consequences of my decisions, a negative force permeated my life. I didn't participate in activities. I avoided friends and family. I had high anxiety. I would sweat profusely and felt uncomfortable in my own skin. I had depleted my sense of self-worth to the point I couldn't make eye contact when interacting with others.

I felt helpless.

Your situation may not be as dramatic as mine. It may be similar. Or your challenges may be even bigger. I want you to know that no matter how hard your current struggle is, you're not alone. Our culture doesn't pay enough attention to the real challenges that are behind health issues like obesity. We love looking at dramatic before and after pictures. We obsess over a number on the scale, or how much weight someone lost. But we don't talk enough about why we have these health issues in the first place, and why it's so hard to correct them. The formula for weight loss is pretty straightforward, but why is it so hard for so many of us to achieve? There are years—if not decades—of history that manifest themselves in our behaviors, in our habits, and in how we show up for ourselves. That's what I ultimately had to explore and understand before succeeding in changing the trajectory of my life.

GROWING UP

Although I was born in the United States, my family and I moved back to Iran when I was three, and we lived there until I was ten. We then immigrated to Canada for three years before finally moving back to the U.S. when I was thirteen. It was a lot of change. There was a confluence of cultures, beliefs, and identities I needed to constantly process and reconcile from a very young age.

In Iran, we lived a good life by Iranian standards. My dad was a well-regarded professor, a profession that was treated with an incredible level of respect in that culture. He worked very hard and traveled between Tehran, Ahvaz, Mashhad, and Shiraz about three weeks out of each month. Meanwhile, my mom stayed at home with me and my siblings and ensured that we took advantage of every possible opportunity to learn and grow beyond the opportunities provided by the Iranian public school system. But no matter what, living in Iran was a life sentence of sorts, and my parents were looking for any opening to get us out, no matter what it took.

That opportunity miraculously presented itself in 1997, when my parents learned of an opportunity to immigrate to Canada. We had no reason to move to Canada specifically. We had no family there. My parents didn't have any job prospects, just hope for a better future. We packed our bags and moved to Halifax, Nova Scotia.

My parents emigrated from Iran with practically no money. Iranian money was nearly worthless in the Western world, and we didn't have much to begin with anyway. My mom took the public bus system to work at the employee cafeteria at the Sheraton hotel, and then worked as a cashier at Walmart when we moved to the United States three years later, ultimately working her way up to leading human resources at that store location. At fifty, my mom started to take English courses at a community college so that she could better support us.

Money was tight, but my parents were committed to turning the tide and setting us up for success. My parents delivered newspapers and weekly sales flyers, and we even collected cans and bottles.

This focus and humility had unexpected consequences on me at an early age. Because my dad couldn't find an academic position around Halifax, he ultimately resorted to flying back and forth between Iran and Canada to support us. I have a large age disparity with my older siblings (eight years with my sister and nine years with my brother), so I was somewhat on my own through all this change. My dad was working in Iran, my mom

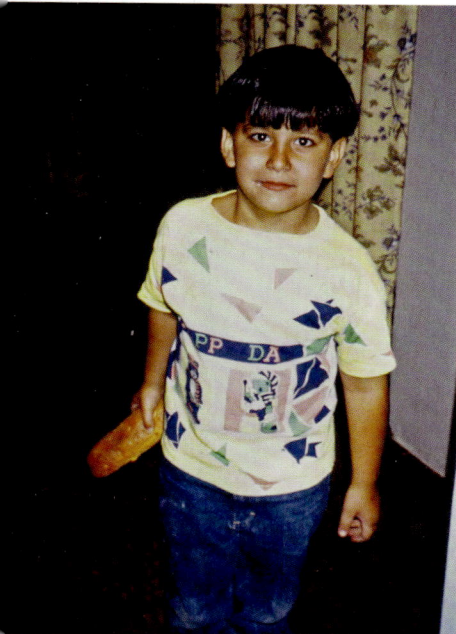

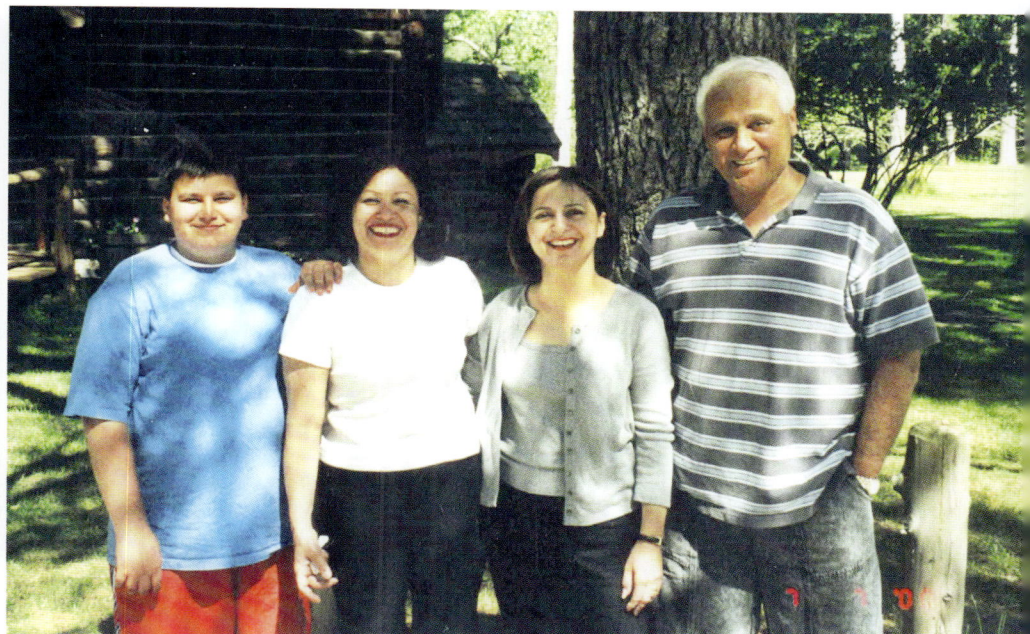

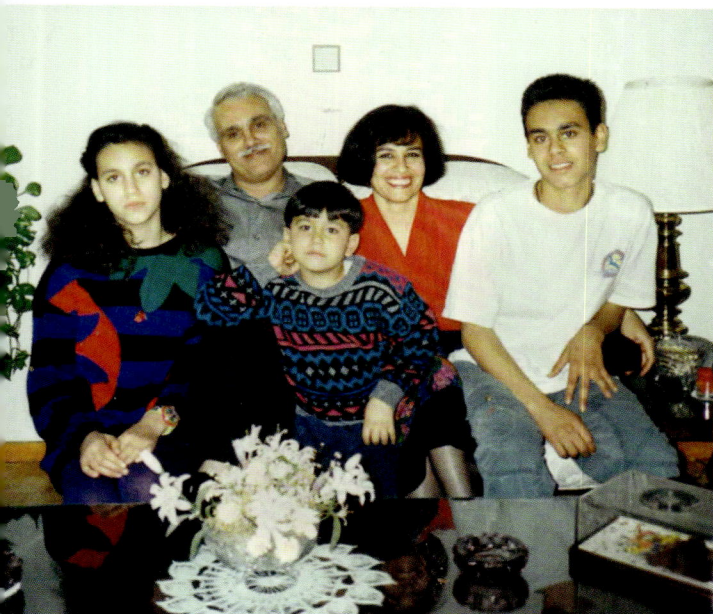

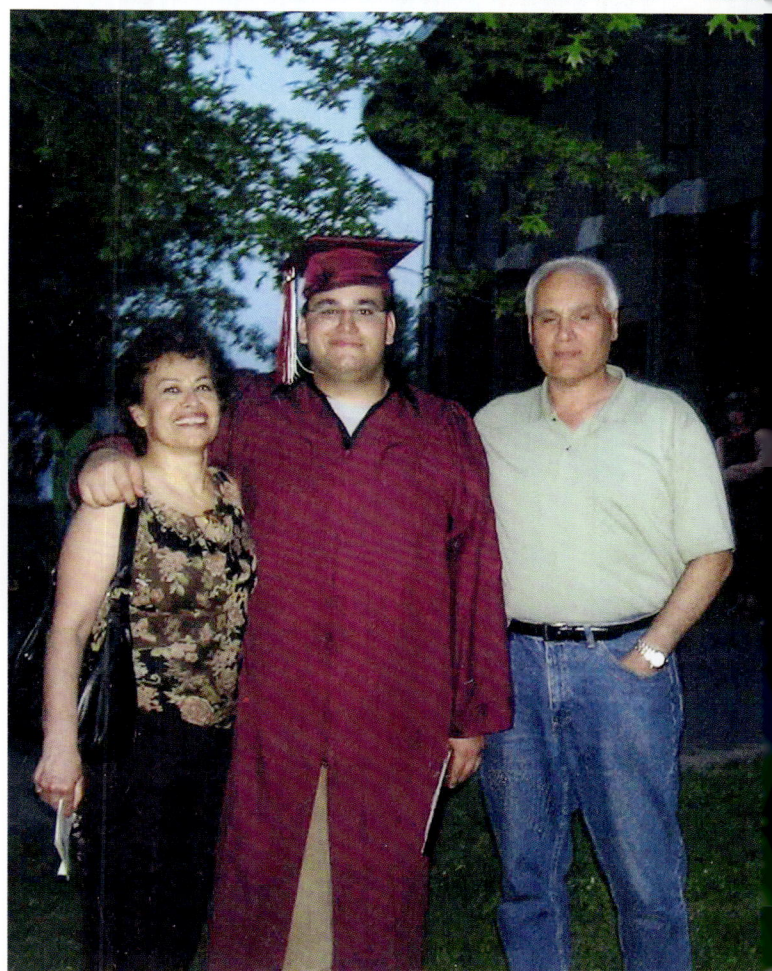

(TOP LEFT) *Growing up in Iran. You can tell I loved carbs at an early age!*

(ABOVE) *With my parents, sister Sara, and brother Ali*

(TOP RIGHT) *I moved with my parents to the United States in the summer of 2000 with my mom (right) and dad (far right). At age 13, I already weighed more than 220 pounds.*

(RIGHT) *At my high school graduation with my parents*

was working nonstop, and my siblings were either at school or working themselves.

To cope with this constant change, anxiety, and boredom, junk food and fast food became my steadfast companions in life. And it didn't help that they were marketed so appealingly in the Western world. They became my sanctuary, a source of comfort and familiarity amid the constant change in my life at home.

As I grew up, this dependence stubbornly carried on, and it became an unconscious habit. I found myself choosing food as my escape mechanism when challenges presented themselves. I reached for candy, fast food, pre-packaged brownies (I had an affinity for Swiss rolls!) when I felt anxious or overwhelmed, or just needed a moment of solace. For others it's drugs, alcohol, or another vice. But for me, it was food.

We finally moved back to the United States in 2000, when I was in eighth grade. My dad was able to find a position at UMass Amherst as a researcher that was aligned with his academic background. It didn't pay much, but it gave him the foundation he needed

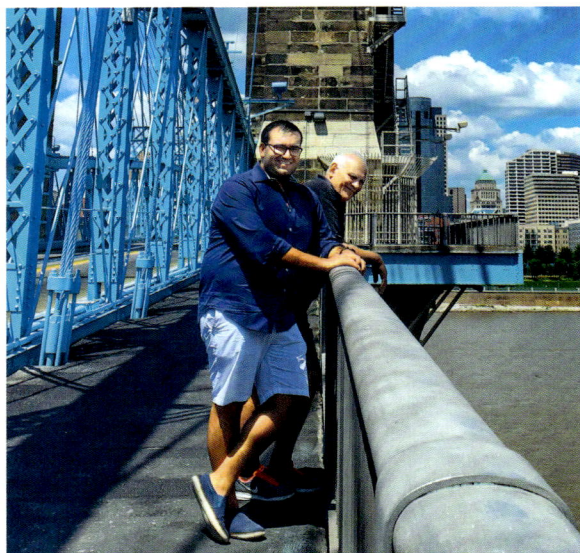

With my dad in Cincinnati just a few weeks before leaving my corporate career to focus on my health

to ultimately work his way up to being a professor at UMass as I write this today. We lived modestly, in university housing, but it felt like we had won the lottery.

In college, my environment somewhat changed, but my relationship with food remained a constant challenge. I was now eating more processed foods, with more frequency, and at more unusual times. The late-night pizza, chicken wings, and calzones ultimately brought me to well over 330 pounds and rock bottom. During this period, I finally experienced my first relationship and, very shortly thereafter, my first heartbreak. It wasn't until that moment that I began to understand the importance of self-worth. A light bulb went off that I needed to start taking care of myself. I started to take control over my weight by focusing more consciously on my food choices. I started cooking healthier meals for myself instead of relying on delivery or fast foods. This period was the first turning point, as I felt real momentum for the first time: I lost some weight, I felt more energetic, and my confidence started to come to life. It seemed like I had finally broken the cycle, and I focused on the little wins instead of the big goal of losing x pounds. I started to acknowledge and celebrate my little decisions instead of obsessing about the final destination. I didn't need to reach a certain number on the scale to feel the momentum, but instead focused on everyday actions. I was in a groove.

MY LIFE IN THE CORPORATE WORLD

Then I graduated and dove headfirst into the fast-paced, fiercely competitive corporate world. The stressors were different there: tight deadlines, high expectations, and an incredibly competitive atmosphere. Initially, I managed to maintain my somewhat healthier habits. However, as the workload increased and the pressure mounted, old habits crept back in. Late nights at the office often meant regularly ordering takeout. Stressful meetings were followed by overindulging in the snack drawer or overeating.

Despite my weight struggles, my time in the corporate world was a transformational period for me both professionally and personally. I met my wife, Madalina, while on an assignment in Atlanta in 2012. We were both part of a program that traveled one hundred percent of the time, auditing GE's businesses globally and providing operational support on some of the company's most strategic initiatives. We got exposure to the most critical initiatives and business leaders. And we got to live in some incredible locations, like Nigeria, Egypt, the United Arab Emirates, Italy, and Kenya. In each of these locations, I realized how much I enjoyed connecting with people, their culture, and their way of thinking. Since GE is such a global company, I learned how to be a leader, and how to connect meaningfully with others in order to drive initiatives forward. But after some introspection, I realized that while I had built valuable leadership skills, I wasn't being a leader for myself.

In 2017, I realized that my weight challenges and dependency on food were going to be my lifelong challenge. That no matter how much control I seemed to have gained, the underlying issue with food was always lurking, ready to surface during times of stress. It wasn't healthy, and it was a wake-up call.

I looked at Madalina and knew it was time for a drastic change in how I lived my life. Fortunately, she is an incredible partner, who has been supportive in every endeavor from the very beginning. Together, we made a bold, uncomfortable decision: I would leave my corporate career to fully focus on my health. It was frightening and required several adjustments, but we trusted that we would ultimately figure out an alternative path for me.

This decision led us to downsize. We sold belongings, letting go of things we had amassed just for the sake of accumulating more things. I leaned into my entrepreneurial skill sets—renting out my car and even thrifting and selling items on eBay to compensate for the income I was losing. It was a drastic change, but necessary for what I aimed to achieve. My parents taught me to do whatever it takes, and I did just that.

When I announced my departure from the corporate world, my managers and mentors were completely baffled. They thought I was crazy and tried to reason with me. I left under the pretense of pursuing a new business venture, but whenever questioned, I was evasive. The truth was, there was no business. I just wanted to dedicate myself to becoming healthy and make healthy eating the cornerstone of my lifestyle. It was wildly uncomfortable, but I had to do it. As the saying goes: "Choose your hard."

MY NEW APPROACH

The first change that I made was around what I was eating. I started my journey by taking inventory. I began journaling my food intake, and quickly realized how many times in a day I was reaching for or thinking about food. It was quite scary, actually. I started tracking my daily caloric intake and aimed for a certain number. The act of recording my intake and being cognizant of what I was eating was a critical behavioral shift for me. It helped me understand my choices. It helped uncover my reliance and emotional dependency on food, and it made me much more mindful.

This led me to start measuring the foods I was consuming. A tablespoon of nut butter in reality is far different from what we estimate. This goes for a serving of cheese, butter, oil, or just about anything. We really underestimate portions, whether at home or in restaurants.

Being mindful of my eating was the single most effective change I have ever made. It helped me tune in to not just what I was eating, but when, why, and how.

Last, I realized that I felt more satiated and satisfied when I was eating higher-protein, lower-starch meals. A few months into my weight-loss journey,

I adopted a more high-protein and low-carb diet. But instead of eating lots of bacon, butter, and cheese, I focused on incorporating more protein, healthy fats, lower-glycemic foods, and lots of fresh vegetables and herbs. And I made a rule: While this was my primary way of eating, I wouldn't completely write off foods that I was craving. If I could make a healthier version, I would. If I wanted the "real" thing, I would have some. I had finally found what worked for me.

The second big change I made was in how I viewed my progress. I set small, medium, and big physical goals for myself. When I started my journey, I could barely run a minute, let alone a mile. But I set this huge goal of competing in a half Ironman race. For those of you not familiar, an Ironman and a Half Ironman are long-distance triathlon events, consisting of three disciplines: swimming, cycling, and running. In an Ironman, athletes swim 2.4 miles, bike 112 miles, and then run a full marathon of 26.2 miles. In a row. A Half Ironman covers half these distances—so a 1.2-mile swim, a 56-mile bike ride, and a 13.1-mile run. I had no business competing in a Half Ironman, but decided I was going to shoot for it.

But I broke this big goal down into much smaller goals. I decided to completely ignore the swim and bike portion to start, and focus only on the running. And since I could only run for a few seconds, I decided to make my first goal a 5K. Once I completed that, I aimed for a 10K, then another, then a half-marathon, and so forth.

Through this journey, I realized the importance of taking small but actionable steps toward our big goals. I learned that the big things are the little things, and that the little things really are the big things. Once I felt more comfortable with the running portion of the race, I hired a swim coach and started building my skill set there, and so on.

There's a word in Japanese for this practice of continuous improvement in small steps: kaizen.

I believe in it so much that I ultimately named my healthier-pasta company after it. It's a daily reminder that to achieve any of the big things in life, we need to focus on the little things over time.

My journey has been a constant learning process. Recognizing that my relationship with food is something I will always have to devote intentional energy to has been both a challenge and an opportunity for growth.

Which is why this book is so personal. Because food is personal. Our relationship to food is personal, and I want you to reflect on your cravings, patterns, and triggers as you start making these recipes. What emotions are behind your cravings? How do you feel after you eat different kinds of food? How can you satisfy your cravings in ways that also support your healthiest, most thriving life?

THIS COOKBOOK

This book is several things.

First, it's a culmination of my favorite ingredients, foods, and flavor combinations. My journey has helped me realize the importance of creating diverse, satiating, and comforting foods that keep me nourished and, more importantly, excited to eat. Without feeling deprived, feeling like a diet, or feeling like I am missing out on anything. I've come to appreciate the power of incredible spices, fresh produce, and satiating protein.

Second, it's a collection of healthier versions of my favorite foods. With just some small tweaks, I've been able to enjoy practically all the foods that I love in a flavorful, engaging, and satiating way. This has completely eliminated me feeling deprived or like I'm on a diet. I have taken boring out of the equation, and every bite is filled with experience. Pay attention and savor the flavors, textures, and sensory feelings when you eat. It's not a race. It should be an experience.

Finally, these recipes are reflections of the places I've lived, the places I've been, and the people I love. You'll find dishes and flavors inspired by my background, but also by my travels to incredible countries in the Middle East, Europe, and Asia. You'll experience fragrant spices from around the world. You'll experience Romanian flavors and dishes thanks to my brilliant wife, Madalina, whom I consider my biggest gift in life. This collection of recipes is my take on the Mediterranean diet. These recipes embrace the region's wholesome abundance of herbs, vegetables, legumes, healthy fats, and protein. The Mediterranean diet is a lifestyle celebrated for its simplicity and health benefits. From the vibrant colors of fresh produce to the zesty tang of lemons, the richness of olive oil, and the flavorful spices elevating a dish, each bite proves that this way of eating can satisfy anyone, no matter where you live.

I invite you to dive into these recipes, not just to follow them but to make them your own. Experiment with swapping the sauces across various proteins, try something unconventional, and trust your instincts. We all have our unique stories and preferences, and it's through embracing these with confidence that we truly enrich our life.

Perhaps you're here because my social media recipes have caught your eye (and for that, I'm truly grateful!). Or maybe it's your passion for food, a desire to embrace healthier eating, or a determination to regain control of your health. Whatever your reason, my aim is that these recipes will be a valuable ally in your journey. This book presents my most personal, easy-to-make, yet rewarding recipes. Perfect for enjoying yourself, sharing with that special someone in your life, or savoring with friends. Consider this collection more than just recipes; it's a celebration of flavors, health, and community.

I am deeply grateful for the opportunity to have a place in your kitchen. Thank you for giving me this platform.

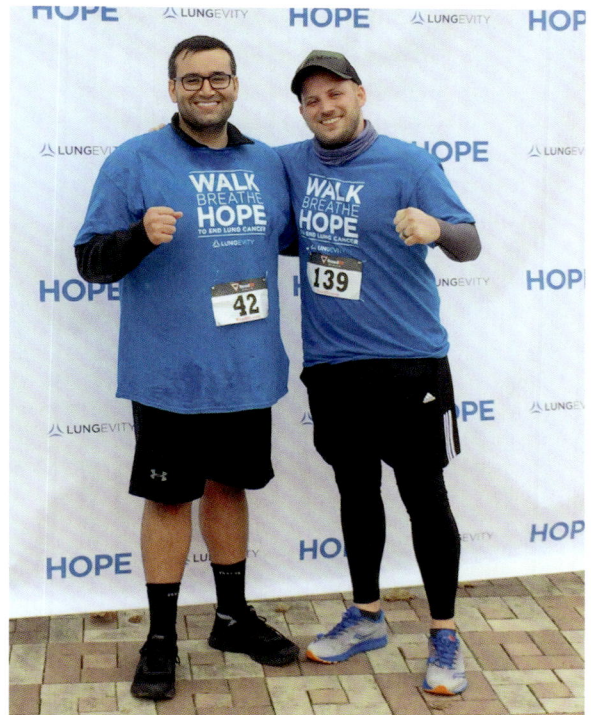

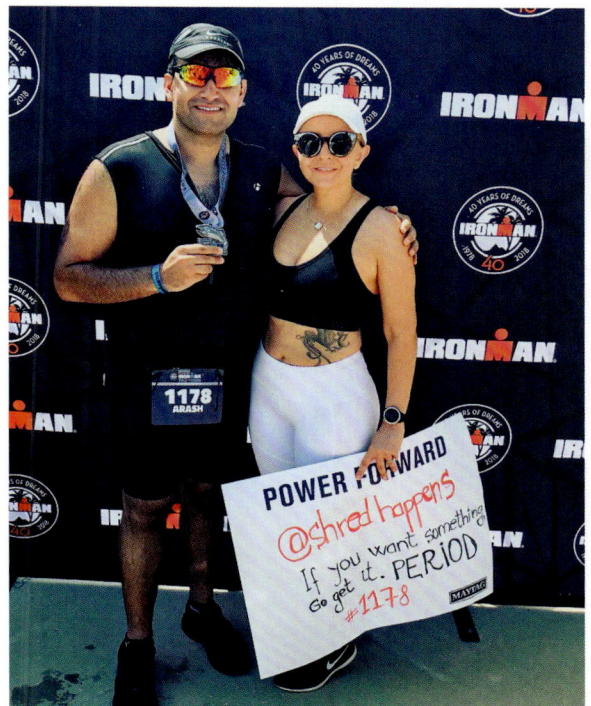

Without any running or athletic background, I decided I wanted to challenge myself by completing a triathlon. I signed up for a Half Ironman race, but knew I had to set smaller goals in pursuit of my big goal. Above, I signed up for my very first 5K. And almost 10 months later, finished my first Half Ironman.

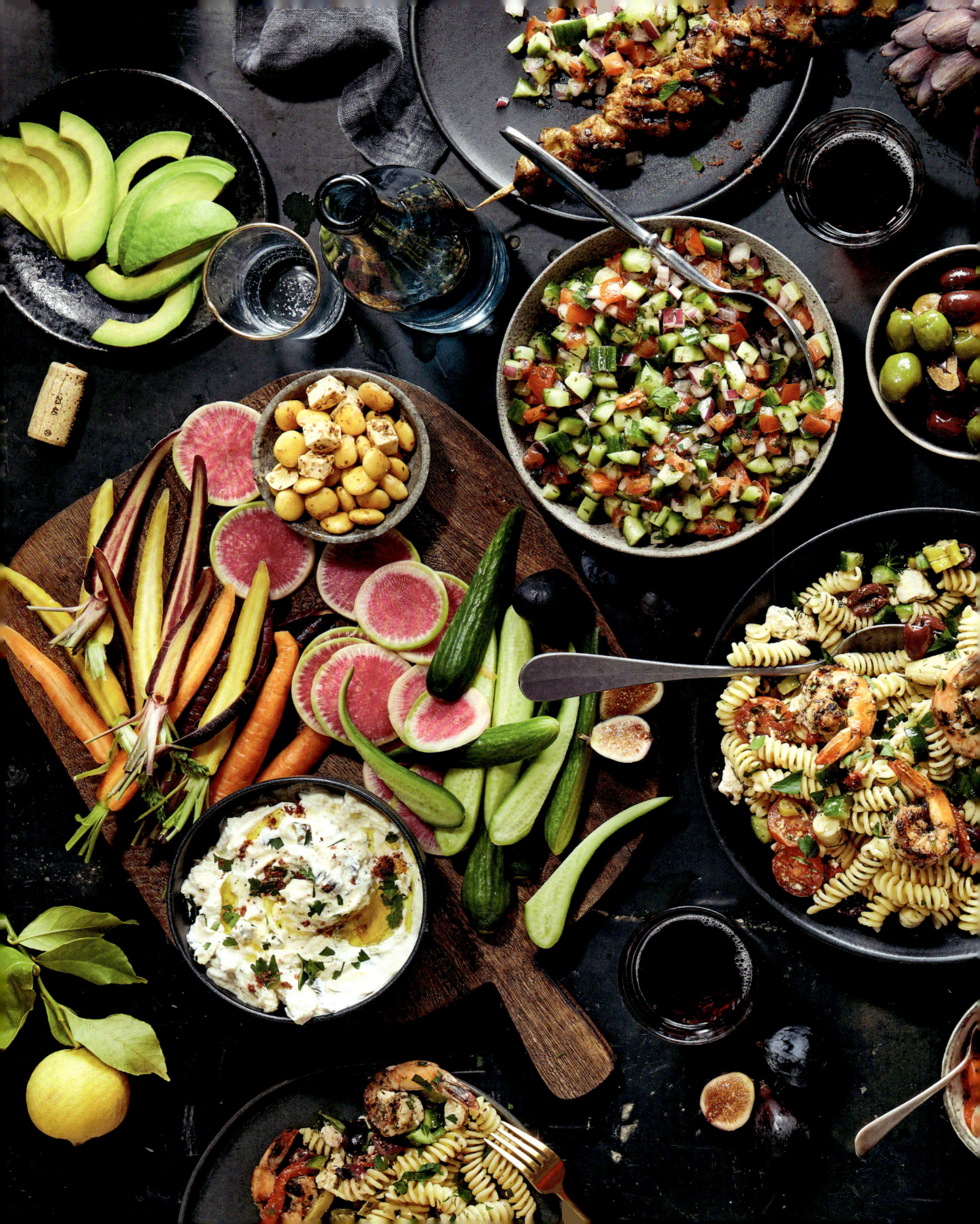

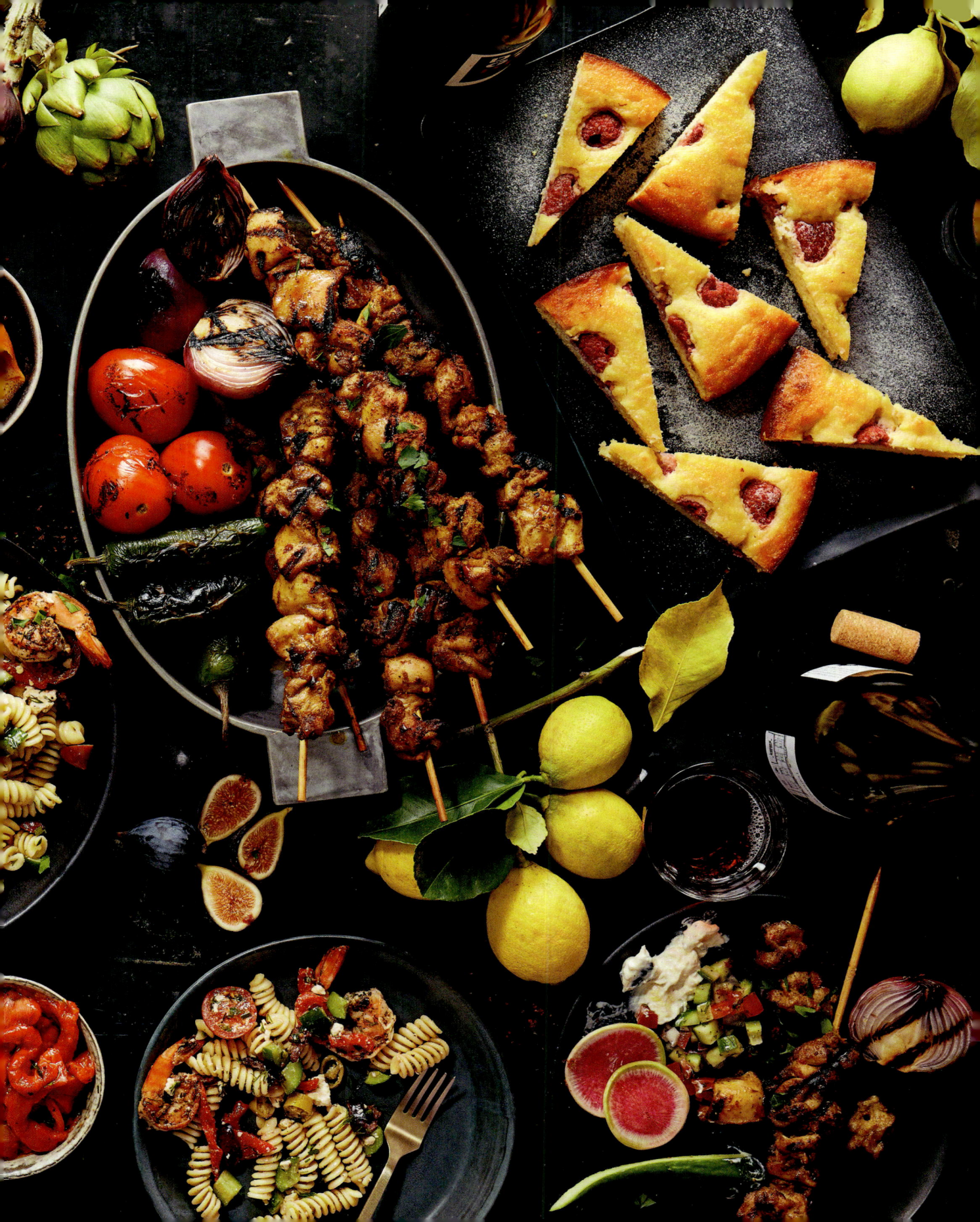

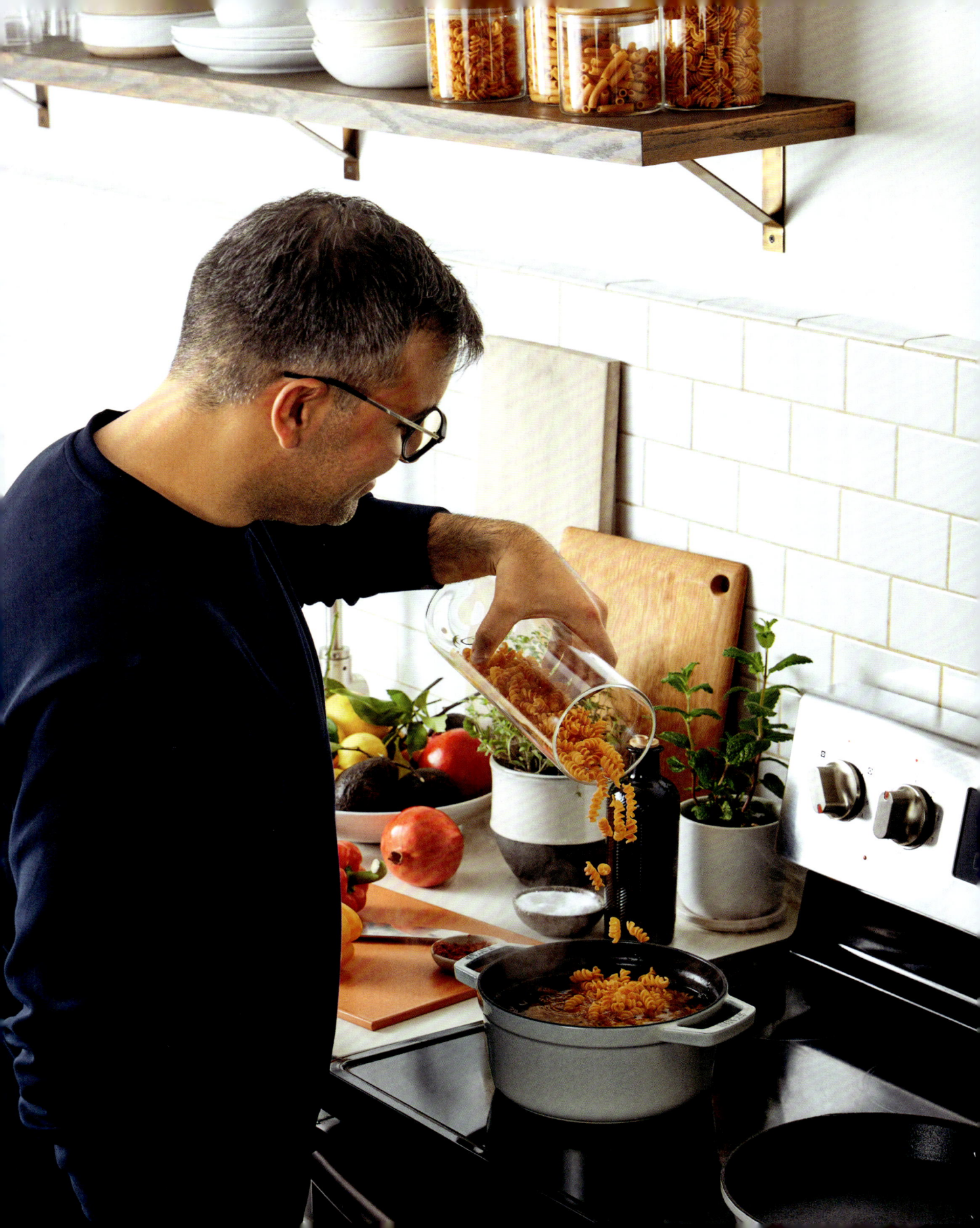

My Food Philosophy: Key Principles

It took me twenty-plus years of yo-yo dieting to realize there wasn't a miracle solution, and to rethink my relationship with food. I finally understood that to make the big change I was looking for, I needed to focus on the little things. But what does that mean?

Here are the key principles that have shaped my new relationship with food. Maybe they'll inspire you on your own wellness journey, or maybe they'll just make your next meal a little more satisfying. Either way, I hope they help you find a deeper connection to the food on your plate and, in turn, to yourself and those around you.

CONSISTENCY VS. INTENSITY

One of the biggest mindset shifts I had to make as I embarked on my transformation journey was to realize that eating healthily and being at a weight I was comfortable with weren't just destinations to reach but required cultivating a lifelong daily practice. I cannot underscore this enough if you are at the beginning stages of your journey. For me, what changed things was not to focus on a strict diet or a quick fix, but rather to make small, sustainable changes that I could maintain day after day. This meant celebrating the little decisions, like ordering the healthier option when dining out, taking time to plate up my full meal instead of constantly snacking, or making a healthier version of a sugary or carb-loaded craving. I had to learn to trust that these small steps would yield the bigger changes that I envisioned.

This meant I had to find joy in the food I ate on a daily basis. Otherwise, it was just another restrictive diet waiting to fail and result in me continuing to go the opposite direction from where I wanted to

go. When you eat food that is nourishing, satiating, and enjoyable, you are more likely to stick with it long term. I ditched the personal mandate to lose *x* amount of weight in *y* period of time, and instead trusted the process.

CONTINUOUS IMPROVEMENT

Continuous improvement has played a key role in my journey, with food at the forefront.

At first, these small improvements will seem insignificant, but over time, they will compound and lead to profound positive change. This approach helped me move away from the trap of fast, aggressive diets and instead embrace gradual change—one dish at a time. It helped me go from barely being able to run for one minute to completing multiple Half Ironman races and a full marathon. It's a powerful principle that will help anyone reach their most aspirational goals.

COMMUNITY

Sharing a meal together should be a celebration, which is why I create recipes that are not just good for you, but delicious and versatile as well. This way, everyone can enjoy a meal together, no matter their dietary restrictions or preferences. This was a dramatic departure from my days at my highest weight, when I was eating multiple fast-food servings in my car while rushing to or from work.

Looking back, I see that one of the biggest constants as I was gaining weight was how I consumed my meals: privately, in secrecy, and away from family and friends. I was using food as an emotional coping mechanism and continuing to feel more lonely and isolated as a result.

Now I aim to celebrate and share my love for food with others, whether it's on social media, hosting dinner parties, cooking with friends and family, or simply enjoying a meal together at the table. Food is meant to be enjoyed together, and it's a beautiful way to bring people closer.

BRING ON THE FLAVOR

Food should be something you crave, look forward to, and enjoy as you're cooking and eating it. Healthy eating doesn't mean you have to settle for bland or boring meals that leave you still feeling hungry. It's about exploring fresh ingredients, new spices, varied textures, and ingredients that bring a burst of flavor and satisfaction to every bite.

For me, this meant experimenting with global cuisine, trying out new recipes from different cultures, seeking new produce, and incorporating all of it into my own cooking repertoire. Each recipe in this cookbook is crafted to ensure that flavor is never sacrificed for health, because food is a celebration, not a punishment.

MAKE IT EASY & ACCESSIBLE

Life is unpredictable, and so are our schedules. Sustainable eating also means cooking with what I have and fitting it into my day-to-day lifestyle—whether I have an hour or only ten minutes. It

feels like we're all strapped for time these days, so I designed the recipes in this cookbook to be ready in less time than it would take for your delivery to arrive. The key is to always have my fridge filled with essential ingredients that I can easily access and use to make quick, nutritious, and delicious meals without feeling deprived. You'll see some essentials in the next section.

I also love experimenting with flexible and versatile recipes that can be easily adapted to fit my mood, my cravings, or what's available in my fridge. This way, I never feel restricted or limited, and it keeps cooking fun and exciting instead of feeling like a chore.

FUEL RIGHT, FEEL GOOD

At its core, my eating philosophy is about fueling our bodies with what they need to thrive. This means a focus on healthy and nourishing foods that provide our bodies with the right balance of macronutrients. It's about listening to our bodies and responding with the nourishment they need to support us in achieving our goals, whether that's weight loss, improved energy, or overall wellness.

It's also about finding the right balance between indulging in the foods we love and nourishing our bodies so we can live our best lives. I believe that healthy eating should never feel restrictive or like a punishment, but rather a way to honor and take care of our bodies.

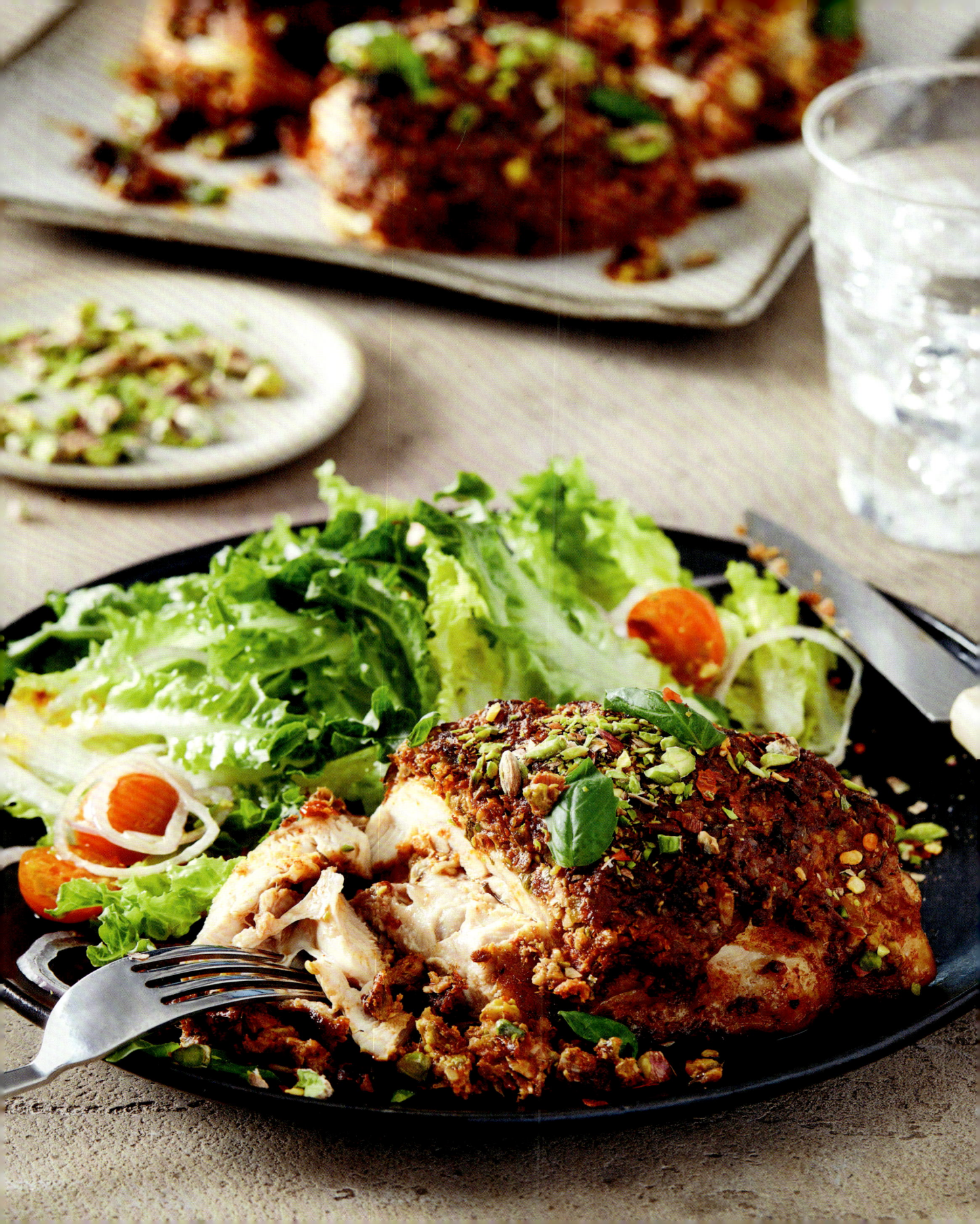

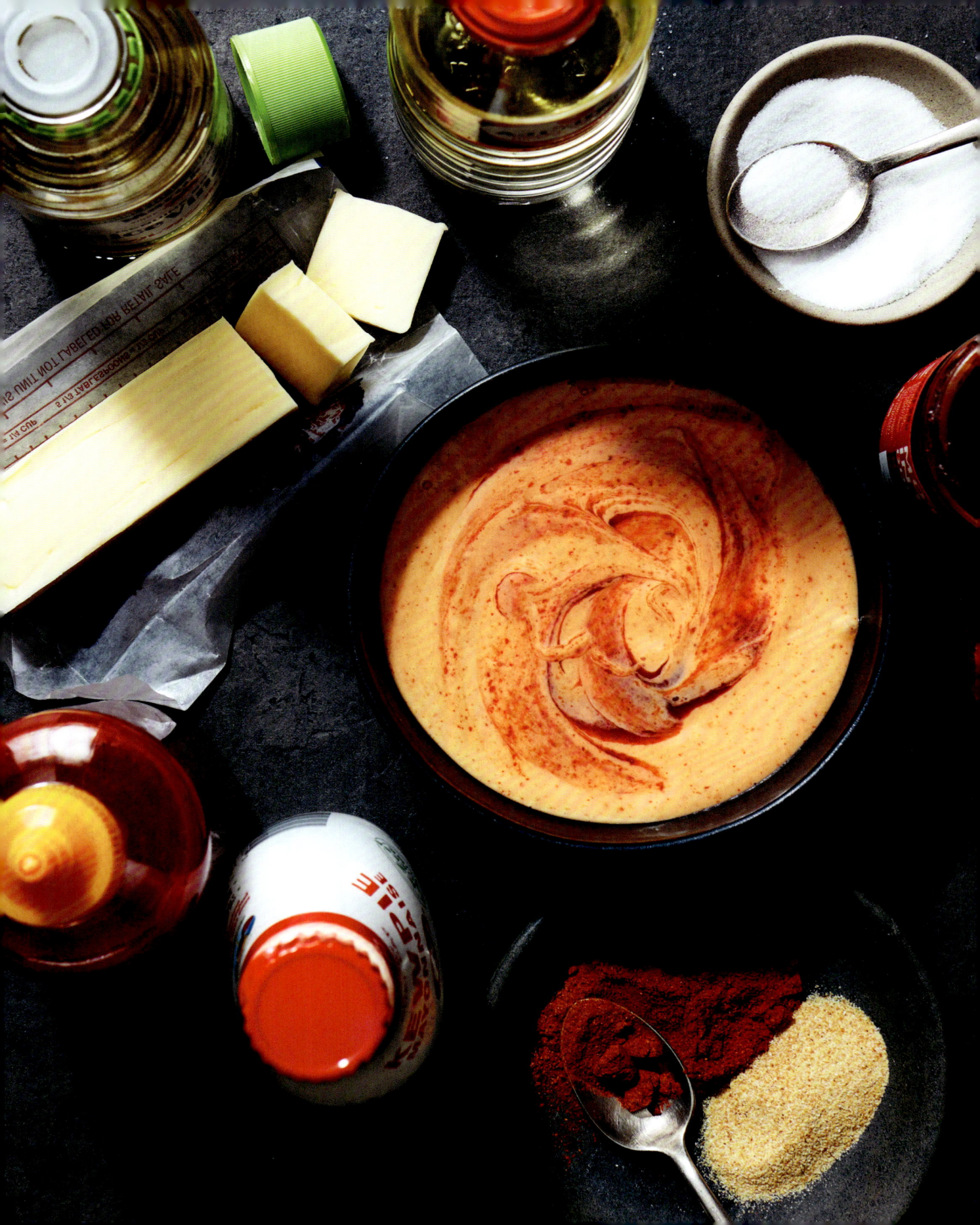

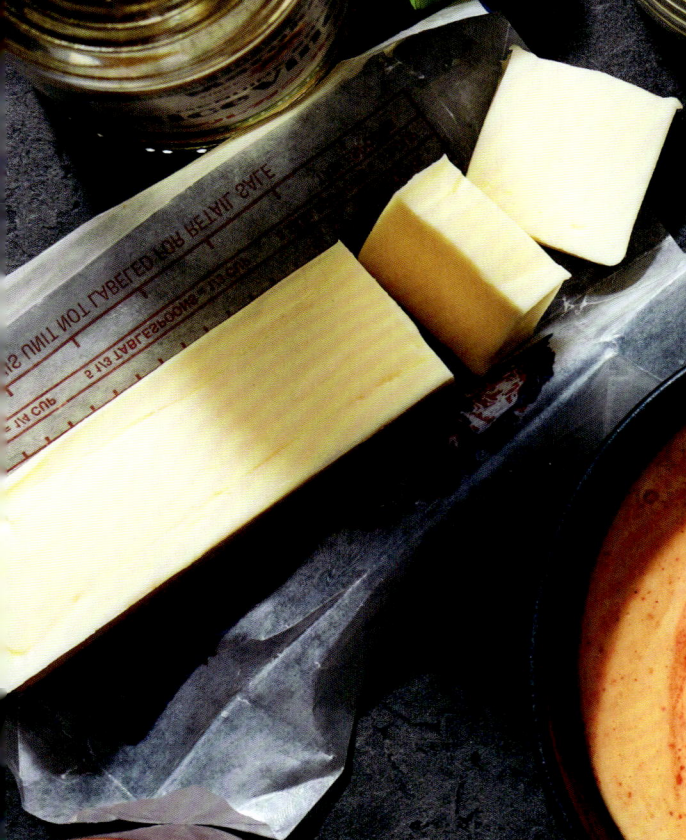

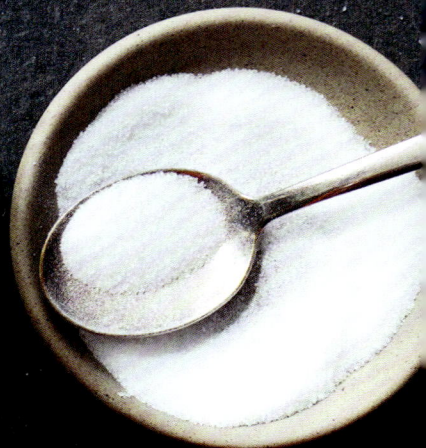

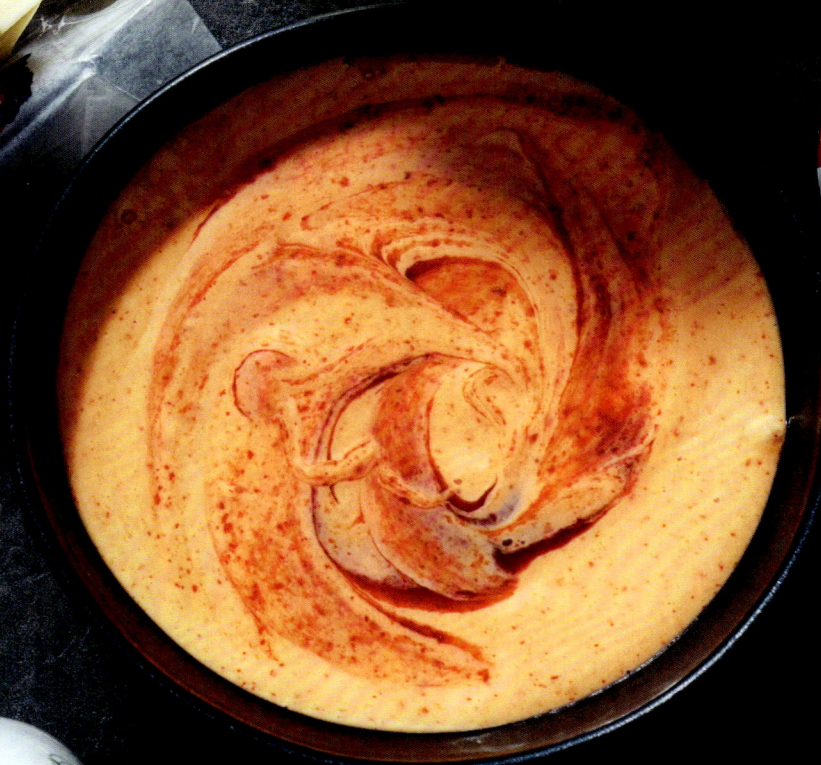

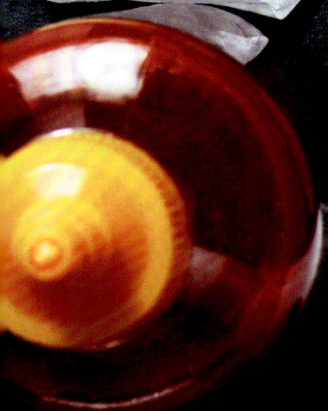

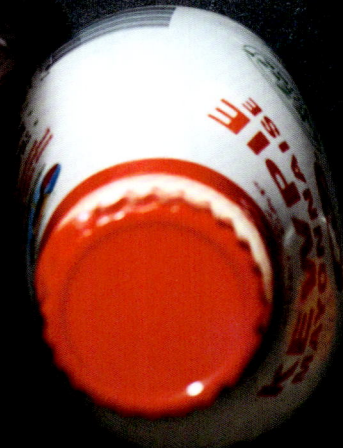

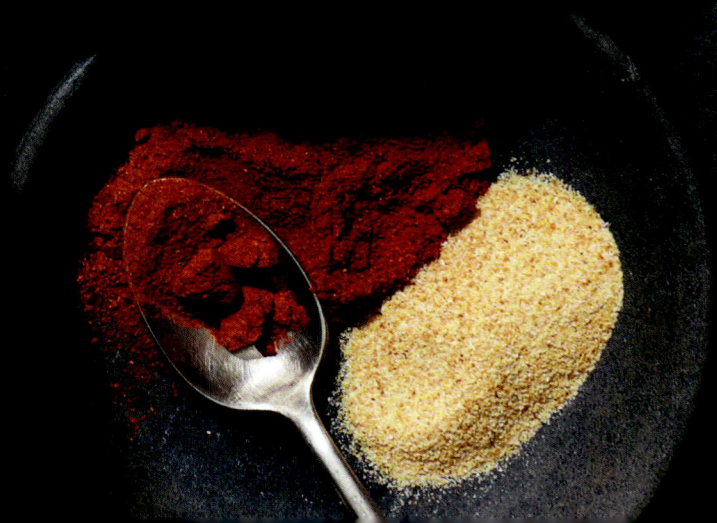

My Food & Pantry Essentials

FRESH HERBS: Fresh herbs add an unmatched aromatic and earthy element to any dish and are nutrient dense, offering plenty of health benefits. They also add flavor and color to your meals without excess calories, fat, salt, or sugar. My go-to herbs are cilantro, parsley, mint, basil, oregano, and thyme.

FLAVORFUL SPICES: Similar to herbs, spices offer a variety of health benefits and elevate the flavor of dishes without extra calories. I like to create my own blends at home to save money and cut down on prep time when cooking. Some of my favorite spices are sumac, paprika, Aleppo pepper, za'atar, onion powder, and cinnamon. These elevate just about any dish.

HEALTHY FATS: Much like the Mediterranean and Middle Eastern diets, my recipes rely heavily on olive oil and various nuts as a source of healthy fats. Olive oil and avocado oil are my staple oils for cooking, while coconut oil is great for baking. I use nuts like walnuts and pistachios, which are low-carb and high in protein and healthy fats. I also use coconut flour, almond flour, and lupin flour in place of traditional flour when making desserts.

SAUCE INGREDIENTS: Sauces add a whole new dimension to dishes and can really tie everything together. Every sauce should have elements of acidity, herbs, spices, aromatics, and fat. For acidity, I often use citrus juice like lemon or lime. For herbs and spices, see above. Aromatics like garlic, ginger, and onion add depth of flavor, while fats like olive oil, tahini, mayonnaise, or yogurt help create a creamy texture. Other key sauce items include Dijon mustard, soy sauce, and harissa paste, depending on the flavor profile I'm looking for.

SIDES: Coming up with side dishes can be one of the trickiest parts of a low-carb diet, as they are traditionally high in carbs. Thankfully, these days you can find plenty of low-carb alternatives to classic sides, such as cauliflower rice instead of regular rice, veggie mashes in place of mashed potatoes, or my Kaizen low-carb rice and pasta made with lupini beans. You can even find chip and cracker replacements, whether it's your favorite low-carb cracker brand or simply some raw veggies to dunk in dips and salsas. Stock up on these low-carb alternatives to have on hand for easy and healthy sides.

PROTEIN SOURCES: Protein is essential for a balanced diet, as it provides us with energy and helps repair and build our muscles. Plus, it helps keep you full and satisfied. You can get protein not just from meat but from many different foods. Here are some of my kitchen staples:

Meats: Chicken thighs, chicken breasts, ground turkey, lean cuts of beef like sirloin or tenderloin, and lamb all make for great protein sources.

Dairy: Greek yogurt, cottage cheese, and cheeses like feta or Parmesan are great sources of protein. I use cream for some of my sauces, and also sometimes use almond milk and coconut milk as alternatives to traditional cow's milk.

Seafood: My recipes often include seafood like salmon, shrimp, and tuna. All three are great sources of lean protein and provide heart-healthy omega-3 fatty acids. I also like using white fish like halibut and sea bass, as they make a great canvas for sauces and marinades and cook up relatively quickly.

Legumes: If you follow a low-carb diet, you're going to be limited in the legumes you can consume. However, peanuts, lupini beans, and edamame are all great low starch and low glycemic options that I use in my recipes. For those not following a super low-carb diet, adding black beans, chickpeas, lentils, and kidney beans to your meals is also a great way to incorporate plant-based protein and fiber.

My Kitchen Essentials

KNIVES: Having high-quality, sharp knives in your kitchen is an absolute game-changer. It makes prepping ingredients a breeze and allows for more precise cuts. I recommend investing in a chef's knife, a paring knife, and a serrated knife as a basic set for all your cooking needs. No specific brand is necessary as long as they are comfortable for you and sharp. Make sure to regularly sharpen your knives for optimal performance. It makes a huge difference.

CUTTING BOARDS: I always have multiple cutting boards on hand to avoid cross-contamination when preparing ingredients. I like to have a large wooden board for chopping fruits and vegetables, and both a small and a large silicone board for meats and fish. Again, nothing fancy or expensive is needed; just make sure they are sturdy and easy to clean. And don't forget to season your wooden boards regularly to keep them looking and performing their best.

GADGETS AND TOOLS: You really don't need every fancy kitchen gadget out there to create delicious and healthy meals! I keep my kitchen pretty simple and accessible: My must-haves include a food processor, a hand mixer, an outdoor grill (or grill pan), an air fryer, and various chopping/slicing tools like a veggie peeler, a grater, and a mandoline.

PANS AND POTS: I make sure to have a variety of pans and pots for different purposes. A large pot or a Dutch oven is great for boiling pasta and making soup, while a medium skillet is ideal for sautéing vegetables and proteins. A large skillet or cast-iron pan is perfect for one-pan meals, and a small saucepan comes in handy for making sauces or reheating leftovers.

SERVING TOOLS: It goes without saying that you'll need serving tools like plates, bowls, silverware, and glasses in your kitchen. However, many overlook the impact that colorful, visually appealing plates and bowls have on the overall eating experience. I love having different plates and bowls to choose from depending on my meal. I recommend investing in some simple yet aesthetically pleasing serving dishware to elevate your meals in both taste and presentation. They really help bring the whole meal together and can be purchased from local discount stores or department stores. I also recommend having a variety of serving spoons, tongs, and spatulas for cooking and plating dishes. It's a simple technique that can elevate the presentation of your meals with ease.

TECHNIQUES

MARINATING PROTEIN: Often overlooked, marinating your protein is a small time investment that reaps big rewards. With the right marinade, you can turn the most basic of cuts into a gourmet experience. There are three vital elements to include in your marinade to ensure that your meat comes out tender, flavorful, and juicy every time. The first is an acid, like citrus juice or vinegar, which helps break down the protein fibers and tenderize the meat. The second is fat, whether it's olive oil, mayo, yogurt, etc. This helps keep the meat moist during cooking and adds richness to the flavor. The third is herbs, spices, and aromatics to bring depth of flavor to the marinade. For best results, let your protein marinate for at least 30 minutes (or up to 24 hours) before cooking.

GRILLING: Grilling your meat or veggies over charcoal creates a smoky and charred flavor that you can't really replicate on the stovetop. Make sure your grill is clean and preheated before adding your protein or vegetables, and don't overcrowd the grates, as you want the heat to circulate evenly. You can close the lid for more intense heat or leave it open for quicker cooking times. Always use tongs or a spatula to flip the food, as using a fork will make punctures that release the juices. I like to use a meat thermometer to ensure that the protein is cooked to the right temperature.

SEARING: Searing is a cooking technique that involves browning the surface of meat or fish quickly over high heat. This not only gives the food a delicious crispy exterior but also seals in moisture and adds a whole other layer of flavor. To sear, make sure to pat your protein dry with paper towels before placing it on a hot skillet with oil. Don't move the meat around too much, and give it enough time to form a crust before flipping.

SAUTÉING: Sautéing is a quick and easy way to cook your vegetables and proteins on the stovetop. Start by heating oil in a large skillet or pan over medium-high heat. You'll then usually add aromatics like chopped onions, garlic, or ginger to the pan and cook for a few minutes, until fragrant. Next, add the protein (chicken, beef, seafood) and cook until golden brown before adding the vegetables. Finish with greens, herbs, and spices for added flavor.

ROASTING: Roasting gives vegetables and meats a crispy outer crust while maintaining tenderness on the inside. You can also broil at the end to make things extra crispy! It's a relatively hands-off and easy cooking method that I like to use for simple one-pan meals or when I want to cook a large batch of food at once. Just pop your dish in the oven and let it do the work for you!

CUTTING VEGGIES: Whether you are dicing, mincing, or slicing, each technique adds a different texture and visual appeal to your dish. It'll even impact the flavor and how the veggies cook. For example, larger chunks will take longer to cook and

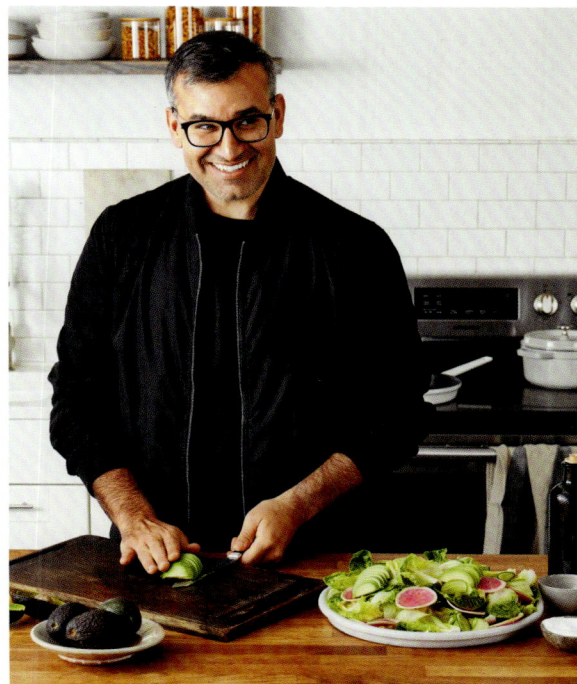

will have a more substantial bite, while smaller diced pieces will cook more quickly and disperse more flavor throughout the dish. Whether you're cutting up a cucumber, a carrot, or an avocado, try slicing them in different lengths, shapes, or on different angles. You'll see how this simple step helps keep things interesting.

PLATING: Plating is the final step in creating a visually appealing and appetizing dish. Now, it doesn't have to look like something out of *MasterChef,* but putting in a little effort to make your plate look nice does make a difference. Start by considering your main focal point (the protein or main ingredient) and build around it, adding smaller elements like grains, vegetables, and sauces. You also can't go wrong with toppings! I like to use fresh herbs, nuts and seeds, a sprinkle of spices, cheese, or a drizzle of sauce to add texture and flavor to the dish. This small step yields huge results.

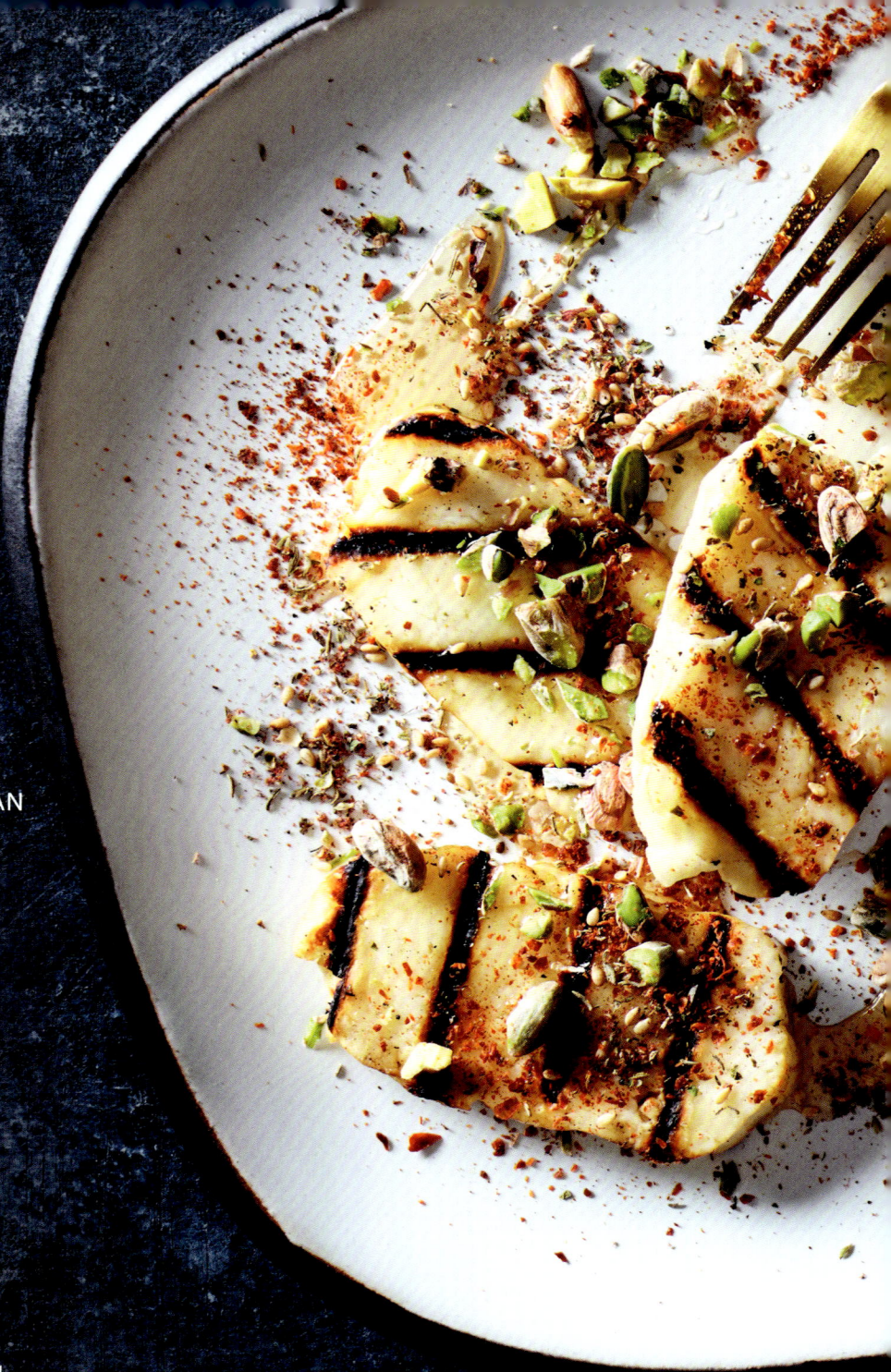

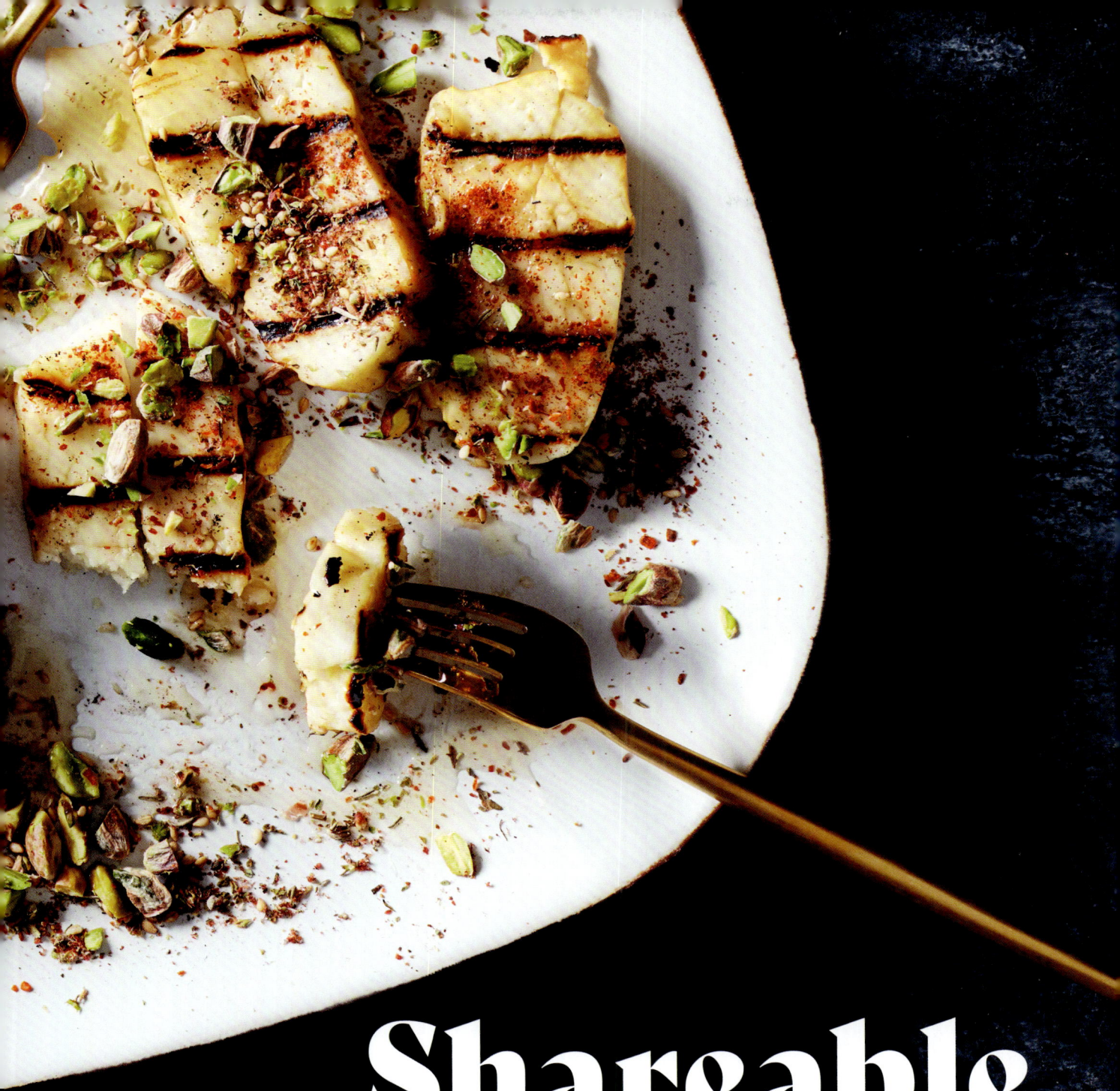

Shareable Plates

These shareable plates were created so that you can connect with the people you care about, whether it's a get-together with family and friends or a cozy dinner for two. In Mediterranean and Middle Eastern cultures, sharing meals is deeply rooted, and I encourage you to break (low-carb) bread with loved ones as often as possible. You're also more than welcome to whip any of these up for yourself—they're just as satisfying solo!

Cooking for others can be stressful, especially when you don't have enough hours in the day and dietary preferences vary. That's why I created these recipes with versatility and practicality in mind.

While these recipes may be low-carb and keto-friendly, they are by no means lacking in flavor. In fact, these dishes will have everyone—including carb lovers—coming back for seconds.

You'll notice that I love using veggies as a vessel (or base) for all sorts of yummy goodness. I also have a lot of fun with toppings, which are my number one secret to elevating any dish! From toasted walnuts and crumbled feta to fresh herbs and sprinkles of sumac or sesame seeds, these toppings provide a boost of flavor and nutrition to each plate. Plus, they add that wow factor for serving to guests.

Spicy Salmon Cucumber Boats

With these spicy salmon cucumber boats, you can enjoy your favorite sushi flavors while staying in your macros. Persian cucumbers make the perfect crunchy and refreshing vessel for the salmon, which is mixed in a delicious spicy mayo sauce. For this recipe, I want you to have the freedom to add whatever toppings you like so you can re-create your favorite sushi-inspired rolls. Ready in just 10 minutes, with no cooking needed, tasty, fully loaded vessels make for an easy lunch, appetizer, or snack.

1. Mince the salmon and toss it into a medium mixing bowl.

2. Add the mayo, soy sauce, rice vinegar, sesame oil, sriracha, garlic chili oil, lemon juice, and salt and pepper to taste. Mix well, taste, and adjust to your liking. Refrigerate for 10 to 15 minutes.

3. Slice the cucumbers in half lengthwise, then hollow out the center using a spoon. Make sure you remove all the seeds.

4. Spoon the salmon mixture into the hollowed cucumber halves. Add your favorite toppings and enjoy!

PREP TIME: 10 MINUTES
SERVINGS: 2 TO 4

---

8 ounces sushi-grade wild salmon

2 tablespoons mayonnaise

2 tablespoons soy sauce or tamari

1 tablespoon rice vinegar

1 tablespoon sesame oil

1 tablespoon sriracha

1 tablespoon garlic chili oil or garlic chili crunch

1 tablespoon freshly squeezed lemon juice

Salt and freshly ground black pepper

6 Persian or mini cucumbers

OPTIONAL TOPPINGS

Mashed avocado

Chopped scallions, green and white parts

Garlic chili oil

Soy sauce

Sesame seeds

Furikake

Baked Whole Cauliflower

This baked whole cauliflower is anything but boring. It requires some advance prep for the overnight brining, but it is well worth the time investment. Since I've followed a low-carb diet, cauliflower and I have gotten quite familiar with each other. It's super versatile and can be used in so many different ways. We're adding my favorite Mediterranean ingredients like feta cheese, Greek yogurt, toasted walnuts, and a delicious green herbs salsa that gives it a gorgeous pop of color. Fork-tender and loaded with flavor, it's definitely a must-try!

PREP TIME: 40 MINUTES, PLUS 14 TO 20 HOURS BRINING AND DRYING
COOK TIME: 30 MINUTES
SERVINGS: 4 TO 6

¼ cup salt

1 medium head cauliflower

1 tablespoon sweet paprika

3 garlic cloves

5 tablespoons freshly squeezed lemon juice

½ tablespoon dried thyme

¼ medium onion, diced

2 tablespoons olive oil

Freshly ground black pepper

FOR THE CHEESE DRESSING

2 ounces feta cheese

½ cup plain Greek yogurt

1 teaspoon lemon zest

Freshly ground black pepper

Salt (optional)

1 ounce raw walnuts

Green Herbs Salsa (page 214)

1. Fill a deep pot or bowl with enough water to cover the cauliflower head fully. Add the salt and mix until it dissolves. Submerge the cauliflower, place it in the fridge, and let it brine for 12 to 18 hours.

2. Set the cauliflower on a plate for a couple of hours to drain and dry. Once it is dry, preheat the oven to 400°F.

3. In a food processor, combine the paprika, garlic, lemon juice, thyme, onion, olive oil, and pepper to taste and blend to a paste.

4. Coat the cauliflower with the paste and place it on a sheet pan lined with parchment paper.

5. Roast for 30 minutes, until the outside is soft and golden but the inside is still firm.

6. For the cheese dressing: In a small bowl, combine the feta, yogurt, and lemon zest and mix with a fork until the feta is fully crumbled and blended with the yogurt. Add pepper to taste. If the feta has not already made the dressing salty enough, add salt to taste.

7. In a small dry pan over medium heat, lightly toast the walnuts for a couple of minutes. Let cool, then chop.

8. Once the cauliflower is roasted, take it out of the oven. Spread the cheese dressing as a base on a serving plate then place the roasted cauliflower on top. Pour over the salsa. Garnish with the walnuts and serve right away.

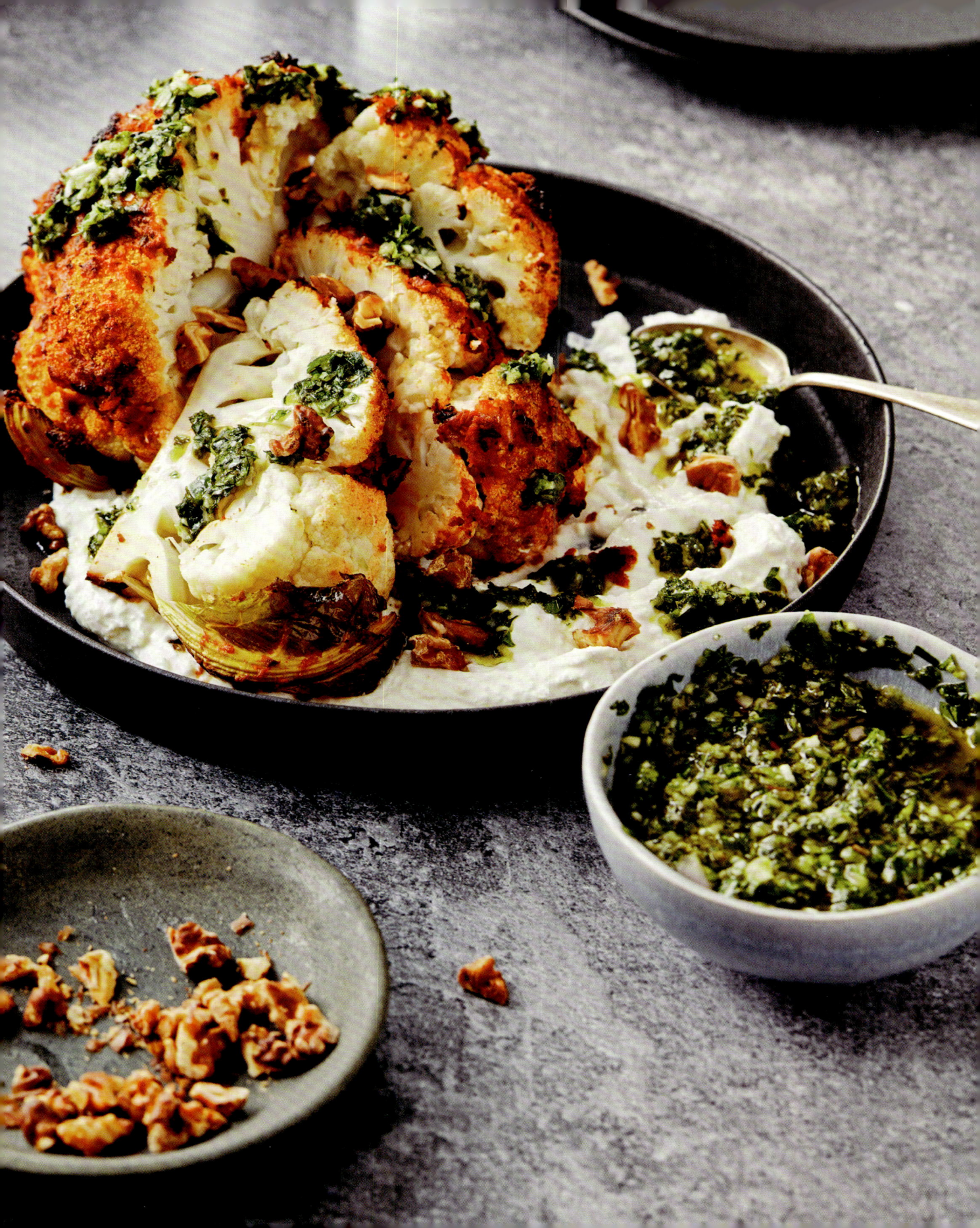

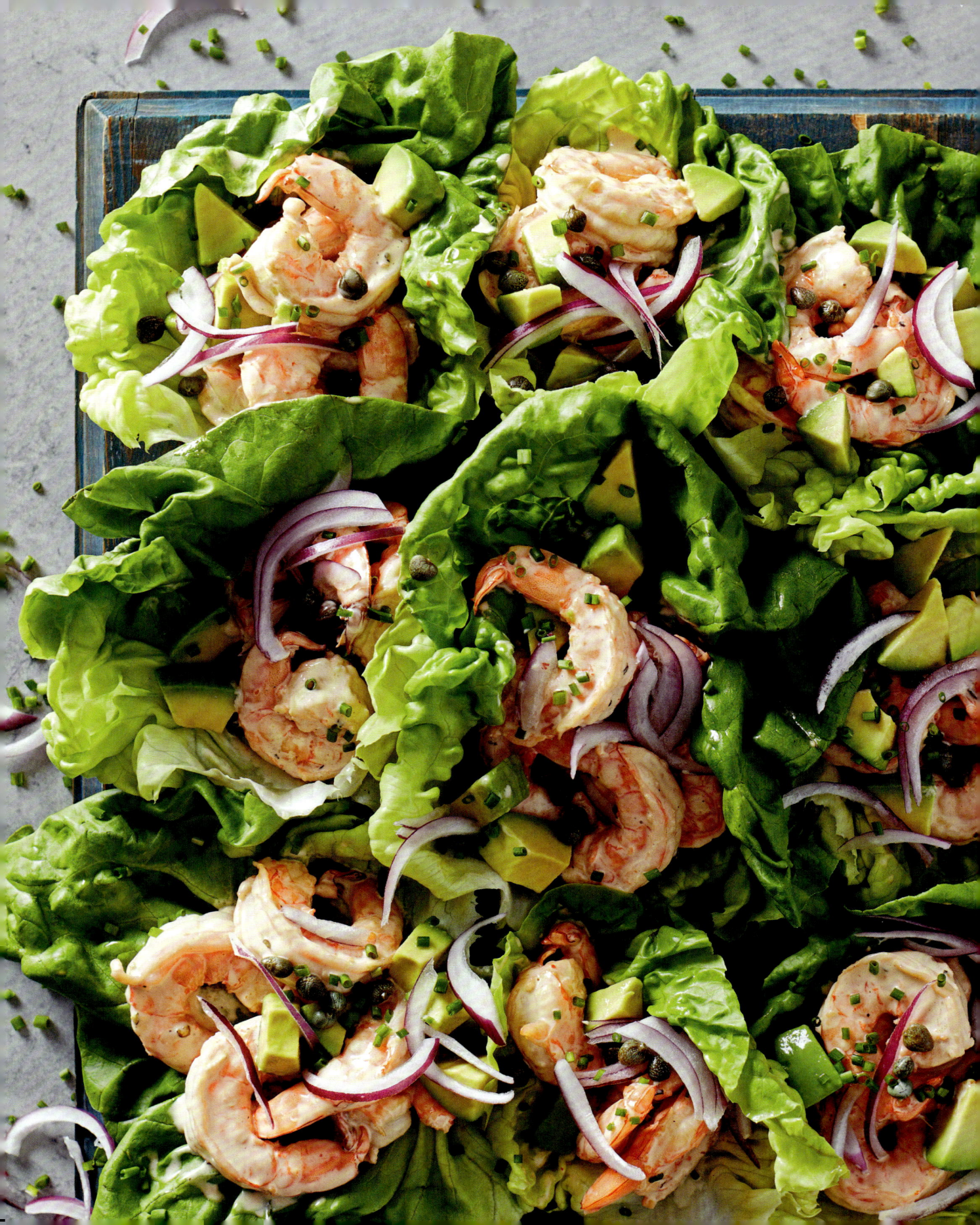

San Francisco Shrimp Louie

Inspired by the classic San Francisco Crab Louie dish, these Shrimp Louie lettuce cups are light, refreshing, and super filling. I use butter lettuce instead of salad and juicy shrimp in place of crab meat. The shrimp is tossed in a zesty truffle mayo dressing with a choice of toppings like avocado, jalapeño pepper, red onion, or whatever tastiness you're craving! The shrimp cooks super quick, so this recipe will be made in a flash. It's one of those flavorful classics for when you are tight on time but want to impress with ease.

1. Bring a medium pot of water to a boil. Add the shrimp, lemon juice, bay leaves, other aromatics (if using), and a couple of pinches of salt.

2. Boil for 60 to 75 seconds, until the shrimp turn orange or pink. Drain and immediately place in a bowl of ice water for 15 to 20 seconds to stop the cooking. Drain the ice water, then dab the shrimp dry with a paper towel. You may leave them whole or slice them into bite-sized pieces.

3. **For the truffle mayo dressing:** In a mixing bowl, combine and add the truffle mayo, lemon juice, chili sauce, Worcestershire sauce, olive oil, and vinegar. Mix well, add salt and pepper to taste, and adjust any of the other seasonings to your liking.

4. Add the shrimp to the sauce bowl and toss gently until they are evenly coated.

5. Place the shrimp onto the lettuce leaves. Add any of your favorite toppings from the suggested list and serve right away.

PREP TIME: 20 MINUTES
COOK TIME: 15 MINUTES
SERVINGS: 6 TO 8

---

2 pounds raw shrimp, peeled and deveined

3 tablespoons freshly squeezed lemon juice

Handful of dried bay leaves

Garlic, ginger, star anise, or other aromatic of choice (optional)

Salt

FOR THE TRUFFLE MAYO DRESSING

½ cup truffle mayonnaise

3 tablespoons freshly squeezed lemon juice

½ tablespoon chili sauce or sriracha

1 teaspoon Worcestershire sauce

1 teaspoon olive oil

1 teaspoon white vinegar

Salt and freshly ground black pepper

6 to 8 butter lettuce leaves, washed and dried, or another wrap of choice

OPTIONAL TOPPINGS

½ avocado, cut in chunks

1 jalapeño pepper, sliced

½ red onion, finely sliced

2 to 3 tablespoons capers

1 tablespoon finely chopped fresh chives

1 teaspoon crushed red pepper flakes

Hasselback Butternut Squash WITH PISTACHIO PESTO

Here's something I wish I'd found out sooner: Butternut squash and pistachios are the ultimate dream-team combo. The rich and nutty flavors of the squash pair perfectly with the crunchy pistachios, creating a dish that is both elevated yet totally comforting. Cooking the squash Hasselback-style brings a delicate texture, making this dish a sure winner on any table. But it wouldn't be nearly as delicious without the pistachio pesto spread underneath, which adds a burst of fresh herbs and zesty lemon to every bite.

PREP TIME: 30 MINUTES
COOK TIME: 60 MINUTES
SERVINGS: 4 TO 6

1 medium butternut squash

3 tablespoons unsalted butter

3 garlic cloves, minced

1 tablespoon chopped fresh thyme

Salt and freshly ground black pepper

FOR THE PISTACHIO PESTO

1 ounce fresh basil

1 ounce fresh parsley

⅓ ounce fresh tarragon leaves

½ cup toasted pistachios, plus extra for garnish

3 garlic cloves

½ ounce grated Parmesan cheese

3 tablespoons olive oil

2 tablespoons freshly squeezed lemon juice

Salt and freshly ground black pepper

1. Preheat the oven to 425°F.

2. Peel the squash, cut it in half lengthwise, and use a spoon to remove the seeds.

3. Place the squash halves face down on a medium baking sheet. Place a chopstick or skewer along each long side of the squash. Hasselback the squash by cutting thin crosswise slices. The chopsticks will prevent the knife from slicing all the way through, creating the Hasselback. Take your time; don't rush through this process.

4. Melt the butter until it is liquid but not hot, less than 30 seconds in the microwave or about 1 minute on the stove on low heat. Add the garlic and thyme, and season with salt and pepper.

5. Using a cooking brush, baste the squash with about two-thirds of the butter by brushing both the tops and between the slices as much as possible without breaking them. Keep the leftover butter.

6. Place the squash in the oven for 30 minutes. Remove it from the oven, baste it with the remaining butter mixture, and then bake for another 30 minutes. Set it aside for 5 minutes to cool.

7. For the pistachio pesto: In a food processor, combine the basil, parsley, tarragon, pistachios, garlic, Parmesan, olive oil, and lemon juice, with 2 tablespoons water and blend until smooth and creamy. Season with salt and pepper. If the mixture is too thick, add more water, 1 tablespoon at a time, until the desired consistency is reached. The pesto should be spreadable, not runny.

8. Spread the pesto on a serving plate and place the squash on top.

9. Garnish with extra crushed pistachios and serve right away.

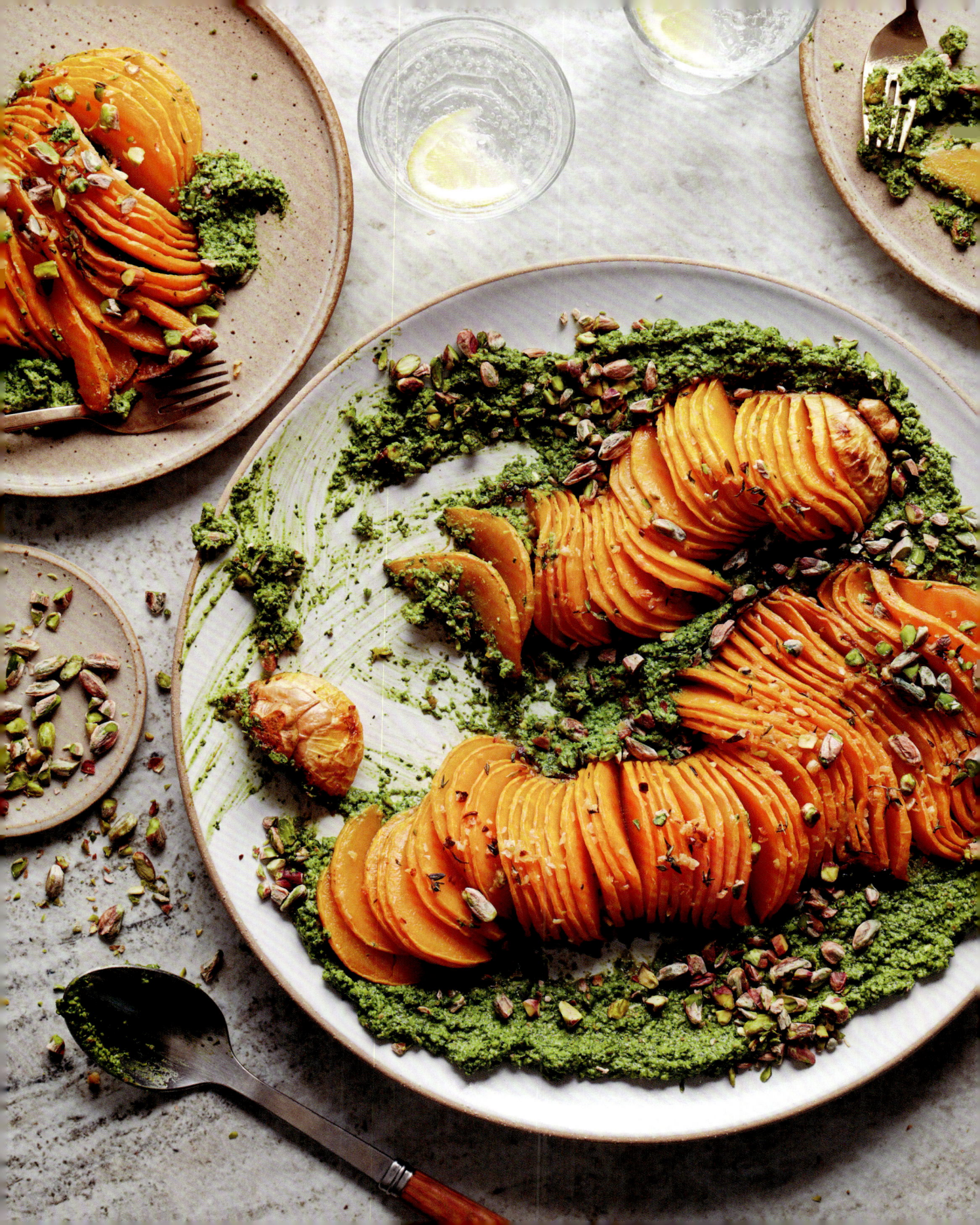

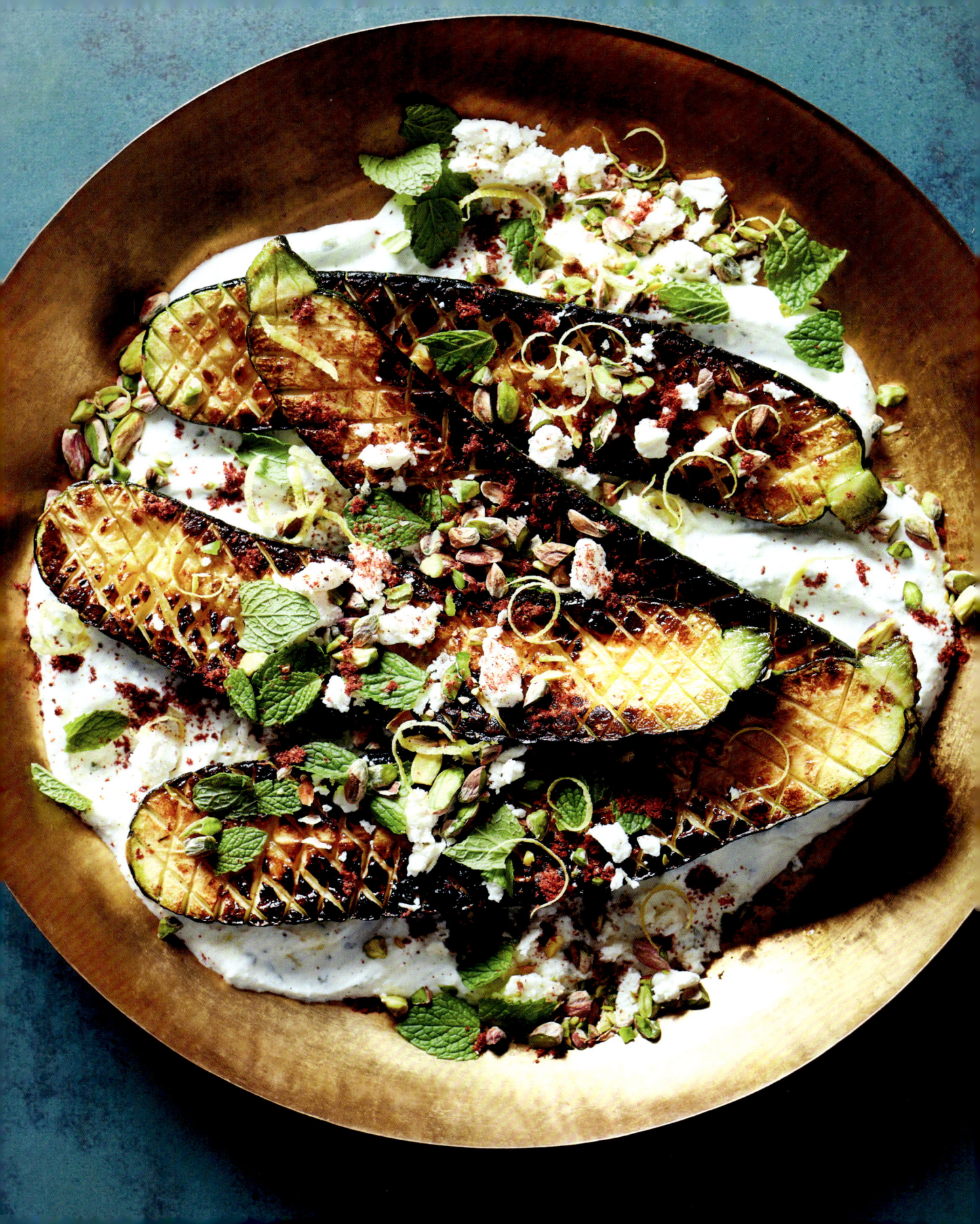

Pillowy Mediterranean Zucchini WITH GARLIC FETA SAUCE

You haven't had a zucchini like this pillowy Mediterranean version. It's my own Mediterranean spin on the viral Thomas Keller Zucchini. You simply cut the zucchini in half and score it so that it absorbs all the amazing flavor from the sauce. I seasoned mine with a simple, creamy garlic, feta, and mint sauce, then topped it with some more feta and mint, along with crushed pistachios, lemon zest, and sumac. It comes together in minutes, making it one of the easiest ways to elevate zucchini. The flavors and textures are simply legendary!

1. Rinse the zucchini and cut in half lengthwise. With a sharp knife, score the cut sides diagonally in both directions to make a crosshatch pattern. Sprinkle them with salt and let sit for 20 to 30 minutes. Remove the excess moisture by dabbing the zucchini with a paper towel.

2. Preheat the oven to 450°F.

3. **For the garlic feta sauce:** While the zucchini drains, combine in a food processor the yogurt, feta, garlic, mint, lemon juice, lemon zest, and salt and pepper to taste. Blend well.

4. Add avocado oil to a medium cast-iron skillet or stainless-steel pan. When the oil is hot, place the zucchini face down, and cook over medium-high heat for 4 to 5 minutes until the zucchini turns golden brown.

5. Transfer the pan with the zucchini to the oven and bake for 5 minutes, flip the zucchini, and bake for another 5 minutes.

6. Remove from the oven. Spoon the sauce onto a serving dish, add the zucchini face up, and garnish with your choice of toppings, such as feta, fresh mint, pistachios, lemon zest, and sumac.

PREP TIME: 30 MINUTES
COOK TIME: 20 MINUTES
SERVINGS: 2 TO 4

---

2 medium zucchini

Salt

FOR THE GARLIC FETA SAUCE

3 tablespoons plain Greek yogurt

1 ounce crumbled feta cheese

1 garlic clove

Handful of fresh mint

¼ cup freshly squeezed lemon juice

½ teaspoon lemon zest

Salt and freshly ground black pepper

¼ cup avocado oil

OPTIONAL TOPPINGS

1 ounce feta cheese, crumbled

1 tablespoon chopped fresh mint

1 tablespoon crushed toasted pistachios

½ teaspoon lemon zest

½ teaspoon sumac

Warm Olives

WITH ORANGE ZEST

When your cheese board or cocktail needs a buddy, these warm olives with orange zest are the perfect match. Olives and oranges may seem like an unusual pairing, but when warmed up together with fresh herbs, the olives become glazy and caramelized to perfection. I use two kinds of olives to give this dish lots of color and dimension. It's so satisfying to serve during the cooler months and easy enough to make that you can prepare it for a dinner party in a pinch. You really can't beat the trifecta of simple ingredients, easy prep, and next-level flavor!

PREP TIME: 10 MINUTES
COOK TIME: 20 MINUTES
SERVINGS: 4 TO 6

1 large orange

5 tablespoons olive oil

1 sprig fresh rosemary

1 sprig fresh oregano

2 garlic cloves

6 ounces black olives or kalamata olives

5 ounces green olives (Castelvetrano)

Pinch of ground fennel, plus extra for garnish

¼ teaspoon crushed red pepper flakes

Fresh bread or crackers, or a cheese board, for serving (optional)

1. With a peeler, remove half the orange peel in thin strips. Zest the other half of the orange and set the zest aside. Finally, squeeze the juice of the whole orange.

2. Set a medium saucepan on the stove over low heat. Add the olive oil and heat for about 1 minute.

3. Add the rosemary and oregano sprigs and stir and fry for 3 to 4 minutes, until the oil becomes fragrant. Make sure the sprigs don't burn, as it will turn the oil bitter. Remove the sprigs from the oil. Keep the leaves and needles from the roasted sprigs for garnishing.

4. Slice the garlic into thin slices and add it to the oil, together with the orange peel, the black and green olives, a pinch of the fennel, and the red pepper flakes. Continue to stir and fry for 5 to 6 minutes.

5. Add the orange juice and cook until the sauce is reduced to a glaze-like consistency, 10 to 12 minutes.

6. Remove the olives from the pan and place them in a serving dish.

7. Garnish with the finely grated zest, another pinch of fennel, and the roasted leaves and needles from the oregano and rosemary sprigs.

8. Serve with fresh bread or crackers, or as a topping on a cheese board.

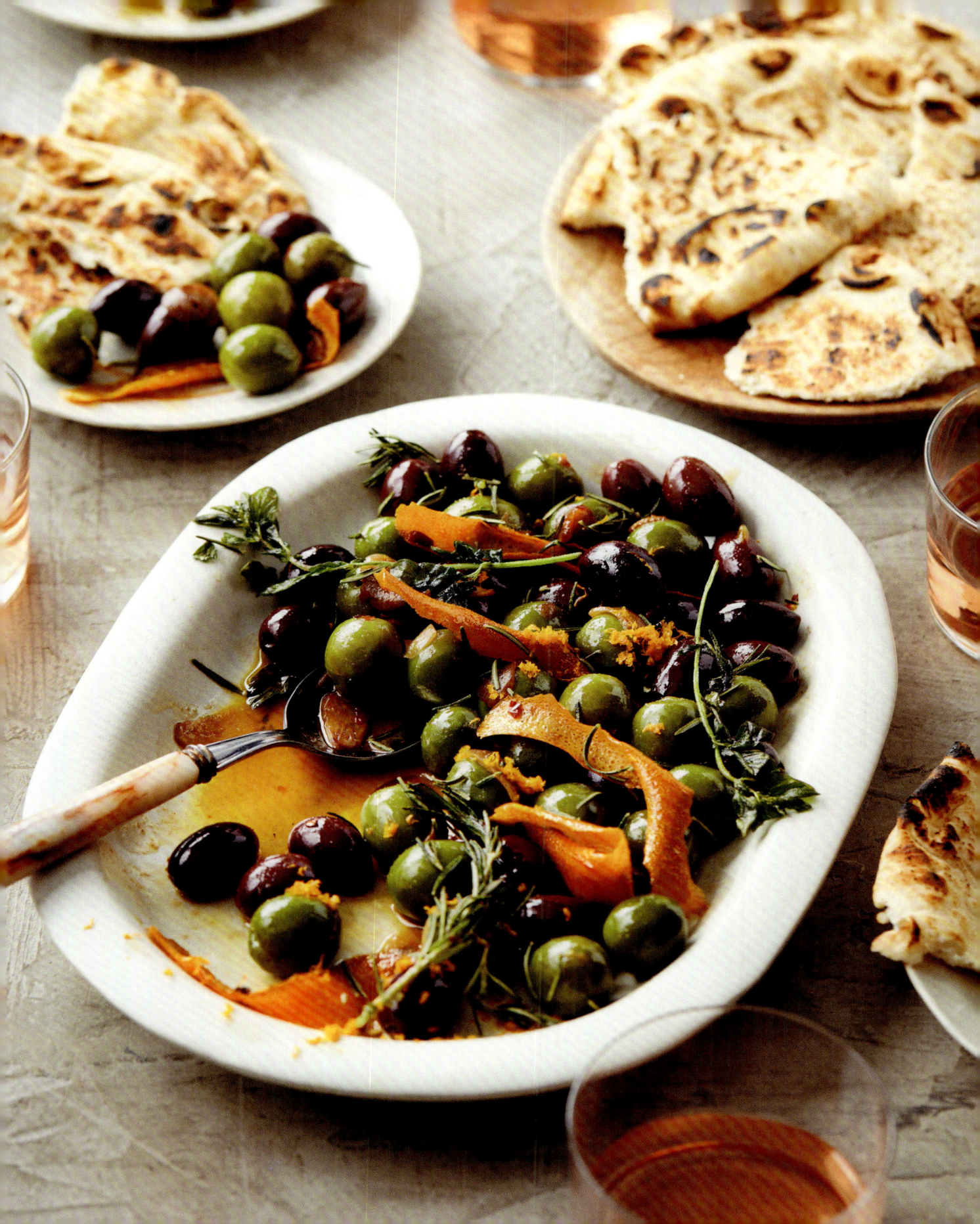

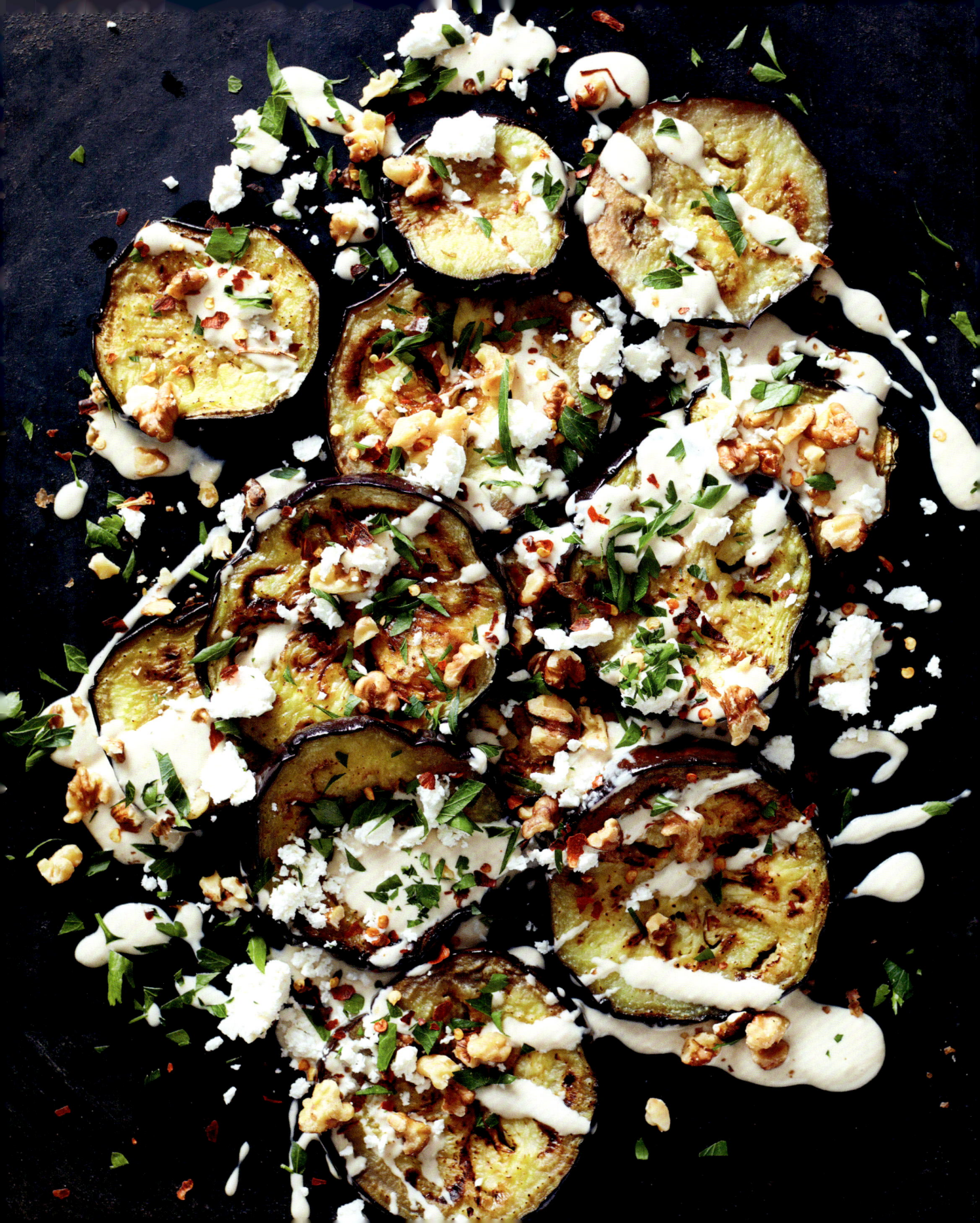

Roasted Eggplant
WITH TAHINI & WALNUTS

This warm roasted eggplant with tahini and walnuts brings all the right textures together. Typically, roasting the eggplant to a crunchy top and creamy middle requires a lot of oil, as the eggplant acts like a sponge. The method below will yield the same results with a fraction of the oil. To connect with my roots, I loaded these delicious eggplants with all my favorite Mediterranean ingredients: tahini, walnuts, parsley, and feta cheese. It's an epic flavor and texture combination that will make you want to lick your plate clean!

PREP TIME: 10 MINUTES
COOK TIME: 25 MINUTES
SERVINGS: 4 TO 6

1 large or 2 medium eggplant

Salt

2 to 3 tablespoons olive oil

1 ounce raw walnuts

2 tablespoons tahini

¼ cup freshly squeezed lemon juice

1 or 2 garlic cloves, minced

Freshly ground black pepper

1½ ounces feta cheese, crumbled

1 tablespoon chopped fresh parsley

1 teaspoon crushed red pepper flakes (optional)

1. Cut the eggplant crosswise into ⅓-inch slices. Sprinkle salt lightly on both sides and set between paper towels or cloth for 30 minutes to absorb the excess moisture.

2. Preheat the oven to 350°F.

3. Brush the eggplant slices with the olive oil using a cooking brush and set in a nonstick pan over medium-high heat. (By brushing the eggplant instead of coating the pan, we reduce the amount of oil.)

4. Sear the slices on each side for 3 to 4 minutes, until the eggplant has light golden-brown spots. Press down occasionally with a spatula to ensure that the entire surface of the eggplant slice touches the pan. The eggplant is not fully cooked yet, but the exterior gets that charred roast.

5. Transfer the eggplant slices to a medium baking sheet and place in the oven for 15 to 20 minutes to allow the eggplant to fully cook.

6. While the eggplant is baking, toast the walnuts in a small dry pan over medium heat, tossing continuously, until the edges of the walnuts look dark brown (about 2 minutes). Remove from the pan, let cool, and chop coarsely.

7. In a small bowl, mix the tahini (stir it first, as it tends to separate), lemon juice, garlic, and salt and pepper to taste. The paste will thicken once mixed; add 1 tablespoon of water at a time and continue whisking until the sauce is creamy, not thick (you should be able to pour it with a spoon).

8. Once the eggplant is cooked, place the slices on a serving plate. Pour the tahini mixture over top, sprinkle with the crumbled feta and toasted walnuts, and top with the fresh parsley. Add red pepper flakes for heat if desired.

Minced Lamb Lettuce Cups

These minced meat lettuce cups with a Middle Eastern flair have converted me into a lettuce wrap fanatic. The crisp lettuce cups provide the perfect vessel to enjoy every bite. To take the flavor to the next level, I added an easy garlic shallot yogurt dip and topped the meat with sumac pickled red onion. It's simple additions like these that really tie everything together and make this dish shine.

1. **For the pickled onion:** In a small bowl, combine the onion, sumac, lemon juice, parsley, and salt and pepper. Give it a quick mix, and set it aside to rest.

2. **For the garlic shallot yogurt dip:** In a small bowl, combine the yogurt, shallot, garlic, and salt and pepper to taste. Set it aside to allow the yogurt to infuse with the flavors.

3. Set a pan over medium heat and add the olive oil. Once the oil is heated, add the onion, garlic, sumac, and Moroccan Spice Blend. Sauté until the onion turns golden brown, then add the ground lamb and beef, continuously chopping it with a spatula or a meat masher to prevent it from clumping. Cook until the meat turns golden brown and all the excess moisture has evaporated, 12 to 15 minutes. Add salt and pepper to taste.

4. Break the lettuce into individual leaves to make the cups. In each cup, spread a couple of tablespoons of the garlic shallot yogurt dip, then add 2 to 3 tablespoons of the cooked meat.

5. Top with the pickled onion and some more fresh parsley, and it's ready to serve.

PREP TIME: 20 MINUTES
COOK TIME: 20 MINUTES
SERVINGS: 6

FOR THE PICKLED ONION

1 medium red onion, sliced into thin strips

1 tablespoon sumac

5 tablespoons of freshly squeezed lemon juice

3 tablespoons chopped fresh parsley, plus extra for garnish

Salt and freshly ground black pepper

FOR THE GARLIC SHALLOT YOGURT DIP

1 cup plain yogurt

¼ shallot, minced

2 garlic cloves, minced

Salt and freshly ground black pepper

½ tablespoon olive oil

½ medium onion, minced

4 garlic cloves, crushed

1 tablespoon sumac

4 teaspoons Moroccan Spice Blend (page 223)

½ pound ground lamb

½ pound ground beef

Salt and freshly ground black pepper

1 head butter lettuce

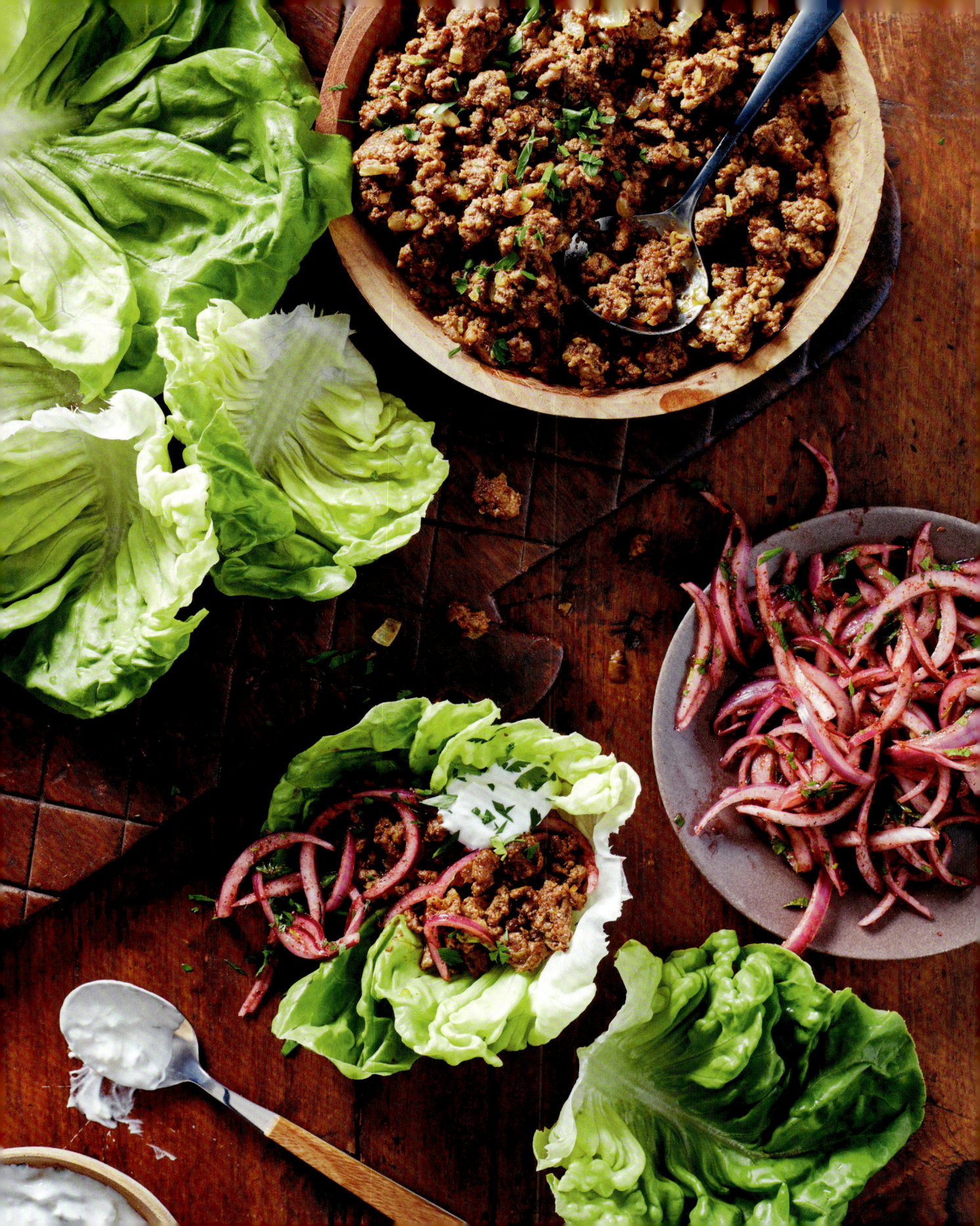

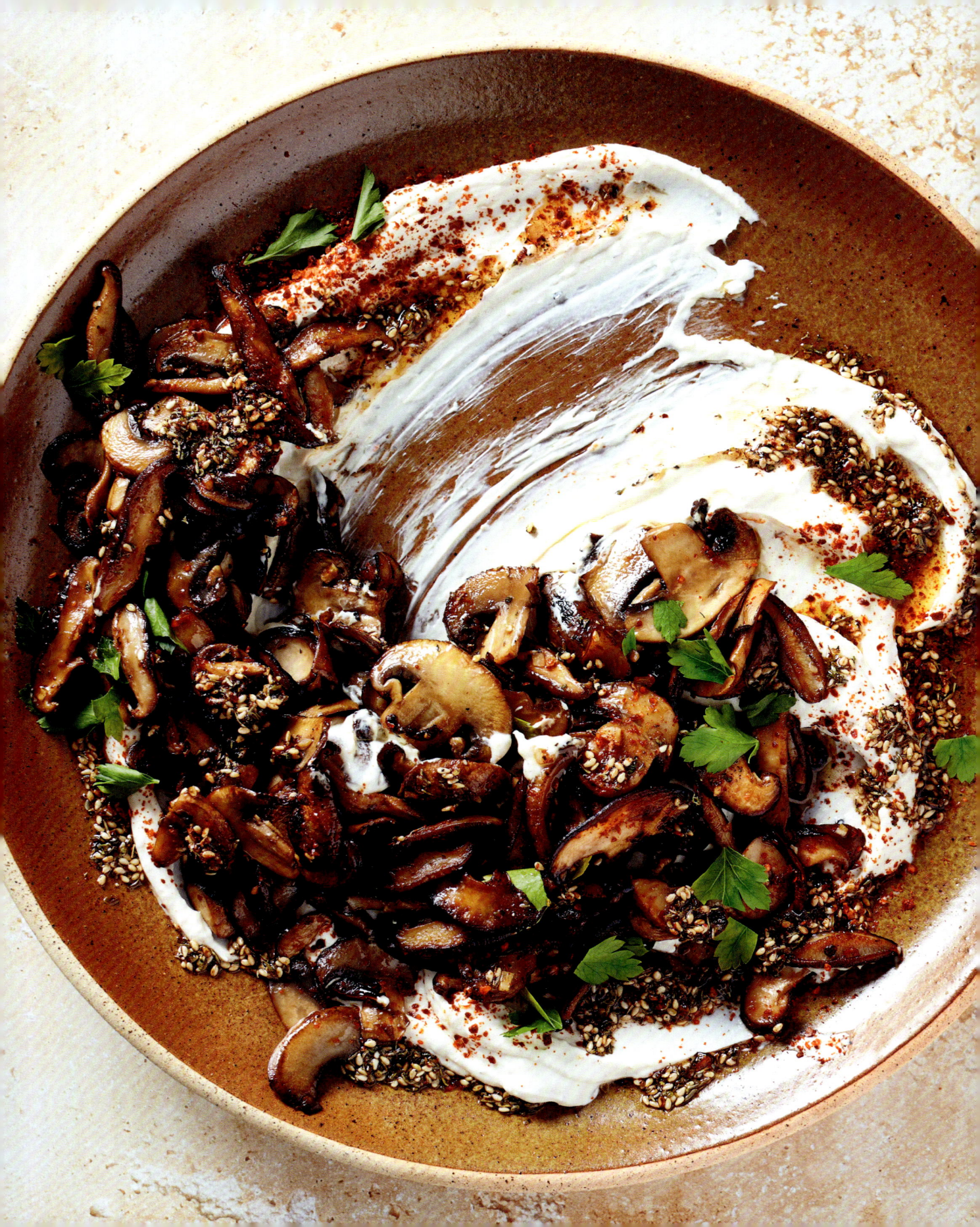

Sautéed Mushrooms

OVER TAHINI LABNEH

This dish of earthy mushrooms and nutty, tangy tahini labneh is equally rustic and bougie. The combination of flavors and textures will make you want to make it again and again, especially because it's so easy to whip up. The dip and oil come together in a matter of minutes, while the mushrooms get seared with a foolproof technique that I've been using for years. It gets them perfectly browned and slightly crisp without any fuss or babysitting. You can also use this labneh as a dip, as a smear on sandwiches, or as a sauce to top off your favorite protein or vegetables.

1. **For the tahini labneh:** In a medium mixing bowl, combine the labneh, tahini, garlic, and salt and pepper to taste. Mix well and set aside.

2. **For the za'atar oil:** In a small bowl, combine the olive oil and za'atar and mix well. Set aside to allow the flavors to infuse.

3. Clean the mushrooms. In order to avoid excess moisture, I recommend lightly brushing the mushrooms with a paper towel instead of washing them. Mushrooms act like a sponge and absorb a lot of water, making them mushy when cooked. If washing, pat them dry with a paper towel. Cut the mushrooms into ¼-inch slices.

4. In a medium dry pan over medium-high heat, sauté the mushrooms. (Dry sautéing eliminates excess moisture and gets that golden-brown sear.) Stirring occasionally, wait for the mushrooms to release their liquid, about 3 to 4 minutes, then sauté until the liquid has reduced, another 2 to 3 minutes.

5. Once the mushrooms are turning golden brown, add the garlic, olive oil, Worcestershire sauce, and salt and pepper to taste. Sauté for another 2 to 3 minutes.

6. Spread the tahini labneh dip on a serving platter. Place the sautéed mushrooms on top and drizzle with the za'atar oil.

7. Garnish with the parsley. For a touch of extra heat, sprinkle on some Aleppo pepper. Serve right away.

PREP TIME: 20 MINUTES
COOK TIME: 15 MINUTES
SERVINGS: 4 TO 6

FOR THE TAHINI LABNEH

10 ounces labneh, homemade (page 66) or store-bought

3 tablespoons tahini

2 garlic cloves, minced

Salt and freshly ground black pepper

FOR THE ZA'ATAR OIL

2 tablespoons olive oil

¾ tablespoon za'atar, homemade (page 222) or store-bought

5 ounces shiitake mushrooms, stems removed

6 ounces cremini mushrooms

2 garlic cloves, minced

1 tablespoon olive oil

1 teaspoon Worcestershire sauce

Salt and freshly ground black pepper

1 tablespoon chopped fresh parsley, for garnish

½ teaspoon Aleppo pepper, for garnish (optional)

Fresh Herb Frittata

Packed with herbs and spices, this frittata is a powerhouse of flavor and nutrition. A traditional frittata features a combination of eggs and cheese, but this recipe takes things to the next level by including fresh herbs like parsley and cilantro and invigorating spices like curry powder, cinnamon, sumac, and fenugreek for a delightfully unique flavor combination you've probably never experienced before. The prep is simple, as all the ingredients get thrown in a blender before being cooked over the stove. The frittata comes out a gorgeous earthy green color, and you can top it with chopped walnuts and slivered almonds for an even more immaculate presentation.

1. In a blender or large food processor, combine the scallions, parsley, cilantro, garlic, curry powder, cinnamon, sumac, fenugreek, almond flour, yogurt, onion, baking powder, eggs, and salt and pepper to taste, and blend together for a couple of minutes.

2. Place a medium pan over high heat and add the olive oil.

3. Test that the oil is hot enough by pouring in a couple of drops from the egg mixture. If they start bubbling right away, add the mixture to the pan and turn the heat to medium-low. Sprinkle in the walnuts (if using) for extra crunch.

4. Cook for 25 to 30 minutes on the first side. To flip, use a flat spatula to gently slide the frittata off the pan and onto a large plate. Place the pan over the frittata plate and flip both together so that the frittata falls face down in the pan.

5. Cook on the other side for about 20 minutes, until the bottom is golden brown. Lightly lift with a spatula to check.

6. **For the onion and nut toppings (optional):** While the frittata is cooking, add the olive oil to a small pan over medium heat. Once the oil is hot, add the onion and the turmeric and sauté until golden brown and crispy. Using a slotted spatula, remove the onion and set aside.

7. In the same pan, using the leftover oil, toast the walnuts and almonds for a minute. Remove the nuts using a slotted spatula and discard the remaining oil.

8. When the frittata is cooked, slide it onto a large serving plate and top it with the sautéed onion, walnuts, and almonds.

9. Serve right away.

PREP TIME: 15 MINUTES
COOK TIME: 1 HOUR
SERVINGS: 6 TO 8

---

4 ounces scallions, white and green parts

4 ounces fresh parsley

4 ounces fresh cilantro

5 garlic cloves

1 teaspoon curry powder

½ teaspoon ground cinnamon

1 teaspoon sumac

1 teaspoon dried fenugreek leaves

2 tablespoons almond flour

2 tablespoons plain yogurt

1 medium yellow onion, chopped

1 teaspoon baking powder

6 large eggs

Salt and freshly ground black pepper

¼ cup olive oil

¼ cup chopped raw walnuts (optional)

FOR THE ONION AND NUT TOPPINGS (OPTIONAL)

¼ cup olive oil

1 medium onion, finely sliced

½ teaspoon ground turmeric

¼ cup chopped raw walnuts

¼ cup slivered raw almonds

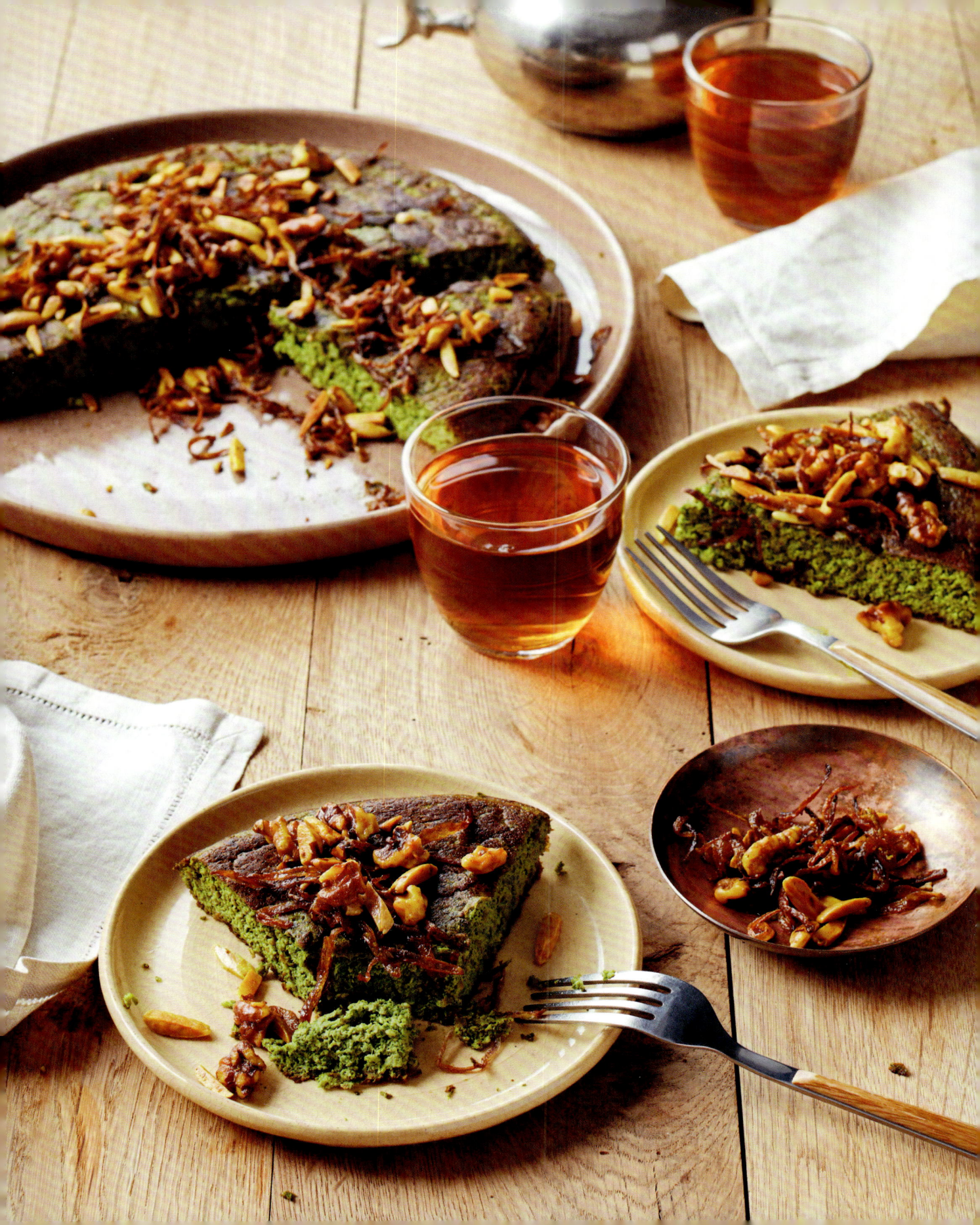

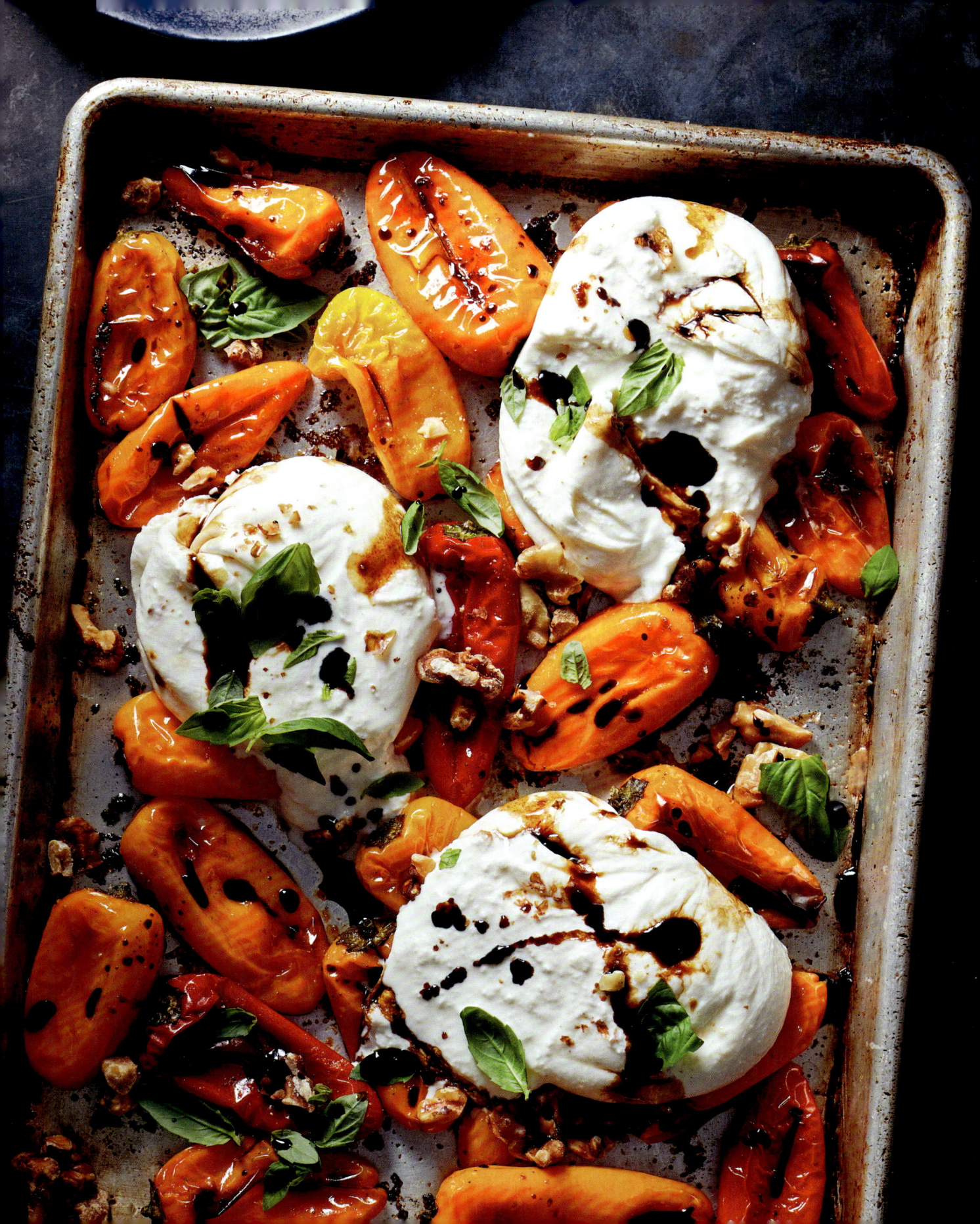

Roasted Red Pepper Truffle Burrata

WITH WALNUTS

This roasted red pepper truffle burrata is a game-changer when it comes to appetizers. The flavor and texture combo of the roasted sweet peppers, truffle burrata cheese, toasted walnuts, fresh lemon basil, and balsamic vinegar is absolute bliss. Just cut and season your peppers, roast them, and top 'em with all the goods. It's one of those easy and delicious appetizers that you can have up your sleeve when you have last-minute guests, a case of the hangries, or the urge to treat yourself to something fresh and tasty.

1. Preheat the oven to 450°F.

2. Rinse the peppers well. Slice them in half lengthwise, and remove the seeds using a small spoon.

3. In a medium bowl, coat the peppers with the olive oil, garlic powder, truffle seasoning, and salt and pepper to taste.

4. Pile the peppers on a large baking sheet and roast for 17 to 20 minutes. Remove from the oven, flip, and add some additional olive oil and salt to taste. Place back in the oven for another 15 to 17 minutes, until thoroughly roasted.

5. Remove from the oven and plate.

6. Tear the truffle burrata and place on top of the peppers. Sprinkle with toasted walnuts and fresh lemon basil and drizzle with balsamic vinegar. Serve as an appetizer or side.

PREP TIME: 15 MINUTES
COOK TIME: 40 MINUTES
SERVINGS: 4 TO 6

---

1 pound mini peppers (Jimmy Nardello peppers are my favorite)

¼ cup olive oil, plus extra

1 teaspoon garlic powder

1 teaspoon truffle seasoning

Salt and freshly ground black pepper

3 3-ounce balls truffle burrata cheese balls

¼ cup toasted walnuts

Handful of fresh lemon basil

1 tablespoon balsamic vinegar

Spicy Marinated Lupini Beans WITH FETA

If you're familiar with my Kaizen low-carb pasta, you may have heard of lupini beans. This healthy bean is ground into a fine powder to make my tasty noodles. So, I figured I could honor this special bean by making these spicy marinated lupini beans with feta! This dish perfectly highlights the beans' rich, earthy flavor in its original form, tossed with feta and a flavorful blend of spices and herbs to make a delicious, high-protein dish that will keep you full for hours. Don't underestimate the power of lupini beans! They're a true gem in the world of low-carb cooking.

PREP TIME: 15 MINUTES
COOK TIME: 30 MINUTES (OPTIONAL)
SERVINGS: 6 TO 8

___

21 ounces lupini beans in brine

1 teaspoon chipotle powder

1 tablespoon garlic powder

½ tablespoon chili lime seasoning, such as Tajín, plus extra for garnish

1 tablespoon fresh oregano, plus extra for garnish

5 tablespoons freshly squeezed lemon juice

3 tablespoons olive oil

Salt and freshly ground black pepper

5 ounces feta cheese, cubed

1. Drain the lupini beans. They come pre-cooked, but if they seem too firm, add them to a pot of boiling water and cook for an extra 30 minutes to soften them up. They should still feel al dente. Drain and rinse with cold water.

2. Place the beans in a bowl and add the chipotle powder, garlic powder, chili lime seasoning, oregano, lemon juice, olive oil, and salt and pepper to taste. Give them a good mix using a spatula.

3. Add the feta cubes to the bowl and gently fold them in so they get coated with the spices but not crumbled or crushed.

4. Serve right away or keep in the fridge for up to 4 days. Garnish with extra chili lime seasoning and fresh oregano.

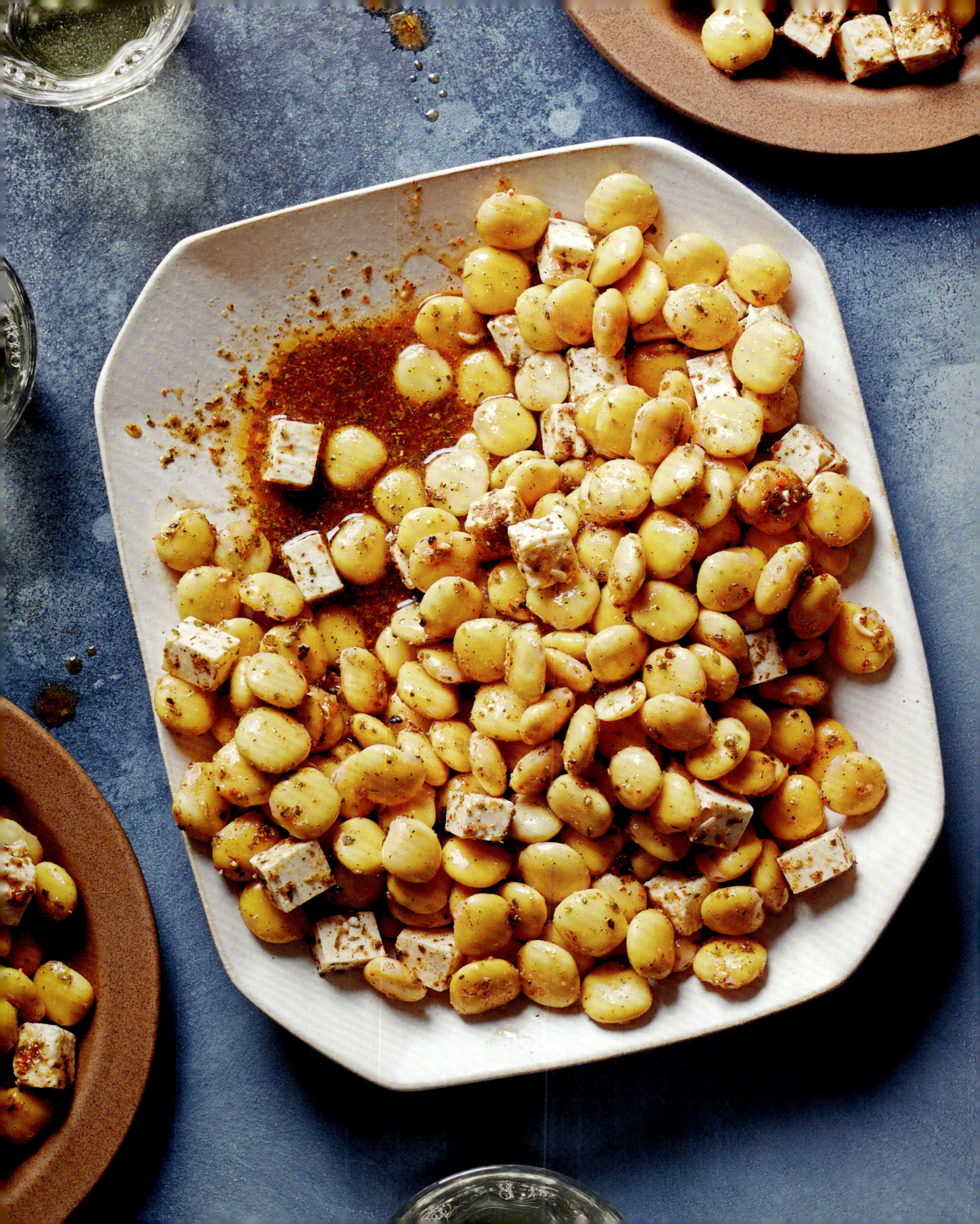

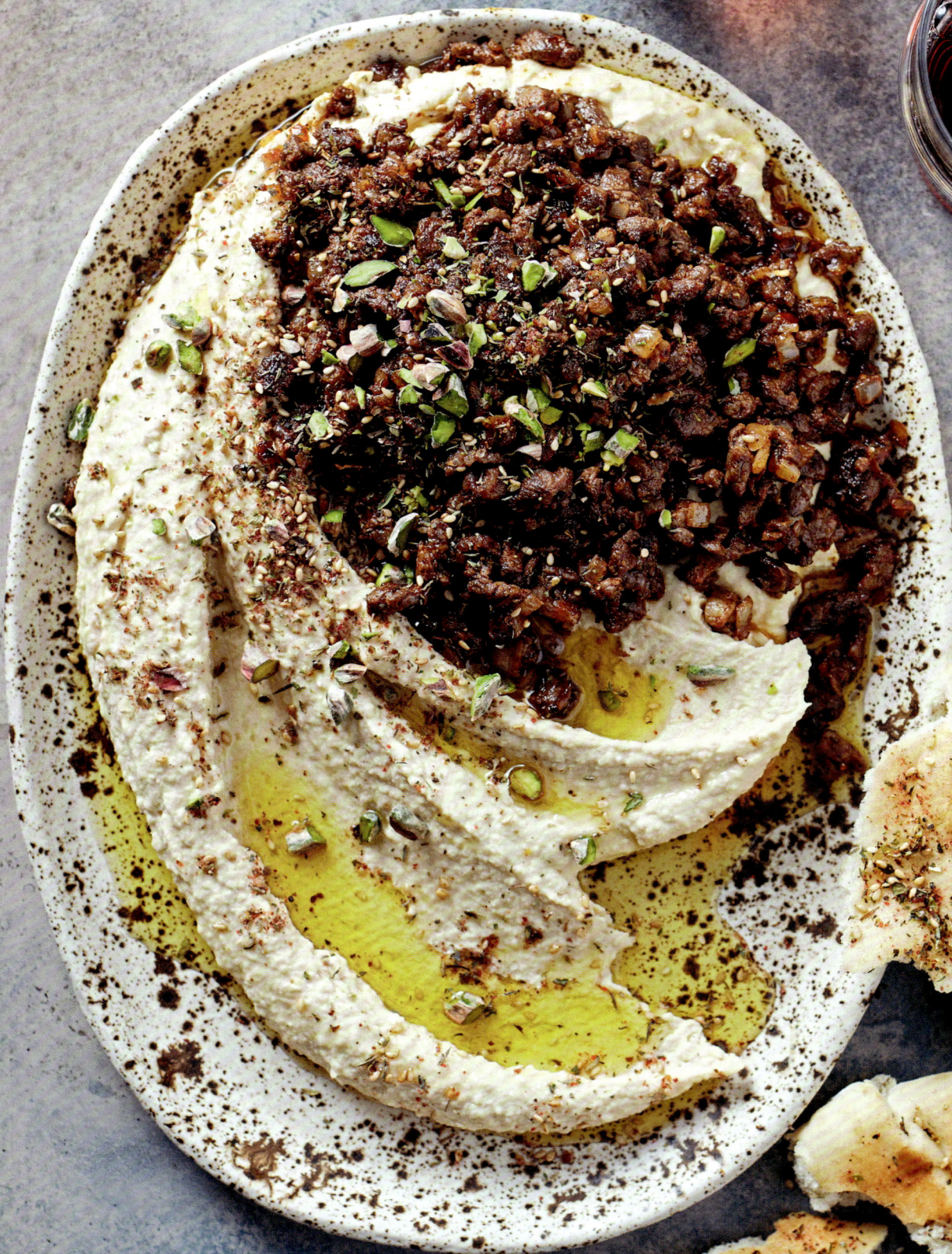

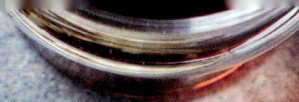

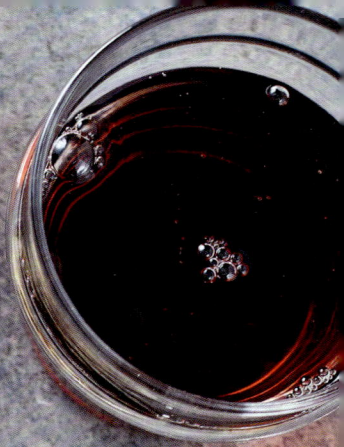

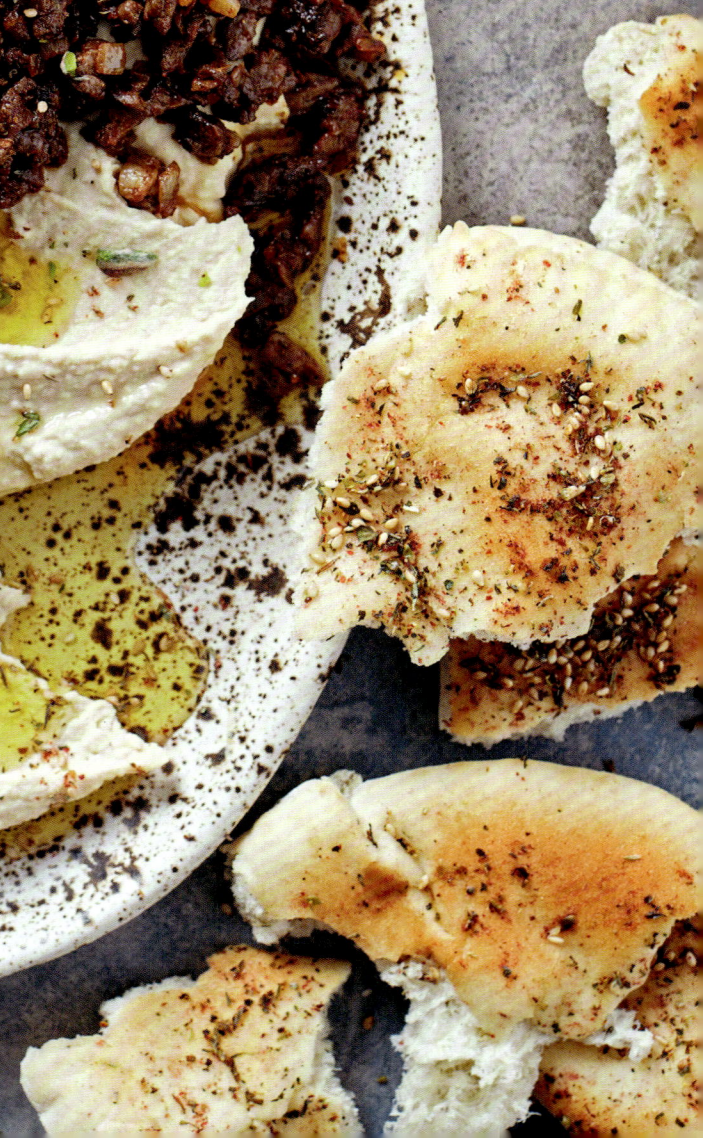

Hummus

WITH MINCED MEAT

Hummus with minced meat is the ultimate shareable. It brings me fond memories of friends and family sharing this dish, making it even more special. It's packed with all kinds of flavor, and the finely diced rib eye adds an exciting element that takes this classic dip to the next level. The marinade is a medley of my favorite Middle Eastern herbs and spices, and the hummus comes out super silky smooth. For extra-special crunch and flavor, top it off with some crushed pistachios and za'atar. You're going to want to dip everything into this hummus—your favorite low-carb chips, fresh veggies, or even good old pita bread if your diet allows.

PREP TIME: 20 MINUTES
COOK TIME: 15 MINUTES
SERVINGS: 6 TO 8

10 ounces rib-eye steak

½ teaspoon sweet paprika

½ teaspoon coriander

½ teaspoon sumac

½ teaspoon dried thyme

¼ teaspoon ground ginger

1 teaspoon ground cumin

½ teaspoon crushed red pepper flakes

Salt and freshly ground black pepper

1 tablespoon olive oil

½ small onion, minced

FOR THE HUMMUS

2 (15.5-ounce) cans chickpeas, drained

3 garlic cloves

6 tablespoons tahini

⅓ cup bone broth or water

4 ice cubes

6 tablespoons freshly squeezed lemon juice, plus more as needed

Salt and freshly ground black pepper

Crushed roasted pistachios, for garnish

Za'atar, homemade (page 222) or store-bought, for garnish

1. Cut the steak into ¼-inch cubes. In a medium bowl, combine the meat cubes, paprika, coriander, sumac, thyme, ginger, cumin, red pepper flakes, salt and pepper to taste, and ½ tablespoon of the olive oil and massage it together. Set aside.

2. Set a medium pan over medium heat and add the remaining ½ tablespoon of olive oil. Once the pan is hot, add the onion to the pan.

3. Sauté the onion for 4 to 5 minutes, until it turns golden.

4. Add the marinated meat to the pan and sauté for 6 to 8 minutes, until the meat is cooked.

5. While the meat is cooking, make the hummus.

6. **For the hummus:** In a food processor, combine the chickpeas, garlic, tahini, bone broth, ice cubes, and lemon juice and blend until you get a smooth, thick paste, 2 to 3 minutes. Add salt, pepper, and more lemon juice to taste.

7. Place the hummus in a deep plate and add the cooked meat on top.

8. Garnish with the crushed pistachios and za'atar.

Honey Grilled Halloumi

WITH PISTACHIOS & ZA'ATAR

This halloumi with pistachios and za'atar is one of my favorite shareable plates with friends and family. Halloumi is a highly versatile cheese that can be sliced and grilled, making a delicious addition to a variety of dishes. In this recipe, I grilled it and topped it with a drizzle of honey and a sprinkling of za'atar and Aleppo pepper flakes. It's a spectacular combination of sweet and salty flavors, with an added crunch when you top it with the toasted pistachios. Make sure you serve it right away, because it tastes the most satisfying when warm and fresh off the grill.

PREP TIME: 5 MINUTES
COOK TIME: 10 MINUTES
SERVINGS: 4 TO 6

3 tablespoons raw pistachios

7 ounces halloumi

2 tablespoons olive oil

2 tablespoons honey or agave syrup or a low-carb substitute such as allulose "honey syrup"

1 to 1½ tablespoons za'atar, homemade (page 222) or store-bought

½ teaspoon Aleppo pepper (optional)

1. In a small dry pan over medium-low heat, toast the pistachios for 3 to 4 minutes, stirring frequently. The pistachios are ready when they become fragrant and slightly golden. Let cool, then chop finely and set aside.

2. Pat the halloumi cheese dry with a paper towel or kitchen cloth. Cut into ¼-inch slices.

3. Heat the olive oil in a medium grill pan over medium heat. Lay the halloumi slices in a single layer and sear for 2 to 3 minutes, until they turn golden brown, then flip and sear for another minute. Drizzle with the honey, sear for 1 more minute, then transfer to a plate.

4. Top with the za'atar, chopped pistachios, and a pinch or two of Aleppo pepper if desired.

5. Enjoy immediately, while still warm.

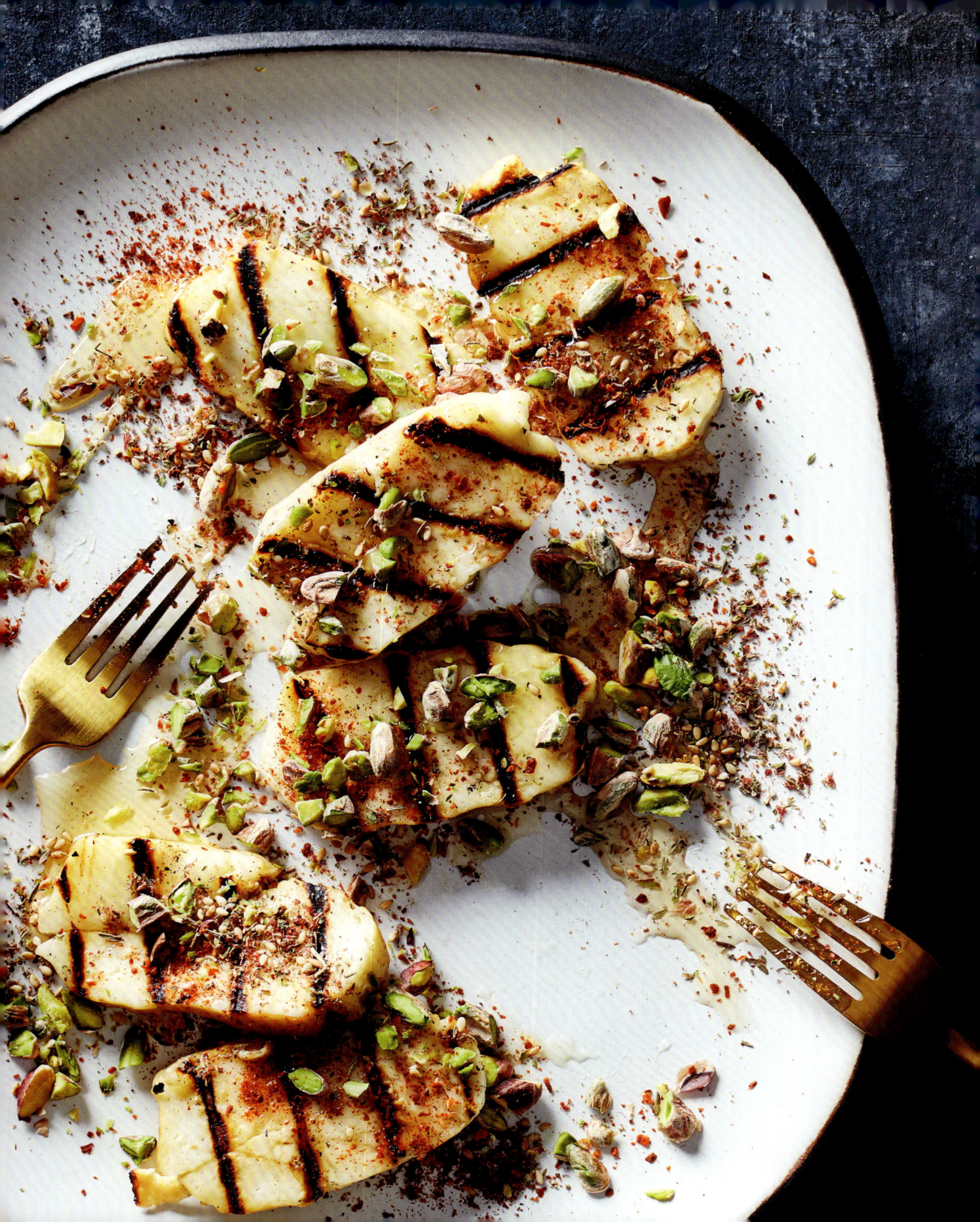

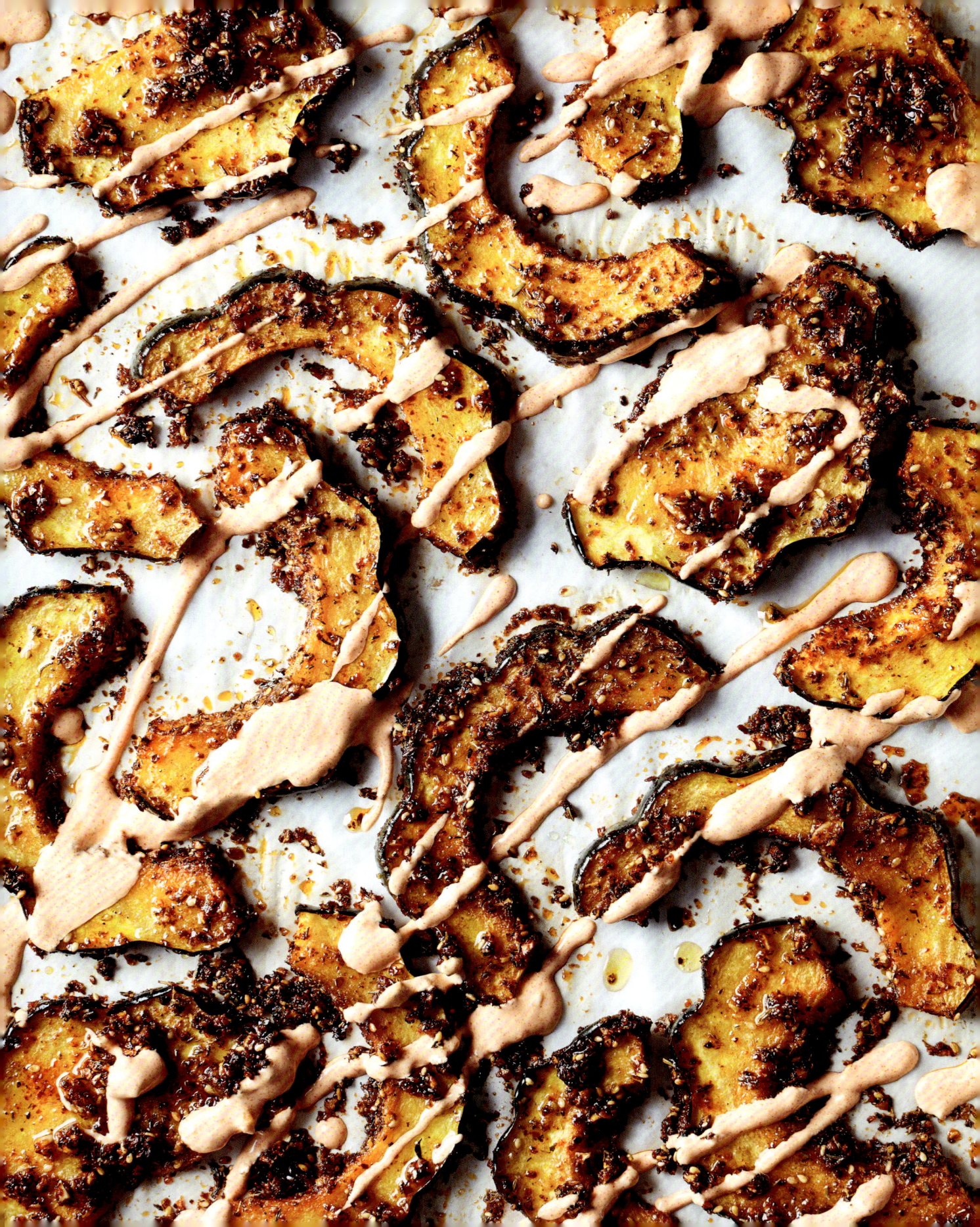

Roasted Acorn Squash

WITH SMOKY GARLIC AIOLI

This roasted acorn squash comes out gloriously tender on the inside and crispy on the outside. I couldn't help but add my own Middle Eastern spin, so I seasoned the squash with staples like Aleppo pepper and za'atar. These flavors, combined with the smoky garlic aioli, really hit the spot—especially during the fall season! It's low-carb and makes a great appetizer or snack, or serve it as a side dish with my Spatchcock Chicken (page 124) or Salmon Skewers (page 151). Just cut and season your squash, pop it into the oven, and you're good to go.

1. Preheat the oven or air fryer to 425°F.

2. Cut the squash in half, remove the seeds, and then cut into slices about ⅓-inch thick.

3. In a large bowl, combine the squash slices, avocado oil, garlic, Aleppo pepper, za'atar, and salt to taste. Toss well.

4. Place the squash slices on a large baking sheet in one layer, and roast for 30 to 35 minutes. Time varies by oven. The squash is ready once the slices are soft and are easily pierced with a fork.

5. **For the smoky garlic aioli:** In a small bowl, combine the mayo, yogurt, garlic, smoked paprika, and lemon juice. Stir well.

6. Remove the squash from the oven and plate. Drizzle the aioli over top or serve it on the side for dipping.

PREP TIME: 20 MINUTES
COOK TIME: 40 MINUTES
SERVINGS: 4 TO 6

———

1 large acorn squash

2 tablespoons avocado oil

4 garlic cloves, minced

2 tablespoons Aleppo pepper

2 tablespoons za'atar, homemade (page 222) or store-bought

Salt

FOR THE SMOKY GARLIC AIOLI

2½ tablespoons mayonnaise

1 tablespoon plain Greek yogurt

2 garlic cloves, minced

1 teaspoon smoked paprika

1 tablespoon freshly squeezed lemon juice

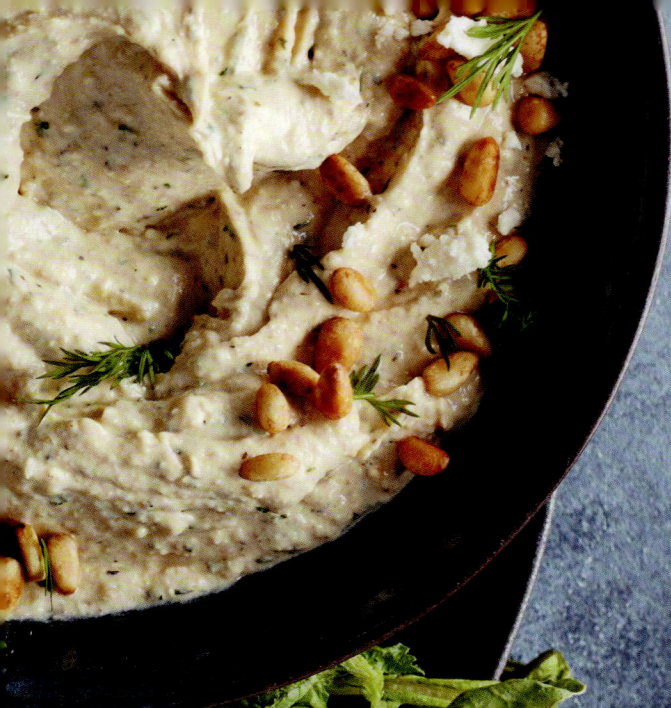

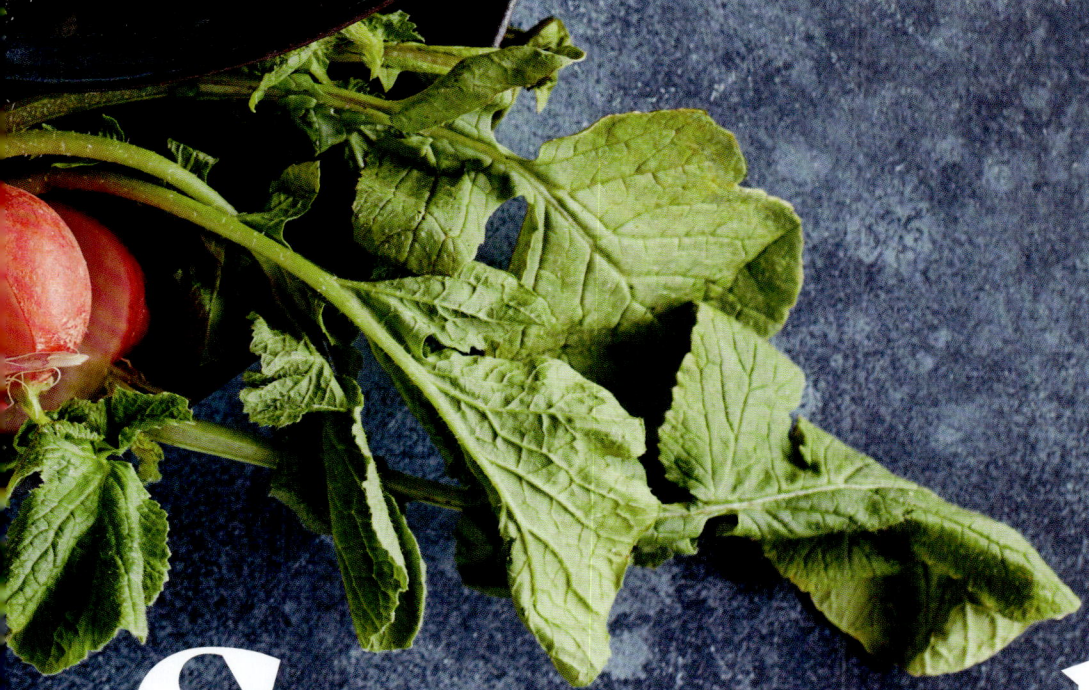

Spreads
& Dips

We all have different preferences for our vessels, or "dippers." Sure, there's chips, crackers, pita bread, or sourdough—and these spreads and dips are delicious with all of those. But some of us (me!) look for lower-carb options. My go-to dippers include fresh veggies like cucumbers, bell peppers, and carrots; crunchy cheese crisps; or low-carb crackers. But don't stop there: You can even dip kabobs into them, dunk in some wings, or spread them over your favorite protein. There are no rules, only delicious possibilities.

Many of these recipes will require a small food processor, so make sure you have one on hand. It not only cuts the prep time in half, it also gets these dips nice and smooth.

Garlic Feta Dip

Garlic, feta, what could be betta? This is every garlic and cheese lover's dream dip, while keeping things fresh, low-carb, and super simple. I used 20 garlic cloves for this recipe, but you can use more or less depending on your tastes. The fresh dill is meant to play a supporting role, as garlic is the real lead act here, so start light and taste as you go! I recommend doubling this recipe because you're going to be eating it by the spoonful before you end up serving it (trust me). This is perfect as a dip with fresh cucumbers and pita chips for a starter or next to your favorite grilled protein such as lamb or beef. PHOTO ON PAGES 58–59

PHOTO ON PAGES 58–59

PREP TIME: 15 MINUTES
COOK TIME: 30 MINUTES
SERVINGS: 4 TO 6

———

20 garlic cloves

¼ cup olive oil

1 tablespoon dried thyme

Salt

9 ounces labneh, homemade (page 66) or store-bought (for a creamier, richer consistency) or plain Greek yogurt (for a more calorie-friendly dish)

8 ounces feta cheese, crumbled, plus extra for garnish

Small handful of fresh dill, plus 1 tablespoon extra for garnish

Sumac, dried thyme, za'atar, or freshly ground black pepper to taste (optional)

2 tablespoons pine nuts, toasted

1. Preheat the oven to 400°F.

2. In an oven-safe dish, toss the garlic cloves with the olive oil. Sprinkle with the thyme and a couple of pinches of salt. Toss again, then roast for 30 to 35 minutes, until golden.

3. Remove from the oven and let the garlic cool completely. Once cooled, remove the garlic and set aside the oil for later.

4. In a food processor, combine the garlic, labneh, feta, and dill. If you'd like, you may add other seasonings like sumac, thyme, za'atar, or pepper, but keep it light. Blend well.

5. Transfer the dip to a bowl. Top with the pine nuts, 1 tablespoon dill, a sprinkle of crumbled feta, and the leftover olive oil from the garlic roasting.

6. Serve as a spread or dip. Keeps well in the fridge for 3 to 5 days.

Grilled Eggplant Dip

(BABA GHANOUSH)

Baba ghanoush is a classic Middle Eastern dish that is both flavorful and creamy. It is made from grilled or roasted eggplants combined with tahini, garlic, lemon juice, and olive oil. It doesn't last very long at the table and is always a staple appetizer for family gatherings. I put my own creative spin on the classic by topping it with pomegranate seeds for a pop of color and a wonderful burst of sweetness. The only time-consuming part of this recipe is roasting and draining the eggplant, but it's necessary to get that smoky-smooth flavor that makes baba ghanoush so addicting. I promise, it's worth it!

PREP TIME: 30 MINUTES
COOK TIME: 1 TO 1½ HOURS, INCLUDING COOLING
SERVINGS: 4 TO 6

2½ pounds eggplant (2 large or 3 small)

3 garlic cloves

¼ cup tahini

1 tablespoon freshly squeezed lemon juice

Salt and freshly ground black pepper

OPTIONAL GARNISHES

1 tablespoon pine nuts, toasted

½ tablespoon olive oil

3 tablespoons pomegranate seeds

1 tablespoon finely chopped fresh parsley

1. The eggplant can either be grilled (highly recommended for that extra smoky flavor) or baked.

2. If grilling: Set the eggplant whole over an open flame (I use my gas burner on medium-high, but you can cook it on the grill too), turning occasionally with a pair of tongs, until the eggplant has fully charred on the outside and the flesh has collapsed and fully softened, 15 to 20 minutes.

3. If baking: Preheat the oven to 450°F. Cut the eggplant in halves lengthwise and place them cut-side down on a lightly oiled medium baking sheet. Bake the eggplant for about 40 minutes, until the eggplant is very soft and cooked through. About 10 minutes before removing from the oven, change the setting to broil to get the skin of the eggplant slightly charred.

4. Set the eggplant aside in a container with a lid for 10 to 15 minutes to cool down. (Covering the eggplant will help steam it and make the peel come off much faster.)

5. While the eggplant is still warm, peel off the charred skin and set the clean eggplant in a colander for 15 to 20 minutes to allow it to drain. (This is an important step. Draining the eggplant properly will keep your dip creamy instead of watery.)

6. Once the eggplant has drained, place it in a food processor and add the garlic, tahini, lemon juice, and salt and pepper to taste. Blend it for about a minute to get a thick paste.

7. Pour the dip into a serving bowl and garnish, if desired, with the toasted pine nuts, olive oil, pomegranate seeds, and parsley. Keeps well in the fridge for up to 5 days.

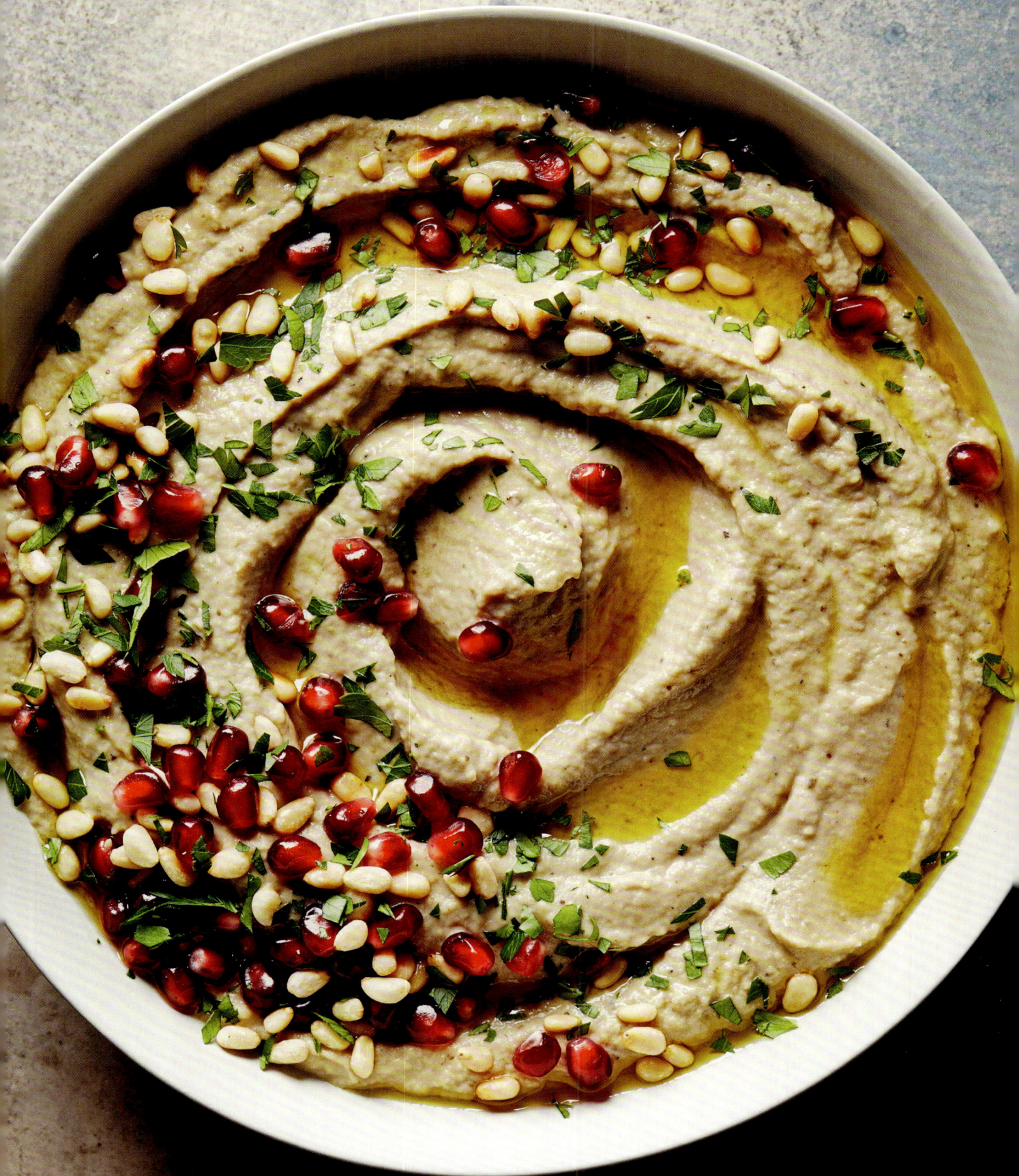

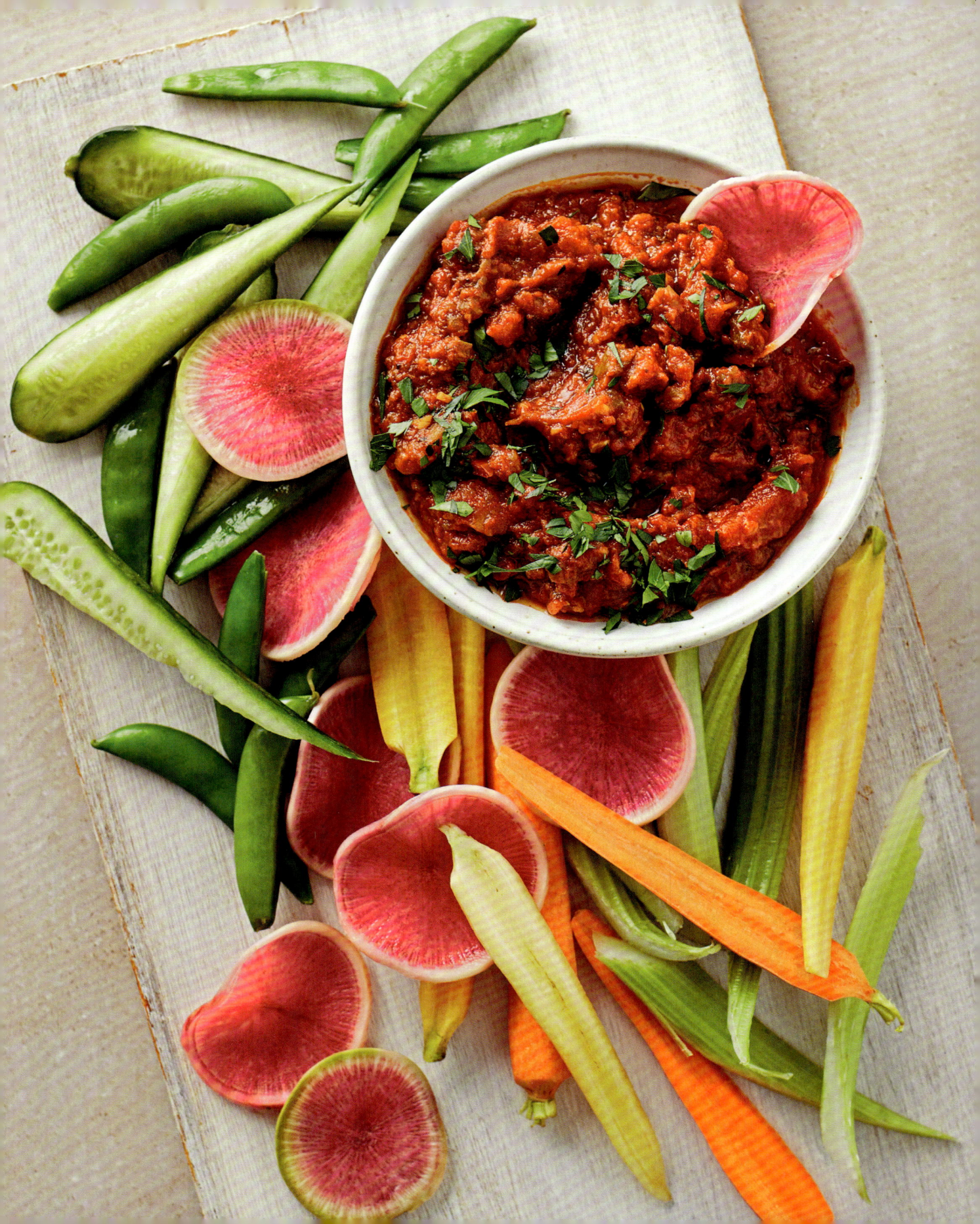

Moroccan Tomato Spread

(MATBUCHA)

Traditionally known as matbucha, this sweet and savory spread is a concoction of roasted peppers, garlic, spices, tomatoes, monk fruit, and balsamic vinegar. I use monk fruit sweetener instead of sugar as a low-carb alternative, and balsamic for an extra kick of flavor. It's a recipe that'll come in handy for all sorts of occasions and can be used in a multitude of ways. Whether you need a shareable spread, a pasta sauce, or a stew base, it has got you covered. I recommend making a large batch so you can store it for use later!

PREP TIME: 30 MINUTES
COOK TIME: 90 MINUTES
SERVINGS: 4 TO 6

2 green bell peppers

1 medium jalapeño pepper

¼ cup olive oil

4 garlic cloves, minced

1½ teaspoons crushed red pepper flakes

1 tablespoon sweet paprika

1 tablespoon dried oregano

1 teaspoon ground cumin

2 (28-ounce) cans diced tomatoes

1 ounce sun-dried tomatoes

2 tablespoons monk fruit sweetener or regular sugar

½ teaspoon balsamic vinegar

Salt and freshly ground black pepper

OPTIONAL GARNISHES

1 tablespoon chopped fresh parsley

1 tablespoon chopped fresh tarragon leaves

1. Preheat the oven to 400°F.

2. Place the bell peppers and jalapeño on a large baking sheet lined with parchment paper. **For the bell peppers:** Roast on each side for 20 to 25 minutes, in total 40 to 50 minutes. **For the jalapeño:** Roast on each side for 8 to 10 minutes, in total 16 to 20 minutes. The skin of the peppers should be charred, soft, and easy to peel off, and the peppers should look slightly collapsed.

3. Once the peppers are cooked, place them in a covered bowl for 15 to 20 minutes. As they cool, the peppers will steam from their own heat and the skin will loosen even more.

4. Once they are cool enough to handle, remove the skin and seeds and chop the peppers into small cubes.

5. Set a medium pot over medium heat and add the olive oil. Once the olive oil is hot, add the garlic, red pepper flakes, paprika, oregano, and cumin and sauté for 1 to 2 minutes, until the garlic turns gold.

6. Add the roasted peppers, diced tomatoes, sun-dried tomatoes, monk fruit sweetener, and balsamic vinegar, and salt and pepper to taste.

7. Bring the mixture to a boil, then reduce the heat to medium-low and simmer for 45 to 60 minutes, until the mixture turns to a paste. Make sure to stir periodically once the liquid starts to reduce, especially in the last 10 to 15 minutes, to avoid burning.

8. Once the spread is ready, either serve in a bowl garnished with your favorite herbs (I use parsley and tarragon) or store in a container if using it as a base for later. Store in the fridge for up to a week or freeze it. For inspo, check out Shrimp Matbucha with Goat Cheese (page 147) and Baked Cheese Matbucha Pasta (page 167).

Homemade Labneh

As a proud Persian, I was practically raised on homemade labneh. Labneh is a popular Middle Eastern dip made from strained yogurt. It's basically a slightly softer, more tart cream cheese. It has become increasingly easy to find labneh in grocery stores, but there's something special about making it at home. It is also highly cost-effective and easy to prepare, which definitely adds to its appeal. This set-it-and-forget-it recipe only calls for two ingredients: yogurt and salt! Spread it on a bagel, dip your veggies in it, or use it as a base for sauces and dips to elevate any dish.

PREP TIME: 10 MINUTES, 24 TO 48 HOURS REFRIGERATING
SERVINGS: 8 TO 10

32 ounces plain whole-milk yogurt

1 teaspoon salt

1. In a large bowl, mix the yogurt and salt.

2. Line a large fine-mesh strainer or colander with cheesecloth or a clean kitchen towel, then place over a larger bowl to catch the liquid that will drip out.

3. Pour the salted yogurt into the lined strainer. Make sure the yogurt is evenly spread, then cover the top with the cheesecloth.

4. Place in the fridge for 24 to 48 hours. The longer you leave it, the thicker the labneh will become. While 24 hours may be enough for some, I leave it for 36 to 48 hours for a thicker consistency.

5. Transfer the labneh from the cheesecloth to a clean container and store in the fridge for up to a week.

6. You can have it as is, serve it as a dip by spreading it out over a large serving dish topped with olive oil, za'atar, everything bagel seasoning, olives and herbs, or use it to make other recipes such as the Sautéed Mushrooms over Tahini Labneh (page 45), my Garlic Feta Dip (page 61), or the Wild Blueberry Bliss Labneh Cheesecake (page 238).

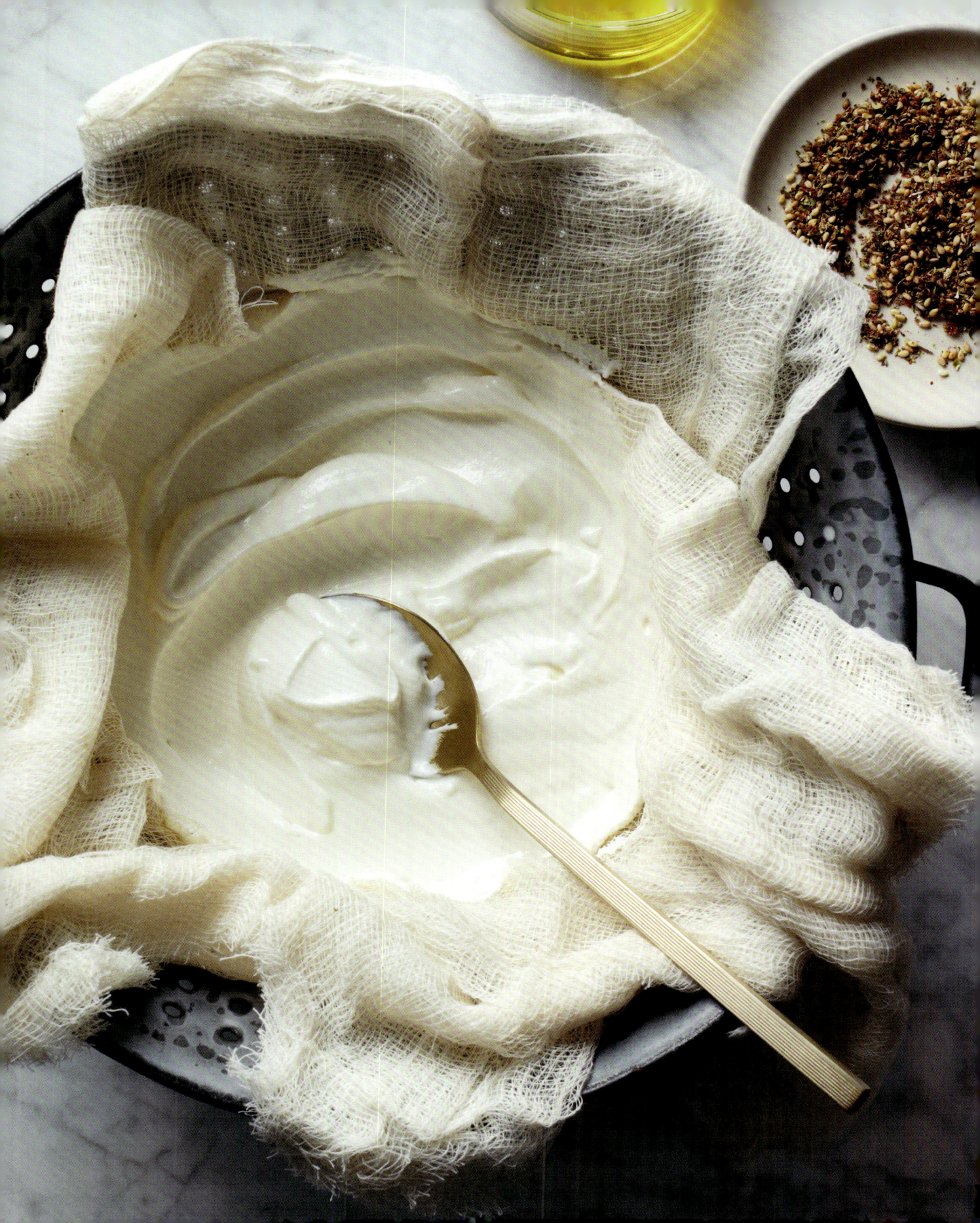

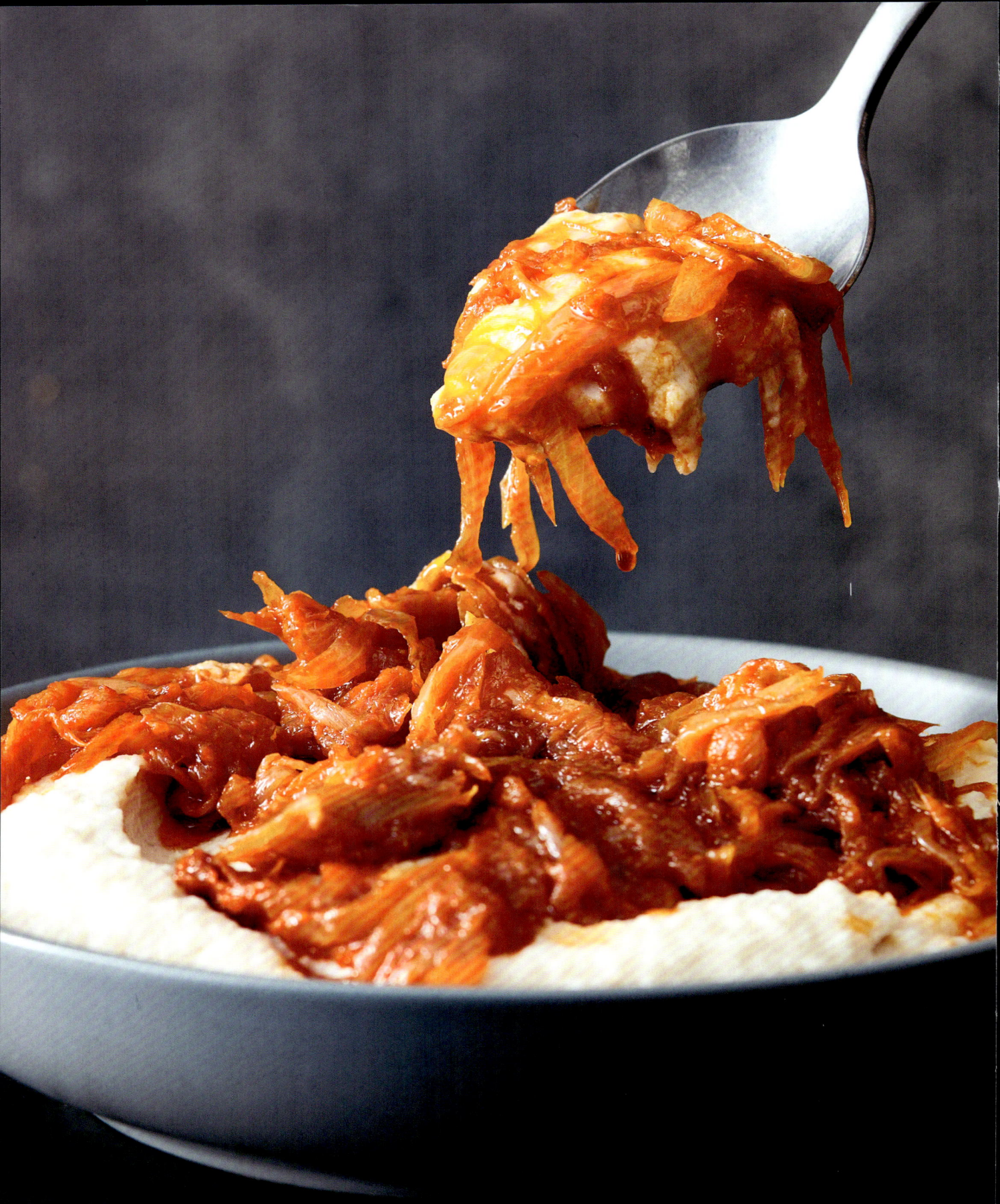

Cannellini Bean Spread

WITH CARAMELIZED ONIONS

Romanian *fasole batuta,* or "whipped beans," is a cannellini bean spread with caramelized onions. It is packed with flavor and protein, and one of my personal favorites when it comes to traditional Romanian dishes. This spread brings out the very best of beans and is proof how they can be the star of the show. The tomatoey caramelized onions, of course, bring everything together beautifully! But you can't underestimate the power of those cannellini beans. They come out creamy, rich, and super satisfying.

1. Drain the cannellini beans and place them in a medium pot with the onion, carrots, celery, bay leaves, and salt and pepper to taste. Cover with water (about 8 cups), bring to a boil, and simmer for 20 minutes.

2. Drain the beans, reserving 1 cup of the water for making the caramelized onions, and discard the carrots, onion, celery, and bay leaves.

3. With an immersion blender, blend the beans into a smooth paste. Add the garlic, olive oil, mustard, and more salt and pepper to taste. Blend for another minute and set aside.

4. **For the caramelized onions:** Place a medium pan over medium heat and add the olive oil. Once the oil is hot, add the sliced onions and 2 tablespoons of the reserved water to allow the onions to soften. Cook until the onions are golden brown. Add the tomato paste and cook for another minute. Gradually add 3 to 4 tablespoons more water to allow the paste to fully cook and blend with the onion. Cook for another 3 to 4 minutes. Add salt and pepper to taste.

5. Place the cannellini bean dip on a plate and top with the caramelized onions.

6. Serve hot.

PREP TIME: 15 MINUTES
COOK TIME: 40 MINUTES
SERVINGS: 6 TO 8

---

3 (15.5-ounce) cans cannellini beans

½ medium onion, untrimmed

3 medium carrots, unpeeled

4 celery stalks, untrimmed

2 bay leaves

Salt and freshly ground black pepper

3 garlic cloves, minced

1 tablespoon olive oil

½ teaspoon Dijon mustard

FOR THE CARAMELIZED ONIONS

2 tablespoons olive oil

2 medium onions, sliced into thin strips

2 tablespoons tomato paste

Salt and freshly ground black pepper

Green Goddess Dip

In my mind, any classic flavor combo can be turned into a delicious dip with the right ingredients, and this includes the beloved green goddess dressing. This creamy, herbaceous dip is a crowd-pleaser and perfect for parties, picnics, or simply snacking at home. It's also incredibly versatile—enjoy it as a snack with veggies and pita chips, use it as a spread to elevate a classic BLT sandwich, or pair it with rotisserie chicken or wings on game days. The options are unlimited. All you need is 15 minutes to whip up this flavorful masterpiece, and trust me—you're going to want to put it on everything.

1. In a food processor, combine the dill, mint, parsley, scallions, garlic, basil, lemon juice, olive oil, yogurt, and feta and blend until creamy.

2. Taste the mix and add salt if needed. Depending on the feta used, the dip might already be salty enough. If salt is added, mix for another 10 to 15 seconds.

3. Pour the dip into a serving bowl and serve right away with your favorite veggies and pita chips, or keep in the fridge for up to 4 days.

PREP TIME: 15 MINUTES
SERVINGS: 6 TO 8

1 ounce fresh dill

½ ounce fresh mint leaves

1 ounce fresh parsley

3 scallions, white and green parts

4 garlic cloves

1 ounce fresh basil

1½ tablespoons freshly squeezed lemon juice

⅓ cup olive oil

½ cup plain Greek yogurt

2½ ounces feta cheese

Salt

Greek Cucumber Yogurt Dip

(TZATZIKI)

Tzatziki is one of the most popular Greek dips. With its refreshing and tangy flavor, this versatile dish can be used as a dip for pita bread and vegetables or paired with your favorite grilled meats, gyros, and souvlaki. To make it, all you need to do is grate and strain some cucumbers, then combine them with fresh ingredients like Greek yogurt, lemon juice, garlic, and fresh herbs. It's super easy to make and is a true crowd pleaser for a reason.

PREP TIME: 30 MINUTES
SERVINGS: 4

6 Persian or mini cucumbers (about 1 pound)

Salt

2 cups plain Greek yogurt

1 tablespoon olive oil

5 tablespoons freshly squeezed lemon juice

3 garlic cloves, minced

2 tablespoons finely chopped fresh dill, plus extra for garnish

2 tablespoons finely chopped fresh mint, plus extra for garnish

1 teaspoon sumac, plus extra for garnish

1 teaspoon white vinegar

Freshly ground black pepper

1. Using a box grater or a mandoline, finely grate the cucumbers or slice them into short, thin pieces. Sprinkle with salt and place in a strainer lined with cheesecloth or a thick paper towel.

2. Let the cucumbers sit for 30 minutes, then squeeze the cloth or paper towel to extract as much moisture as possible. Discard excess moisture.

3. In a mixing bowl, combine the strained cucumbers, yogurt, ½ tablespoon of the olive oil, lemon juice, garlic, dill, mint, sumac, and vinegar. Add salt and pepper to taste.

4. Mix all the ingredients together and place in a serving bowl. Garnish with more dill, mint, sumac, and the remaining ½ tablespoon of olive oil.

5. Serve chilled. Keeps well in the fridge for 2 to 3 days.

Roasted Zucchini Spread

Simple, delicious, and packed with protein, this roasted zucchini spread has that special "wow" factor. All you have to do is roast the zucchini and garlic in the air fryer or oven, chop it up, and mix it with some Greek yogurt. It's so easy to make and tastes fantastic with just about anything. Serve it as a dip, spread it on meat or fish, or add a dollop or two to your favorite salad.

PREP TIME: 20 MINUTES
COOK TIME: 30 MINUTES
SERVINGS: 2 TO 4

---

1 large zucchini

4 large garlic cloves

Salt and freshly ground black pepper

2 tablespoons olive oil

2 cups plain Greek yogurt

GARNISHES

Drizzle of olive oil

A few sprigs of fresh herbs (I like to use mint)

¼ cup toasted walnuts

Pinch of Aleppo pepper (optional)

1. Preheat the oven or an air fryer to 400°F.

2. Wash and dry the zucchini, then cut it in quarters and add it to an air fryer tray or a medium baking dish along with the garlic cloves. Season with salt and pepper and drizzle with the olive oil.

3. Air-fry or bake for 20 to 25 minutes. Time varies by the oven or air fryer. If you cut the zucchini smaller, it'll cook up faster.

4. Once the zucchini and garlic are roasted, let them cool completely.

5. Chop the zucchini and garlic. If you like a chunkier spread, make larger chunks. If you want the spread to be creamier, you can even blend them.

6. In a medium bowl, combine the yogurt and the chopped zucchini and garlic. Mix the spread well and add more salt and pepper to taste.

7. When you're happy with the result, plate it up and top with olive oil, fresh herbs, toasted walnuts, and Aleppo pepper (if using).

8. Use this as a side, dip, or spread, or enjoy it on its own!

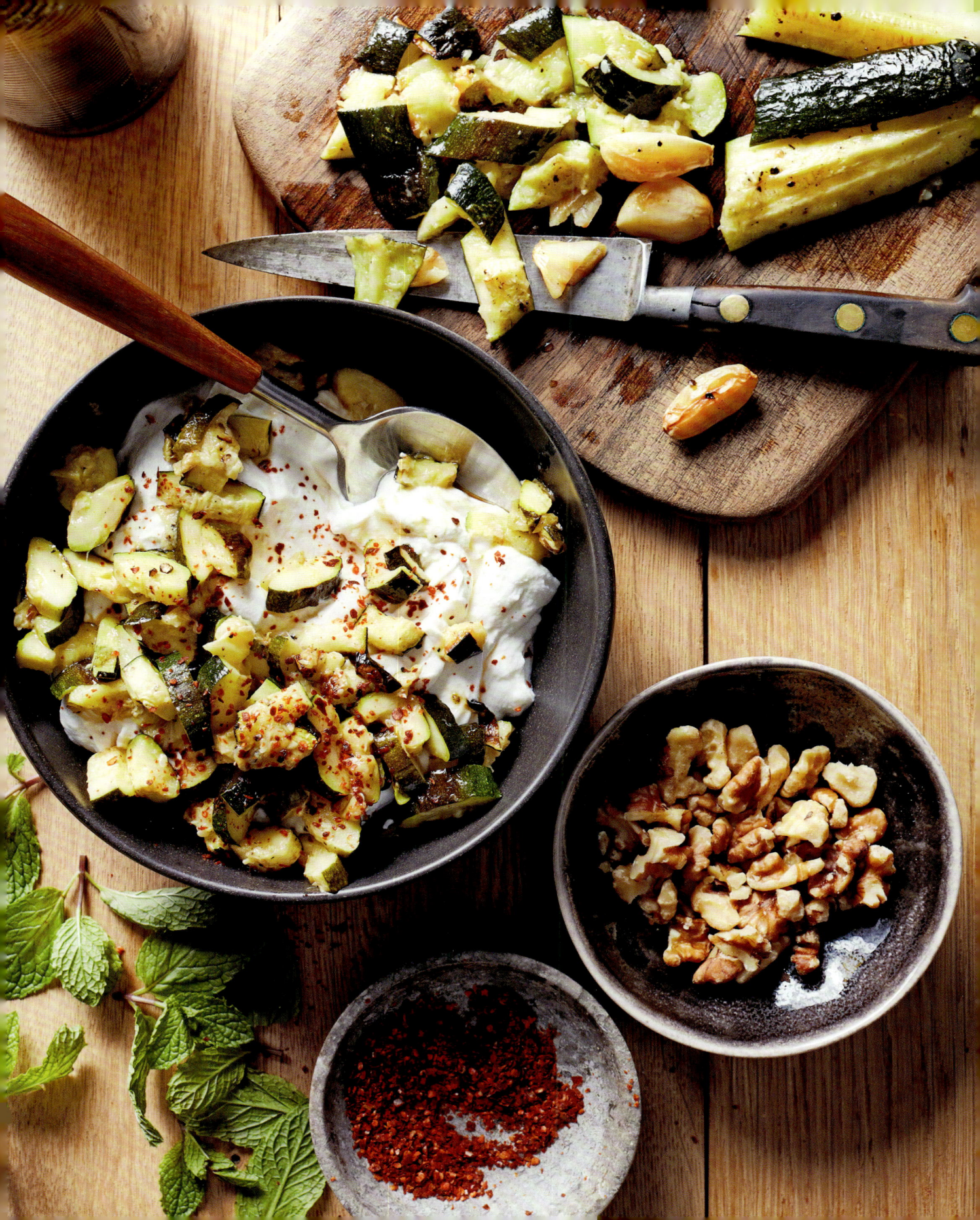

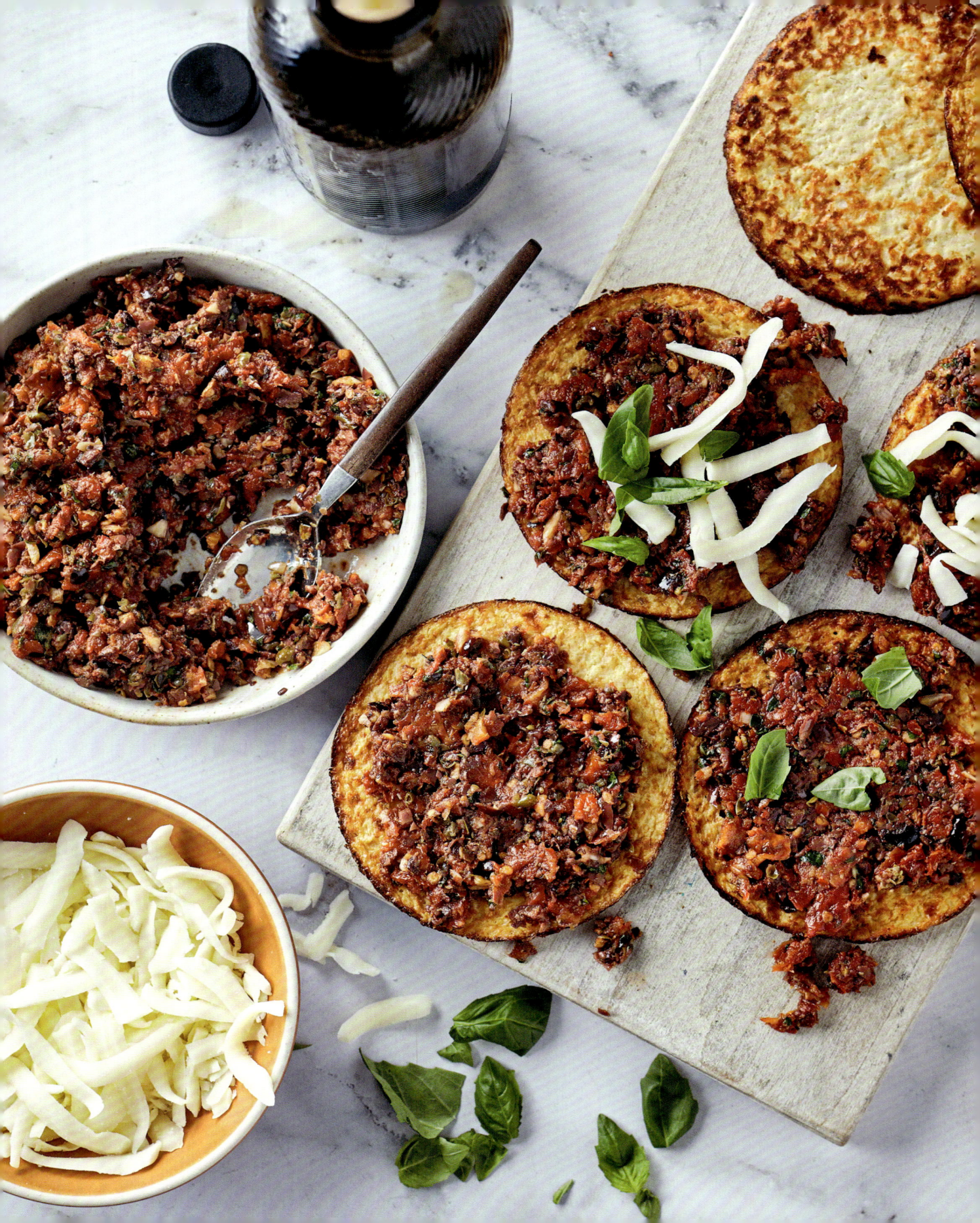

Sun-Dried Tomato Olive Tapenade

This recipe will transport you to the Mediterranean with its bold, vibrant tones at every bite. Flavorful ingredients like sun-dried tomatoes, kalamata olives, capers, garlic, olive oil, and lemon are blended in a food processor and garnished with fresh basil. This will be a party favorite whether served directly with low-carb crackers or bread, added as a centerpiece to a cheese board, or even spread on a low-carb pizza crust topped with fresh mozzarella.

PREP TIME: 10 MINUTES
SERVINGS: 4 TO 6

5 ounces sun-dried tomatoes

5 ounces kalamata olives, pitted

1 ounce capers

2 garlic cloves

2 teaspoons olive oil

1 teaspoon freshly squeezed lemon juice

½ teaspoon lemon zest

10 fresh basil leaves

Salt and freshly ground black pepper

1. In a food processor, combine the sun-dried tomatoes, olives, capers, garlic, olive oil, lemon juice, lemon zest, and 6 of the basil leaves and blend into a paste. Add pepper to taste.

2. Taste the mix and check for salt. Depending on the sun-dried tomatoes and olives used, the paste might already be salty enough. If needed, add salt and mix for another 10 to 15 seconds.

3. Pour the tapenade into a bowl and garnish it with the remaining 4 basil leaves.

4. Use as a dip with freshly toasted bread or crackers, or use it as a base for mini pizzas with fresh mozzarella cheese.

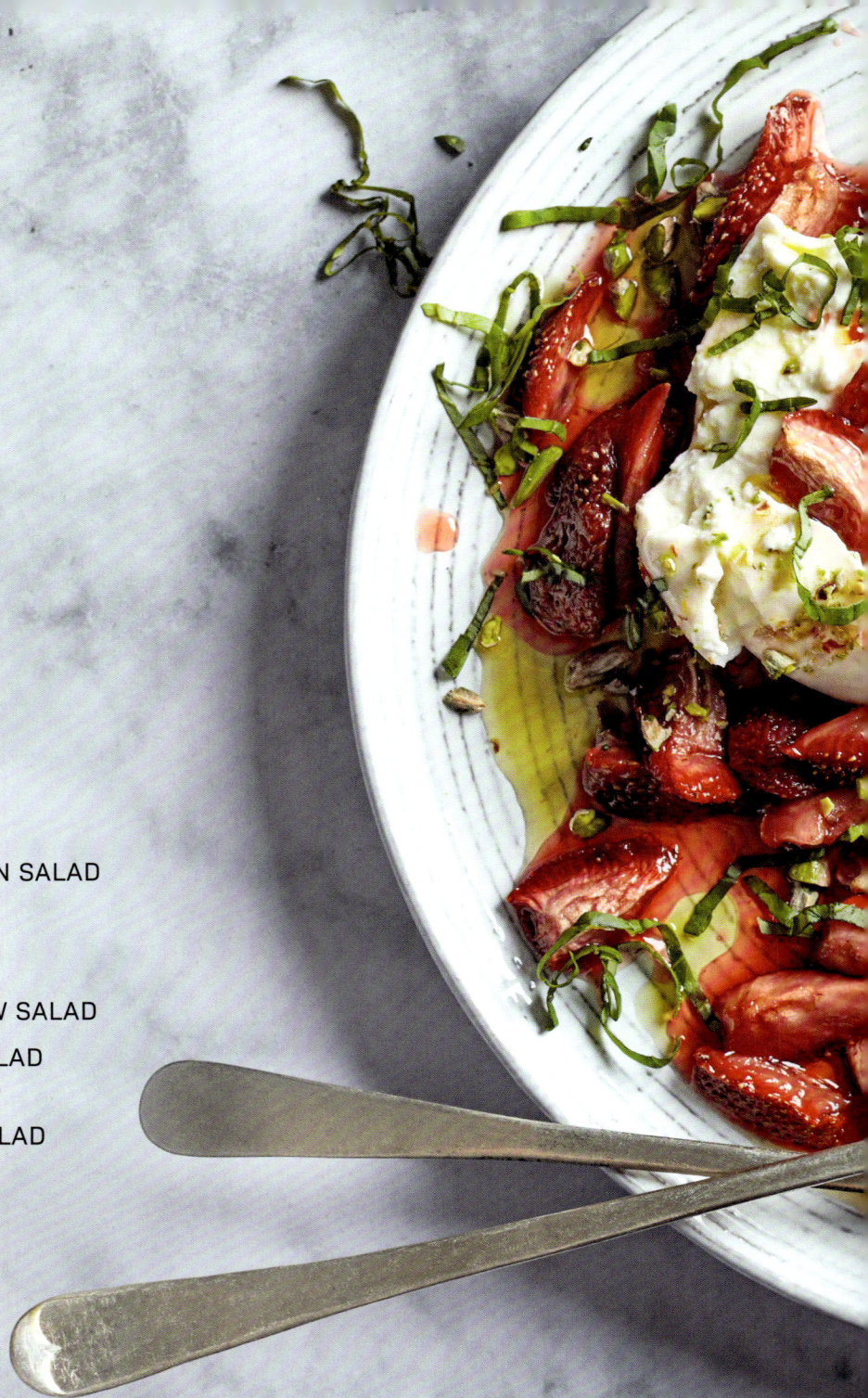

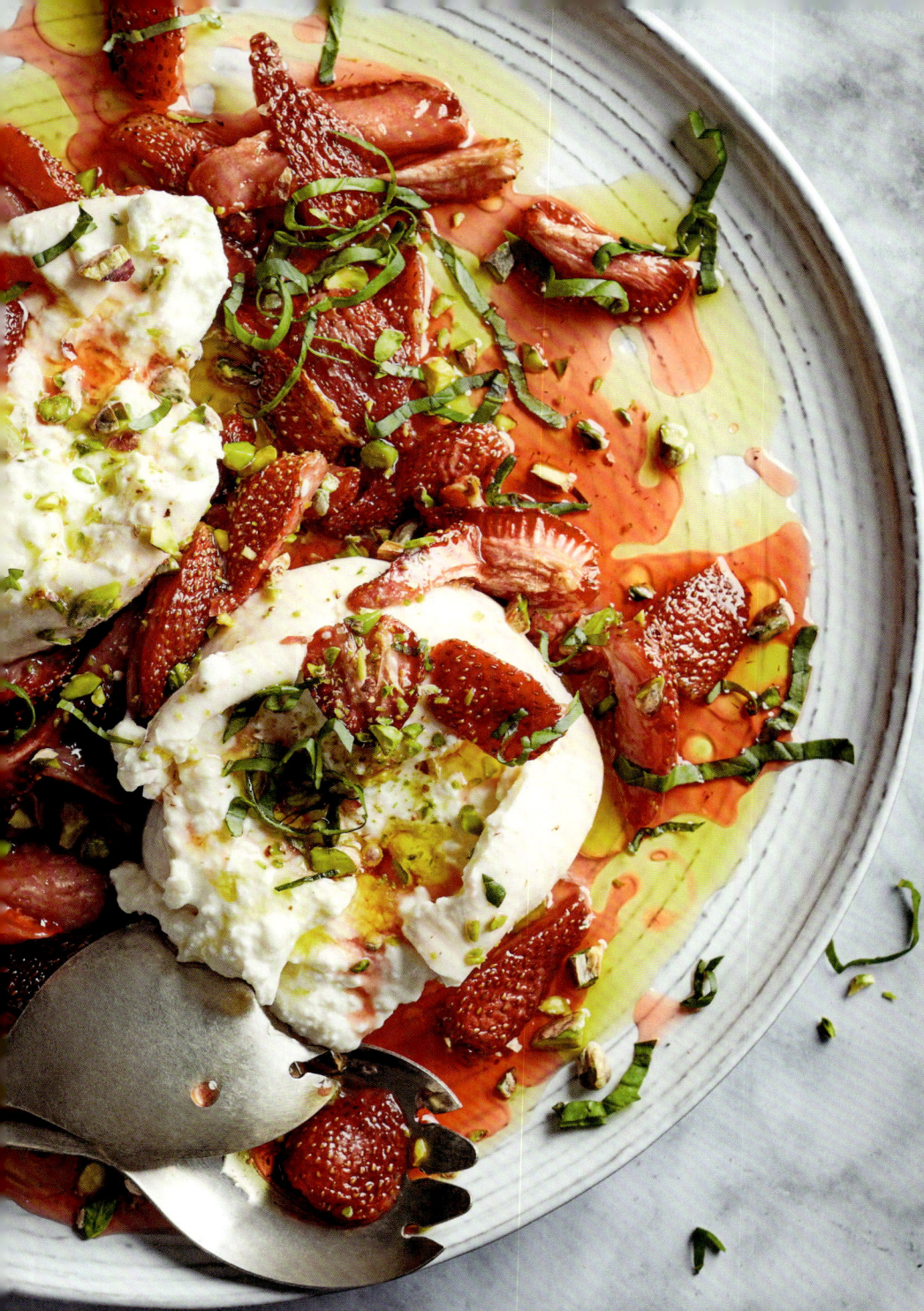

Salads

My goal is to make you fall in love with salads.
We're going beyond the standard lettuce and dressing options and getting into different textures, colors, and flavors. The ones you'll find here are hearty enough to be a meal on their own or make for a bangin' side dish. Not only are they colorful and vibrant, but each is packed with a variety of textures and flavors that'll truly excite your taste buds.

My philosophy for making a good salad is to include something crunchy, something herbaceous, something creamy, and something tangy. This combo creates the perfect balance of textures and flavors that make you *want* to scrape your plate clean. That's why I love adding nuts or veggies for crunch, fresh herbs for an aromatic touch, a homemade dressing or cheese to add richness, and a tangy element like pickled veggies or citrus juice to cut through any heaviness.

And feel free to add or swap ingredients depending on what's in season or what you have on hand. That's the beauty of salads—they're versatile, customizable, and meant to be celebrated.

Spicy Tuna Salad

Everything always tastes better with a little spice in it! This spicy tuna salad only takes 10 minutes to put together and is an excellent source of protein when you're on the go—it's great for meal prep. My homemade yum yum sauce is the star ingredient here. It transforms the most basic of dishes into an explosion of flavor, adding just the right amount of heat and creaminess. Serve this salad with veggie wedges, with low-carb pita crackers, in a wrap, or on top of your favorite salad.

PREP TIME: 10 MINUTES
SERVINGS: 4 TO 6

1 shallot

3 celery stalks

3 gherkin dill pickles

3 (5-ounce) cans tuna
in water, drained

6 tablespoons freshly
squeezed lemon juice

6 tablespoons Spicy Yum
Yum Sauce (page 201)

Salt and freshly ground
black pepper

3 red bell peppers, halved and
cored, for serving (optional)

1 tablespoon finely
chopped fresh parsley,
for garnish (optional)

1. Mince the shallot, celery, and gherkins and place in a medium bowl. Add the tuna, lemon juice, and yum yum sauce and mix with a fork, crushing the tuna into a chunky paste. Add salt and pepper to taste.

2. Serve on red bell peppers or with your vessel of choice, such as low-carb pita chips, bread, or other veggie wedges. Garnish with the finely chopped parsley, if using, and serve right away or store in the fridge up to 3 to days.

Mediterranean Chicken Salad

In this chicken salad, you'll find all your favorite classic Mediterranean ingredients diced into a fresh and flavorful salad that's perfect for lettuce wraps, bread, or crackers, or simply on its own! Shredded chicken and minced artichoke hearts, black olives, dill pickles, and fresh herbs combine with a savory mustard dressing. Use plain Greek yogurt instead of mayonnaise for a lower-calorie version.

1. Shred or mince the chicken and add to a medium mixing bowl.

2. Grab a handful of dill or parsley, finely chop it, and add to the bowl.

3. Mince the artichoke hearts, black olives, and dill pickles. Add to the bowl.

4. Add the yogurt, Dijon mustard, garlic powder, cayenne, and salt and pepper to taste. Mix well.

5. Serve immediately on its own or with lettuce wraps, bread, or crackers. Keeps well in the fridge for 3 to 4 days.

PREP TIME: 20 MINUTES
SERVINGS: 8 TO 10

2½ pounds cooked chicken (rotisserie, grilled, or boiled)

½ bunch fresh dill or parsley

½ cup marinated artichoke hearts

½ cup black olives

½ cup dill pickles

1 cup plain Greek yogurt or mayonnaise

3 tablespoons Dijon mustard

1 tablespoon garlic powder

1 teaspoon cayenne pepper

Salt and freshly ground black pepper

Shirazi Salad

Shirazi salad is a recipe close to my heart, as it's been a staple in my family for as long as I can remember. My mom makes it best, so naturally I had to give her a call. It's fresh, crunchy, and centered on three simple ingredients: Persian cucumbers, tomatoes, and red onions. Super easy, super delicious. Mediterranean salads use the same veggies, but the Shirazi difference is to dice them small and toss them with chopped mint and a glorious dressing made of sour grape juice or lemon juice and olive oil for the perfect side salad on a hot summer day! If eating as a side, I recommend pairing it with my Persian Kabob Koobideh (page 135), Saffron Lemon Grilled Chicken (page 120), or Spatchcock Chicken (page 124).

PHOTO ON PAGES 82–83

PREP TIME: 10 MINUTES
SERVINGS: 4 TO 6

4 Persian or mini cucumbers, cut into ¼-inch cubes

3 Roma tomatoes, cut into ¼-inch cubes

½ large red onion, minced

Handful of fresh mint, finely chopped

2 garlic cloves, minced

¼ cup sour grape juice or freshly squeezed lemon juice

⅓ cup olive oil

2 tablespoons dried mint

Salt and freshly ground black pepper

1. In a medium salad bowl, combine the cucumbers, tomatoes, and onion. (Using small pieces as recommended helps coat the veggies with just the right amount of dressing, but you can chop them larger if you prefer.)

2. Mix in the fresh mint, garlic, grape juice, olive oil, and dried mint, and add salt and pepper to taste.

3. Serve it up with your favorite protein, or eat as is.

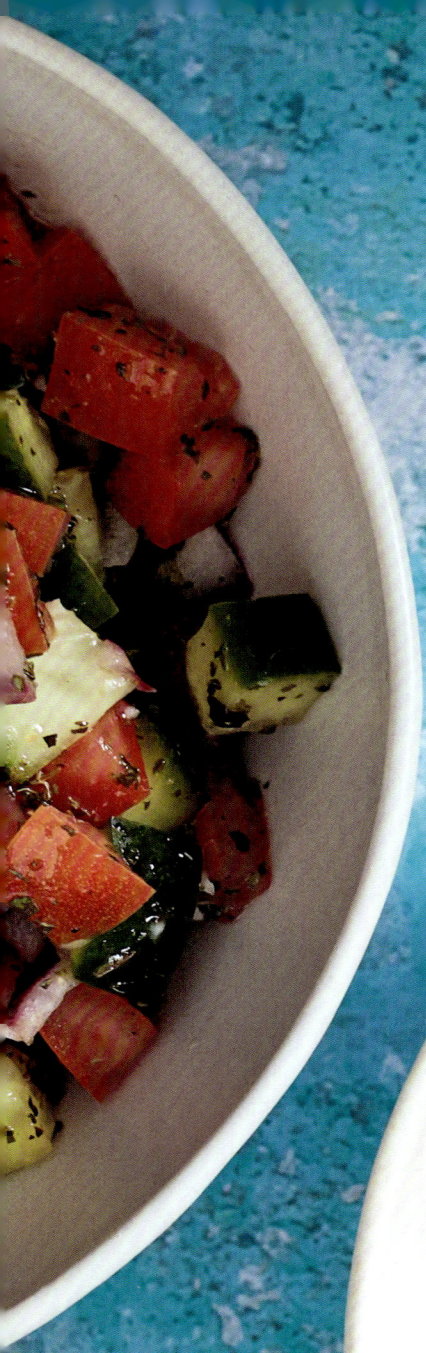

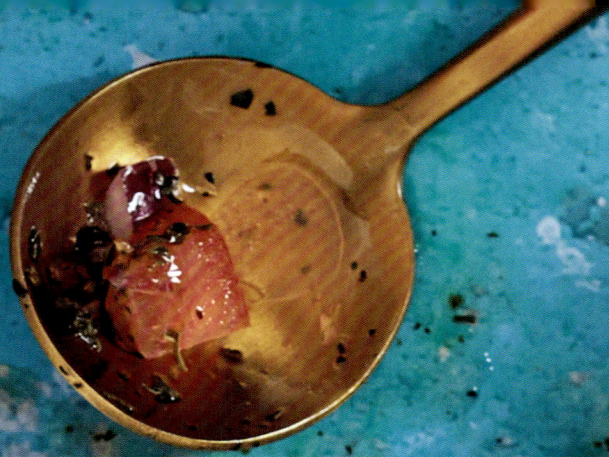

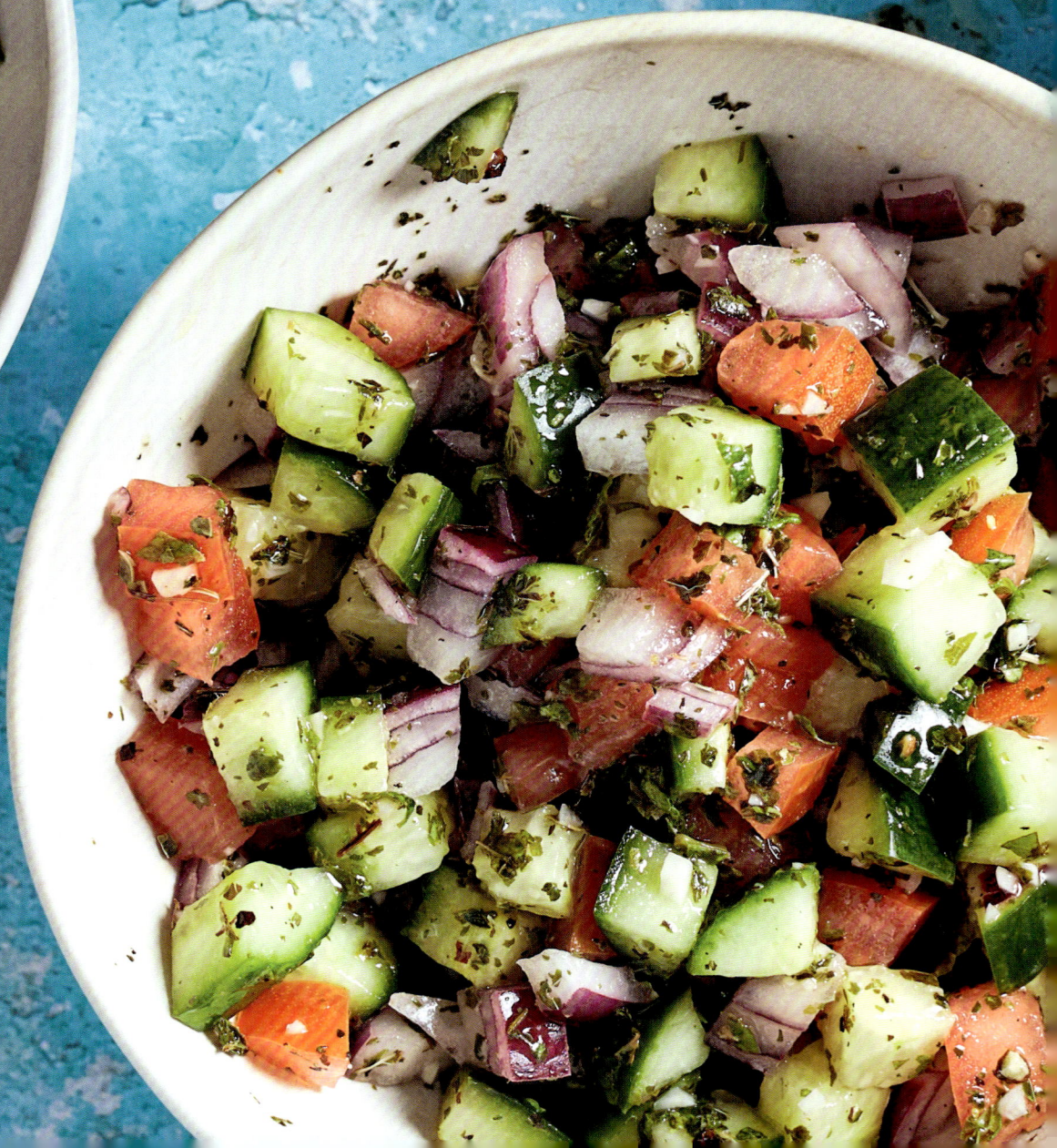

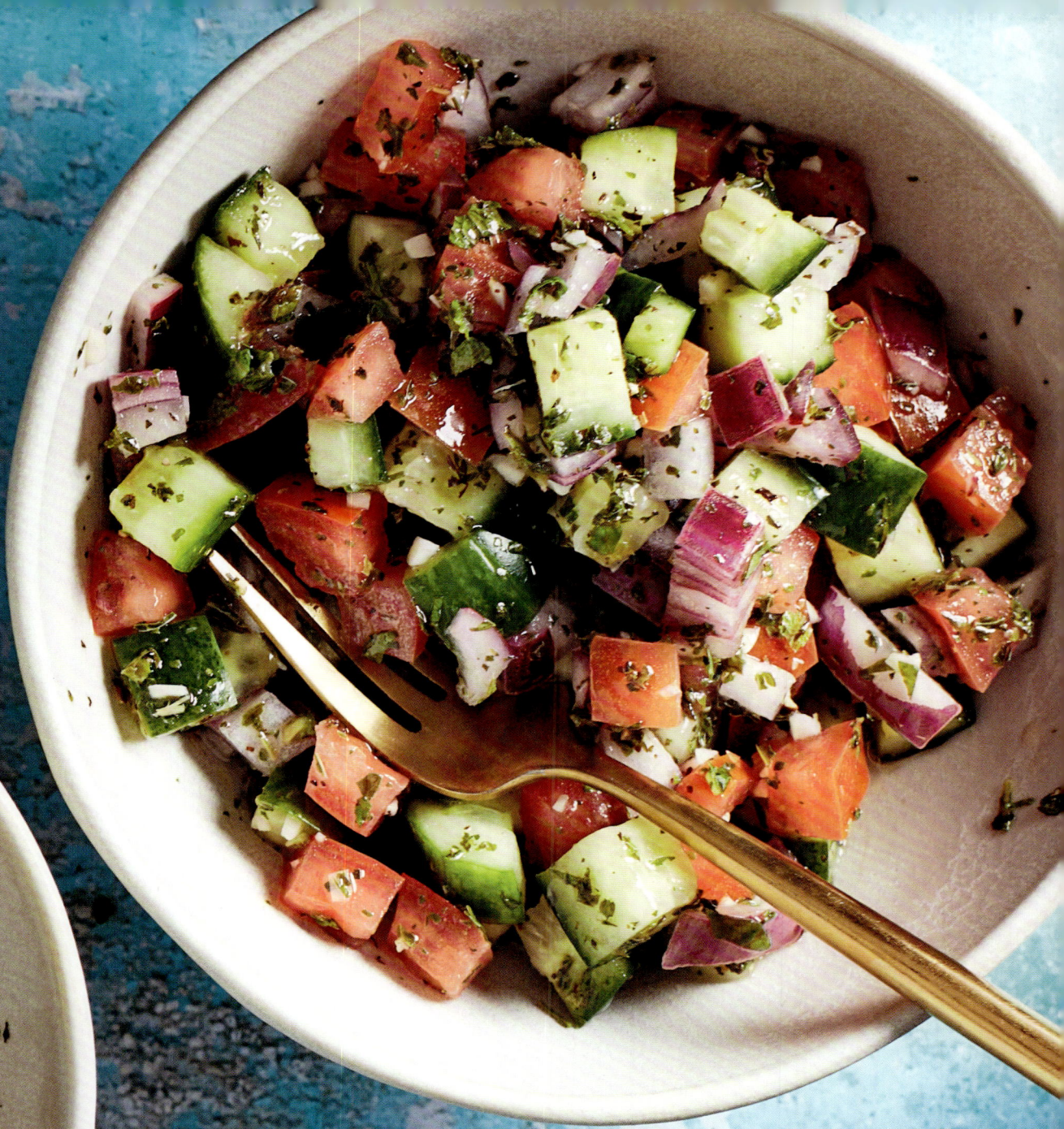

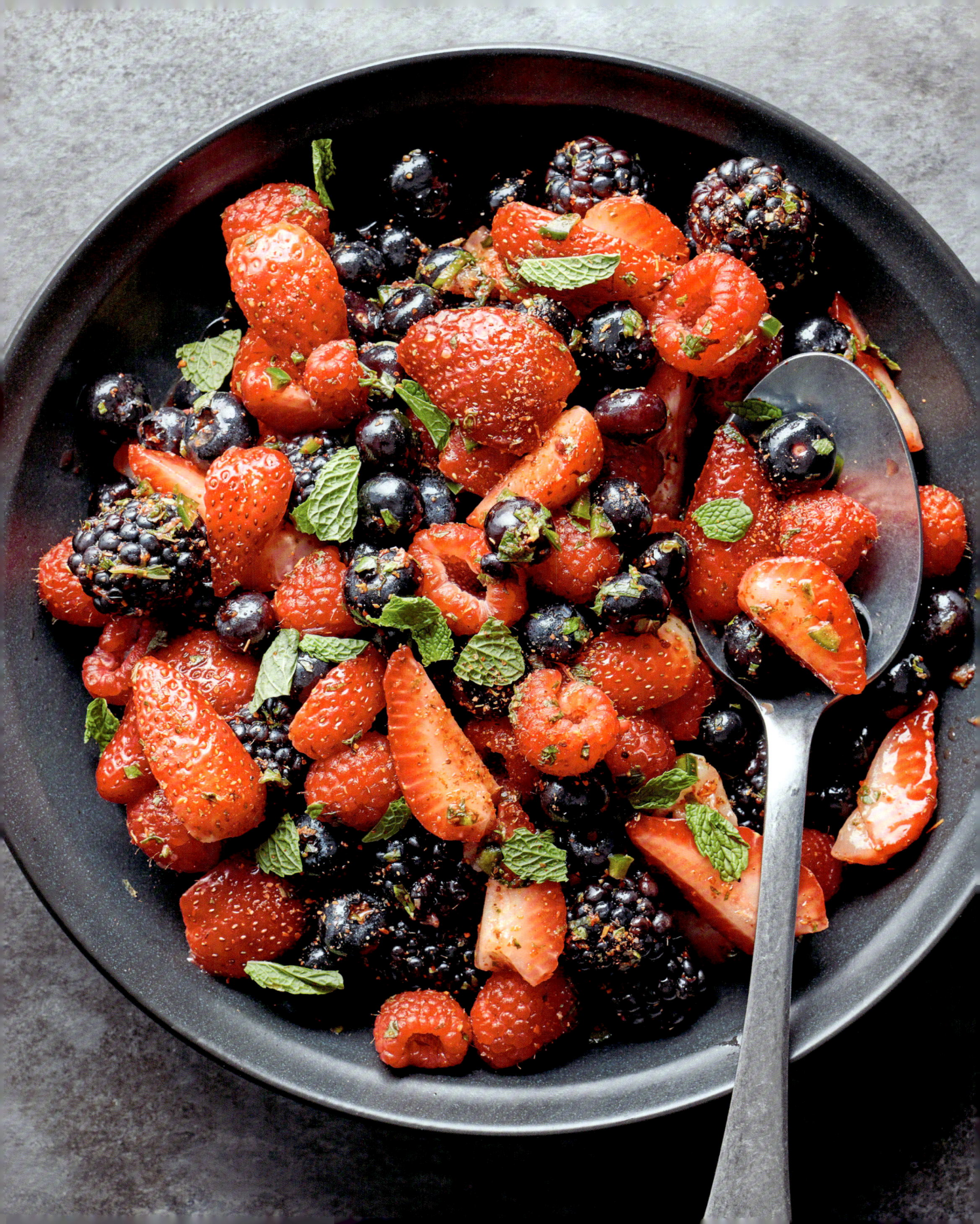

Spicy Berries Salad

A fun and unique twist on the traditional fruit salad, this spicy berries salad is a surprise delight for the taste buds. Sweet berries are combined with a zesty dressing made with jalapeño, hot sauce, lemon and lime juice, monk fruit sweetener, and Tajín seasoning to create a flavorful and refreshing side dish. It uses fresh ingredients, will be ready in a flash, and is the perfect addition to any summer barbecue, potluck, or picnic. Top it with some fresh mint for a pop of color, and enjoy the burst of flavors in every bite.

PREP TIME: 15 MINUTES
SERVINGS: 4 TO 6

FOR THE DRESSING

2 tablespoons finely chopped fresh mint, plus extra for garnish

¼ cup freshly squeezed lemon juice

1 tablespoon freshly squeezed lime juice

2 tablespoons monk fruit sweetener or regular sugar

1 tablespoon chili lime seasoning, such as Tajín, plus extra for garnish

¼ teaspoon lemon zest

¼ teaspoon lime zest

½ tablespoon minced jalapeño peppers

¼ teaspoon plain hot sauce (such as Tapatío or Tabasco)

10 ounces strawberries, cut in quarters

8 ounces raspberries

7 ounces blueberries

7 ounces blackberries

1. **For the dressing:** In a small bowl, combine the mint, lemon juice, lime juice, monk fruit sweetener, chili lime seasoning, lemon zest, and lime zest. Add the jalapeño and hot sauce gradually, tasting until you find your preferred level of heat. (The measurements in this recipe should yield a medium level of heat, but spiciness varies depending on the pepper and the hot sauce.)

2. In a large bowl, combine the strawberries, raspberries, blueberries, and blackberries with the dressing, folding gently until the berries are evenly coated.

3. Garnish with some extra chopped mint and chili lime seasoning.

4. This salad can be served right away, but for an extra kick, I recommend storing it in the fridge for 30 to 40 minutes to allow the berries to marinate with the dressing.

Sesame Ginger Rainbow Salad

This sesame ginger salad is such a vibrant dish, both visually and flavor-wise. Red cabbage, cucumber, carrot, red bell pepper, scallions, and cilantro get chopped into a medley of colors, textures, and flavors. The veggies get tossed in a creamy sesame ginger dressing that ties all the fresh and crunchy goodness together. The fact that you can prep this salad 1 to 2 days in advance is such a bonus perk for me. Just make the dressing, cut the veggies, and store them separately in the fridge. When ready to eat, simply toss everything together and dig in! Serve as is or add grilled shrimp, chicken, or baked tofu for extra protein.

1. **For the sesame ginger dressing:** In a food processor, combine ginger, garlic, mayo, rice vinegar, sesame oil, and sriracha and blend until smooth (1 to 2 minutes). Add salt and pepper to taste and make any adjustments you prefer. This has a powerful ginger and garlic punch, so feel free to dial it down based on your own preferences.

2. In a large bowl, combine the red cabbage, cucumbers, carrot, bell pepper, and scallions. Add the dressing and mix everything well to ensure that all the veggies are coated. (You can change the size of the pieces if you prefer, but using small pieces does help the veggies get coated with just the right amount of dressing.)

3. Garnish with the toasted sesame seeds and cilantro.

PREP TIME: 30 MINUTES
SERVINGS: 4 TO 6

FOR THE SESAME GINGER DRESSING

1-inch piece fresh ginger, peeled

4 garlic cloves

¼ cup mayonnaise

5 tablespoons rice vinegar

3 tablespoons sesame oil

2 tablespoons sriracha or other hot sauce

Salt and freshly ground black pepper

½ red cabbage head, shredded

3 Persian or mini cucumbers, cut into ¼-inch cubes

½ carrot, cut in thin 1-inch sticks

1 red bell pepper, cut into ¼-inch cubes

3 scallions, white and green parts, finely chopped

2 to 3 tablespoons toasted sesame seeds, for garnish

1 tablespoon chopped fresh cilantro, for garnish

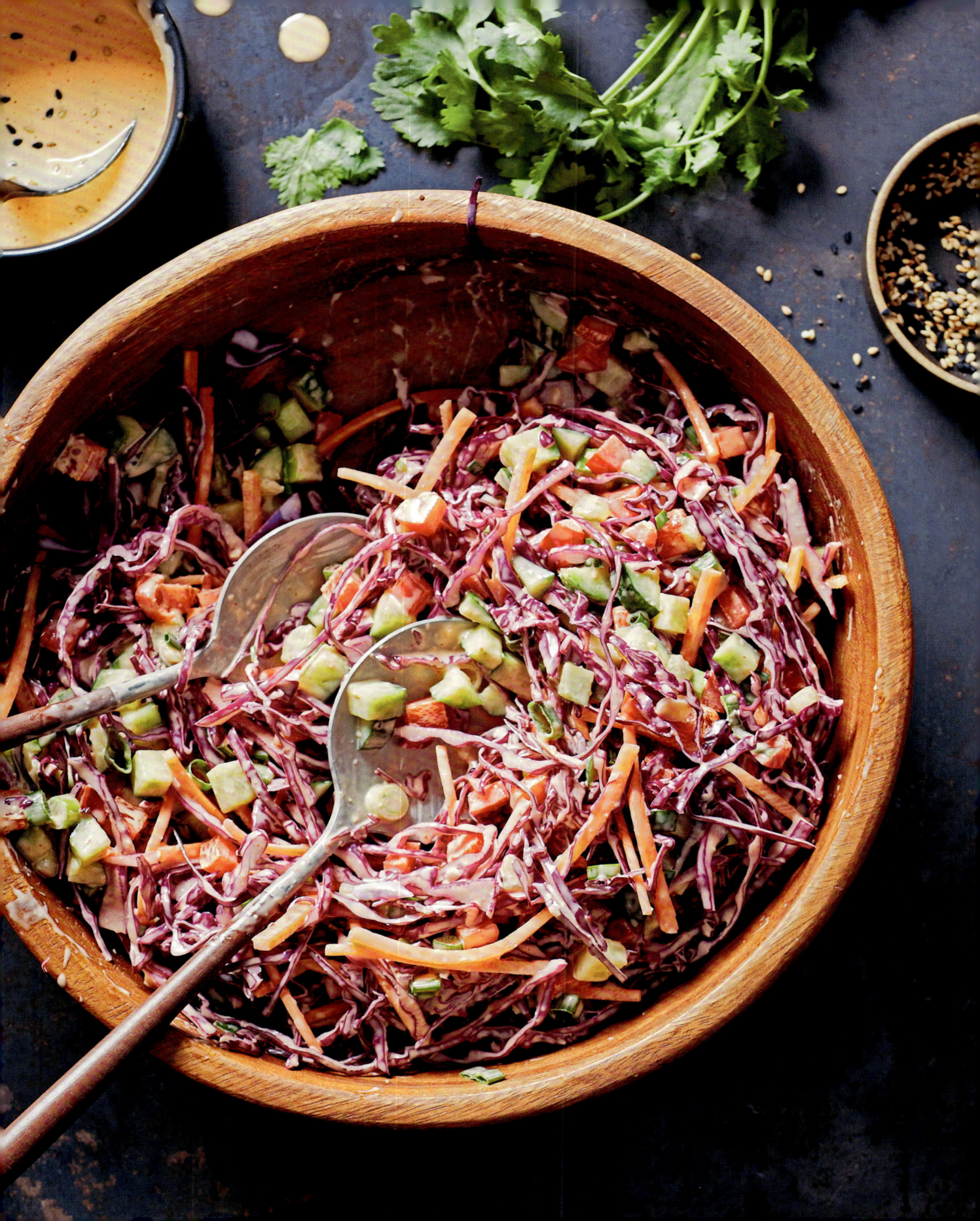

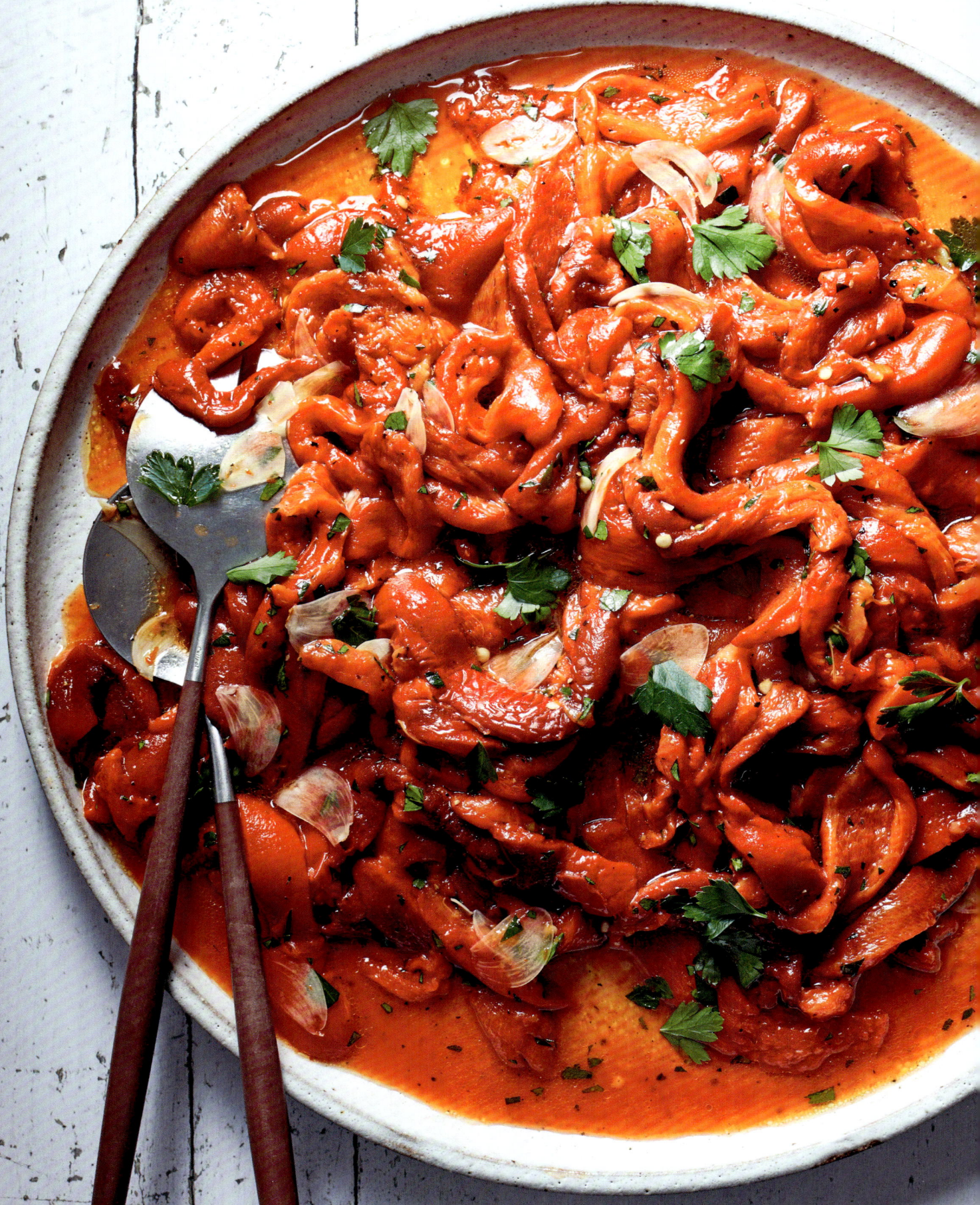

Roasted Red Pepper Salad WITH PARSLEY

Enjoy red peppers in a whole new way with this roasted red pepper salad with parsley. It's a simple and highly versatile recipe that can be eaten on its own or as a side dish for grilled meats. The red peppers are roasted and then steamed, so they come out perfectly charred and tender, while the olive oil, garlic, and red wine vinegar elevate the flavor even further! All you need is some time for roasting and steaming the peppers, and you're good to go.

1. Preheat the oven to 400°F.

2. Line a large baking sheet with parchment paper and arrange the bell peppers, leaving about an inch of space between them. Roast the peppers on each side for 20 to 25 minutes, in total 40 to 50 minutes. The skin of the peppers should be charred, soft, and easy to peel off, and the peppers should look slightly collapsed.

3. Transfer the peppers to a bowl and cover with a lid for 15 to 20 minutes. They will steam from their own heat, which will help with the peeling process.

4. Once they are safe to touch, move them onto a cutting board and remove the peel and seeds. Cut them into ¼-inch strips and place them in a medium bowl.

5. Add the garlic, olive oil, red wine vinegar, and salt and pepper to taste. (Add the vinegar gradually, depending on your taste.) Give them a mix.

6. Garnish with the fresh parsley.

7. The salad is ready to serve right away, but I recommend preparing it at least a few hours ahead so that the peppers marinate further.

PREP TIME: 15 MINUTES, PLUS 3 HOURS MARINATING (OPTIONAL)
COOK TIME: 50 MINUTES
SERVINGS: 4 TO 6

---

10 red bell peppers

4 garlic cloves, thinly sliced

2 tablespoons olive oil

1 to 2 tablespoons red wine vinegar

Salt and freshly ground black pepper

1 tablespoon chopped fresh parsley, for garnish

Effortless Arugula Salad

This effortless arugula salad is a great example of how even the simplest of ingredients can come together to create a delicious and healthy dish. Arugula is combined with toasted pine nuts, freshly shaved Parmesan, and a little salt and pepper before getting tossed in a super easy olive oil and lemon juice dressing. To up the convenience, you can even skip toasting your own pine nuts and pick up a bag of pre-toasted ones at the store. This salad makes a perfect canvas for other tasty additions too, so feel free to switch it up each time you make it!

1. If your pine nuts aren't already toasted, toast them in a small dry pan over medium heat, stirring frequently for 3 to 4 minutes, until they are golden and fragrant. Remove from the pan and let cool.

2. Place washed and dried arugula in a large salad bowl.

3. Drizzle the olive oil and lemon juice over the arugula, and add a pinch or two of salt and pepper. Use your hands or salad tongs to gently toss the arugula, ensuring that the leaves are evenly coated with the dressing.

4. Top the salad with shaved Parmesan cheese and the toasted pine nuts, and any other additions you'd like, and serve immediately.

PREP TIME: 5 MINUTES
SERVINGS: 4 TO 6

¼ cup raw or toasted pine nuts

6 ounces arugula

¼ cup olive oil

2 tablespoons freshly squeezed lemon juice

Salt and freshly ground black pepper

1½ ounces shaved Parmesan cheese

OPTIONAL ADDITIONS

Sliced strawberries

Sliced grape tomatoes

Grilled chicken breast

Grilled shrimp

Curried Egg Salad

Not your typical egg salad! Creamy and full of warm spices, this curried egg salad is packed with protein and all kinds of flavor. The fresh taste of egg, Greek yogurt, and dill mingle with the boldness of curry powder, cayenne pepper, and mustard in this easy, delicious dish. I love prepping it ahead, as it stays fresh and flavorful in the fridge for several days. Serve it as a dip with veggie sticks or pita chips, pile it high on a sandwich, or eat it straight up with a spoon!

1. Bring a 6 cups of water to a boil in a large pot.

2. Place the eggs in the boiling water and boil for 9 to 10 minutes. Drain and rinse with cold water.

3. Once they're cool to the touch, peel the eggs and finely chop them.

4. In a medium bowl, combine the eggs, mayo, yogurt, curry powder, mustard, dill, and cayenne and mix well with a fork. Add salt and pepper to taste. Give it a taste, and adjust if needed.

5. Serve right away with your favorite fresh veggie sticks or pita chips, or store in the fridge for 2 to 3 days.

PREP TIME: 20 MINUTES
COOK TIME: 20 MINUTES
SERVINGS: 4 TO 6

---

8 eggs

¼ cup mayonnaise

6 tablespoons plain Greek yogurt

2 teaspoons curry powder

2 teaspoons Dijon mustard

1 tablespoon finely chopped fresh dill

1 teaspoon cayenne pepper

Salt and freshly ground black pepper

Rustic Walnut Tomato Salad

This is not your average tomato salad. The combination of fresh tomatoes, cucumbers, toasted walnuts, and tangy feta cheese is an absolute dream! For an extra flavor boost, I tossed in a bunch of freshly chopped herbs and drizzled on some olive oil and lemon juice with lemon zest, salt, and pepper for the easiest dressing. It's super simple to make and packed with fresh, vibrant flavor, making it one of my favorite go-to lunches when I'm in need of something quick, healthy, and oh-so-satisfying. It can also be eaten as a side with kabobs or grilled chicken.

1. If your walnuts are already toasted, skip to the next step. Otherwise, toast the walnuts in a dry pan over medium heat for a couple of minutes, tossing continuously to avoid burning. Once cooled, coarsely chop them.

2. In a large salad bowl, combine the cucumbers, mint, oregano, basil, and cherry tomatoes.

3. Add the lemon zest, olive oil, lemon juice, and salt and pepper to taste and give it a mix.

4. Gently fold in the feta and walnuts.

5. Serve right away or store in the fridge for up to 2 days.

PREP TIME: 15 MINUTES
SERVINGS: 2 TO 4

¼ cup raw or toasted walnuts, coarsely chopped

4 Persian or mini cucumbers, halved and cut into thick slices

2 tablespoons finely chopped fresh mint leaves

1 tablespoon finely chopped fresh oregano, leaves only

¼ cup finely chopped fresh lemon basil or regular basil

20 ounces cherry tomatoes, halved

1 teaspoon lemon zest

2 tablespoons olive oil

2 tablespoons freshly squeezed lemon juice

Salt and freshly ground black pepper

2 ounces feta cheese, cubed

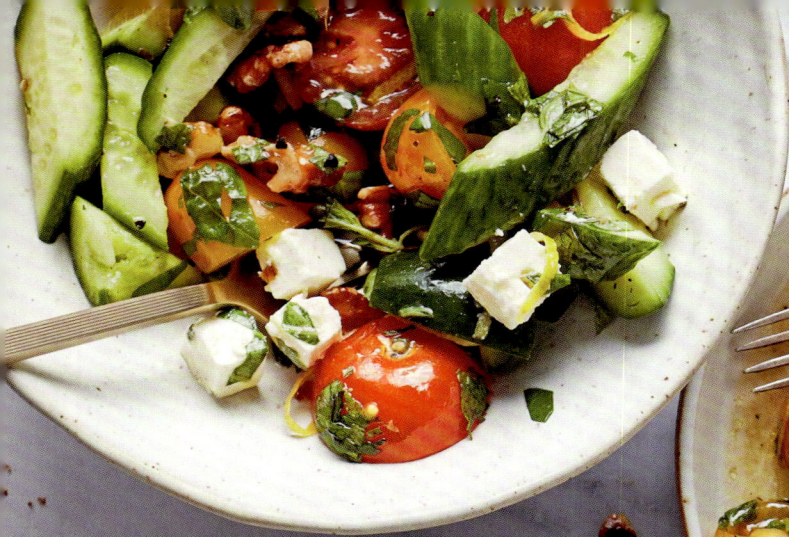

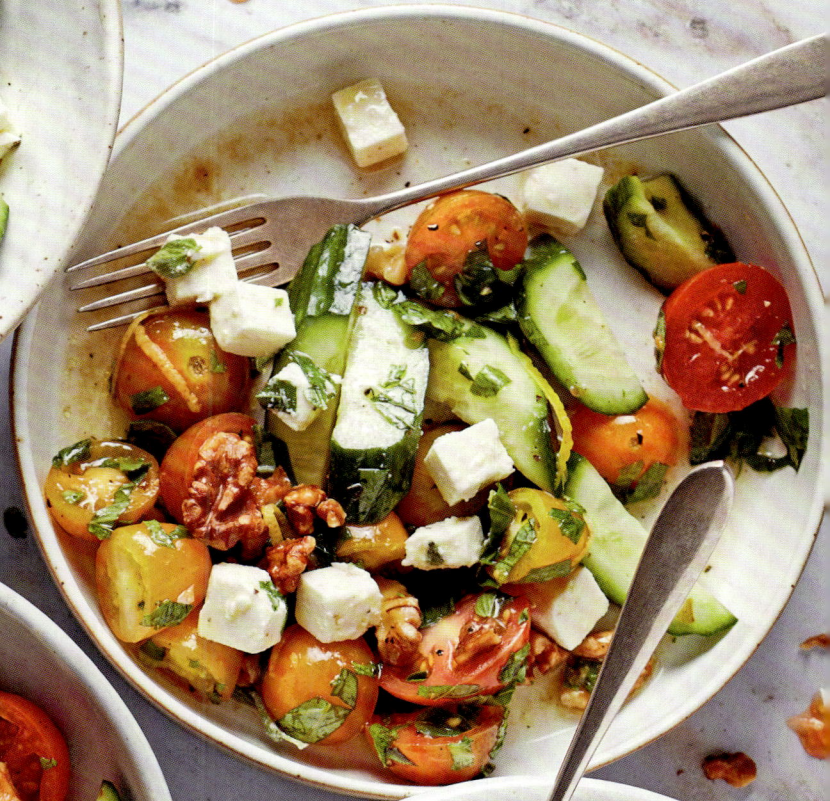

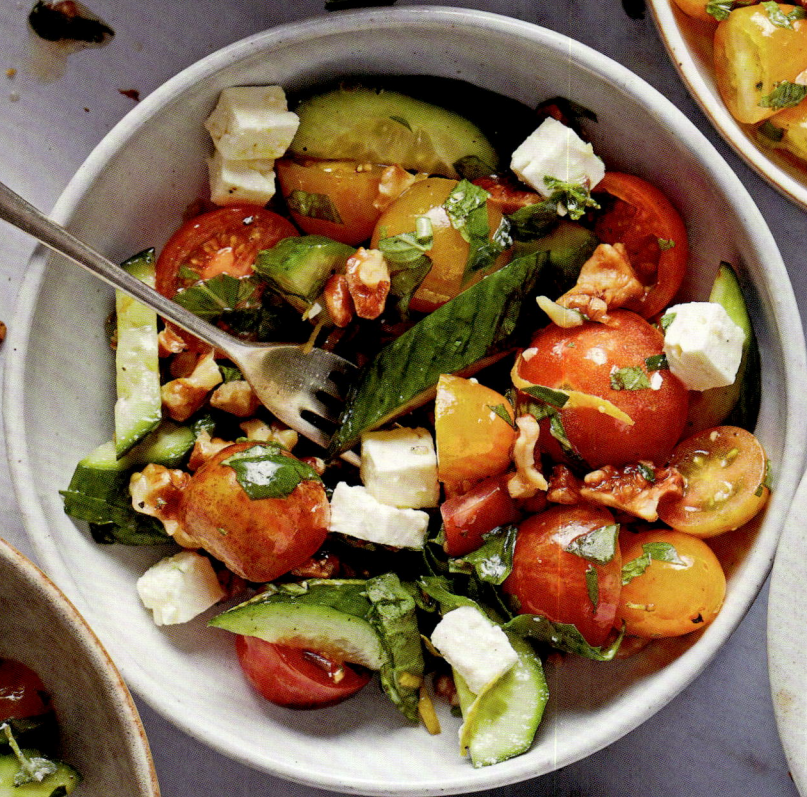

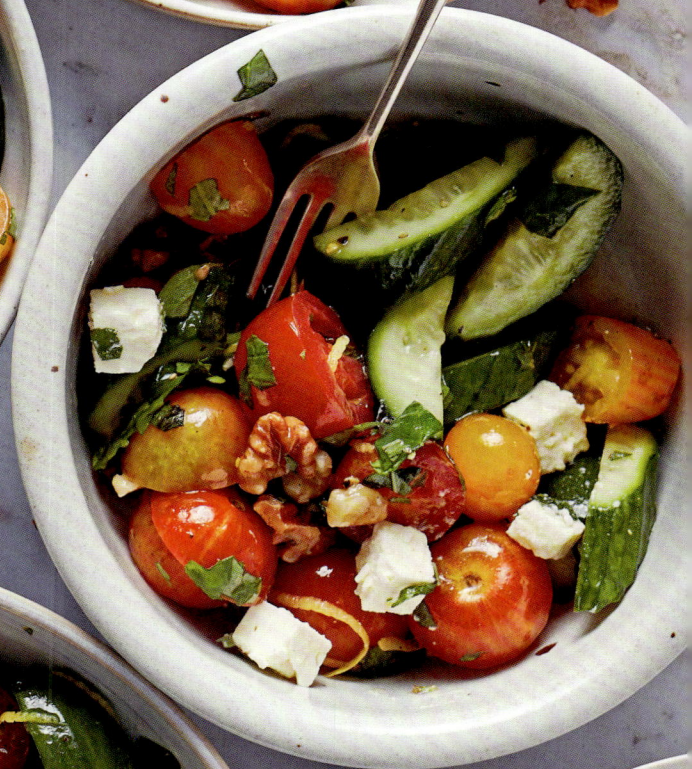

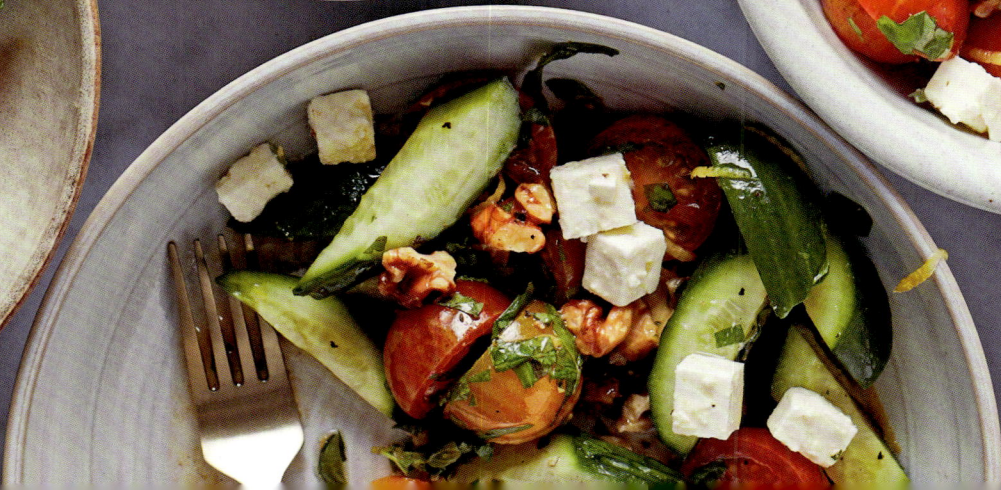

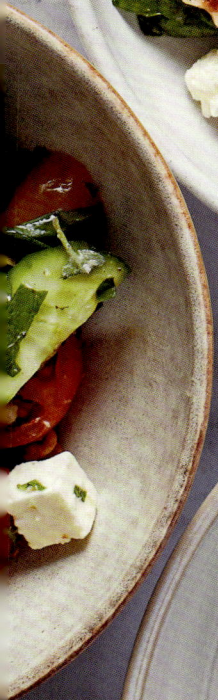

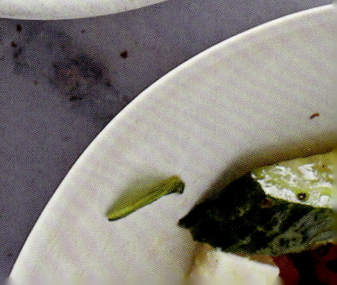

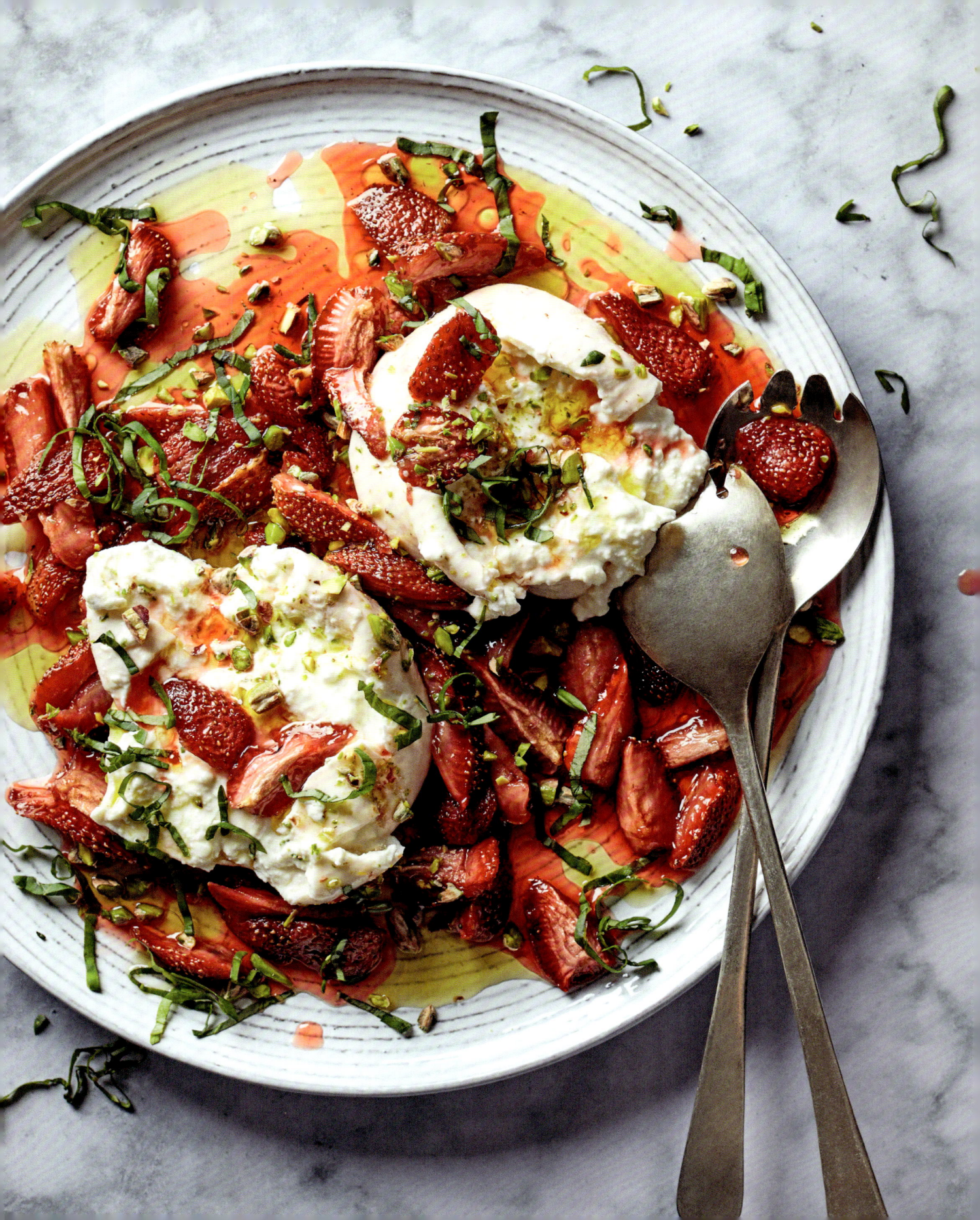

Slow-Roasted Strawberry Burrata Salad

Rich, buttery, and oh-so-sweet, this slow-roasted strawberry burrata salad is healthy decadence at its finest. I'm a big fan of this salad because it requires barely any prep, and the oven does all the cooking for you, making it a super easy, hands-off recipe. The strawberries get roasted until caramelized and syrupy, intensifying their flavor. They then get spooned over the creamy burrata and topped with chopped pistachios for a delightful crunch. It may take a little longer to make this recipe, but the result is incredibly rewarding.

1. Preheat the oven to 300°F.

2. In a medium mixing bowl, toss the halved strawberries with the granulated allulose and mix well until evenly coated.

3. Spread the strawberries in a single layer in an oven-safe medium-size dish. Bake for 2 hours, mixing with a spatula after 1 hour.

4. Thirty minutes before the strawberries are done, remove the burrata from the fridge. Remove it from its liquid, gently pat it dry with a paper towel, and let it come to room temperature.

5. Remove the strawberries from the oven and let them cool slightly.

6. Place the burrata on a serving plate and spoon the roasted strawberries, along with their juices, over and around the burrata.

7. Drizzle the olive oil over the strawberries and burrata. Sprinkle the chopped pistachios over the top. Add a few fresh basil leaves (if using) for a burst of color and freshness, and sprinkle with a pinch of salt.

PREP TIME: 10 MINUTES
COOK TIME: 2 HOURS
SERVINGS: 4 TO 5

---

1 pint fresh strawberries, halved

½ cup granulated allulose, monk fruit sweetener, or regular sugar

2 (4-ounce) balls burrata cheese

GARNISHES

1 tablespoon olive oil

¼ cup toasted pistachios, chopped

Fresh basil leaves, for garnish (optional)

Salt

Sun-Kissed Tomato & Walnut Salad

This sun-kissed tomato and walnut salad has got the crunch factor and flavor punch that you crave for a perfect summer starter or side dish. The shredded romaine, red cabbage, carrot, and cucumbers offer a delightful crunch, while the sweet and nutty dressing brightens everything up beautifully. Just prep your veggies, make the dressing, and toss everything together.

1. In a large salad bowl, combine the cabbage, cucumbers, cherry tomatoes, carrot, lettuce, shallot, and mint. You can add any other shredded or diced veggies you like.

2. **For the tomato walnut dressing:** Toast the walnuts in a dry pan over medium heat for a couple of minutes, stirring from time to time to ensure that they toast evenly and avoid burning. Set aside and let them cool to room temperature. In a food processor, combine the walnuts, sun-dried tomatoes, lemon juice, olive oil, garlic, shallot, basil, tarragon, thyme, and salt and pepper to taste. Blend for a couple of minutes, until the dressing is nice and creamy, no chunks.

3. Pour the dressing on top of the salad and fold gently until the veggies are evenly coated. Top with feta cubes (if using) or other protein.

4. Serve right away.

PREP TIME: 30 MINUTES
SERVINGS: 6 TO 8

½ medium head red cabbage, shredded

3 Persian or mini cucumbers, diced

15 cherry tomatoes, cut in quarters

1 carrot, cut in thin sticks

½ head of romaine lettuce, shredded

1 shallot, minced

2 tablespoons finely chopped fresh mint leaves

FOR THE TOMATO WALNUT DRESSING

¼ cup walnuts

10 sun-dried tomato halves

9 tablespoons freshly squeezed lemon juice

⅓ cup olive oil

4 garlic cloves

1 small shallot

3 tablespoons fresh basil

2 tablespoons fresh tarragon leaves

1 tablespoon fresh thyme

Salt and freshly ground black pepper

3 to 4 ounces feta cheese, cubed (optional)

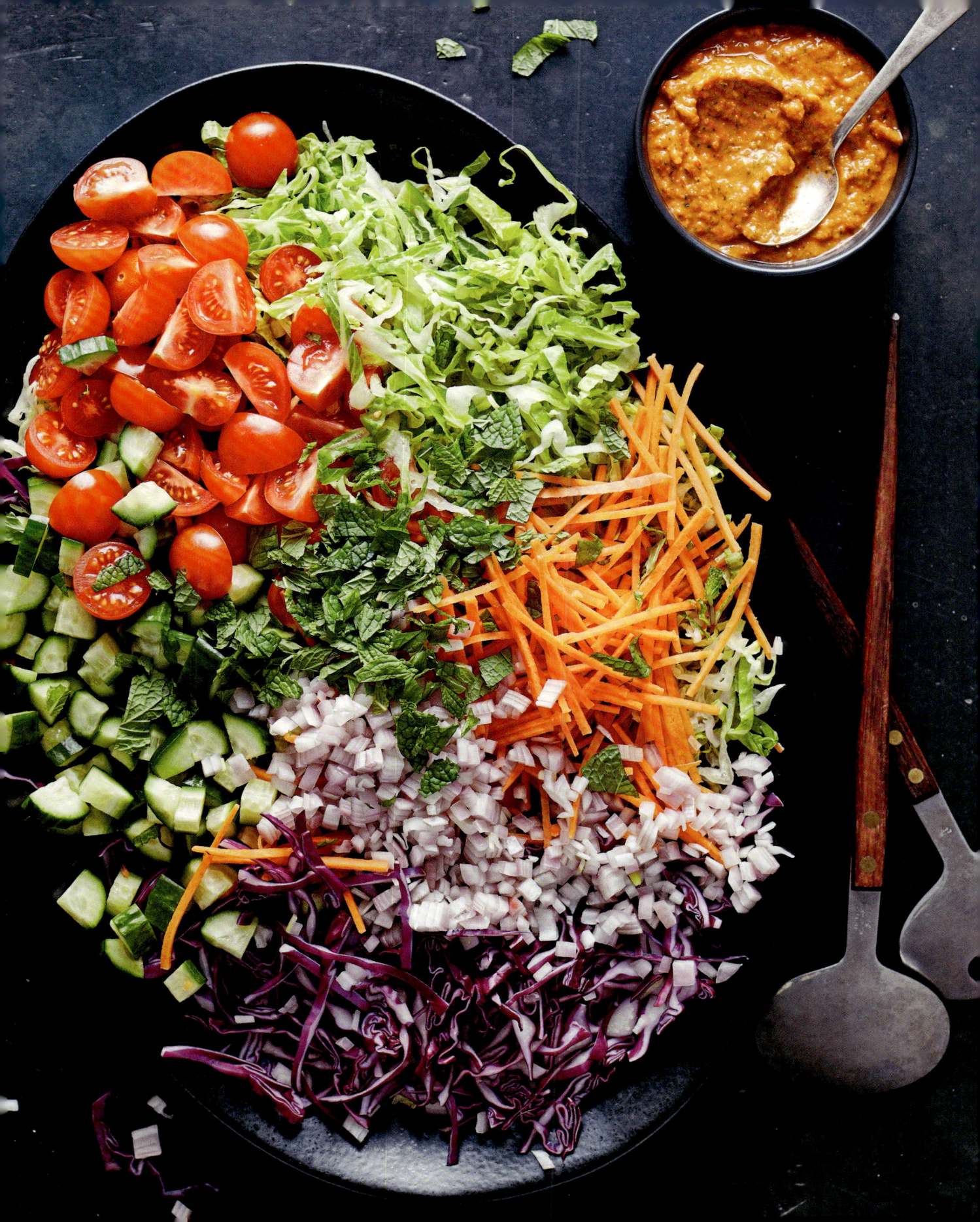

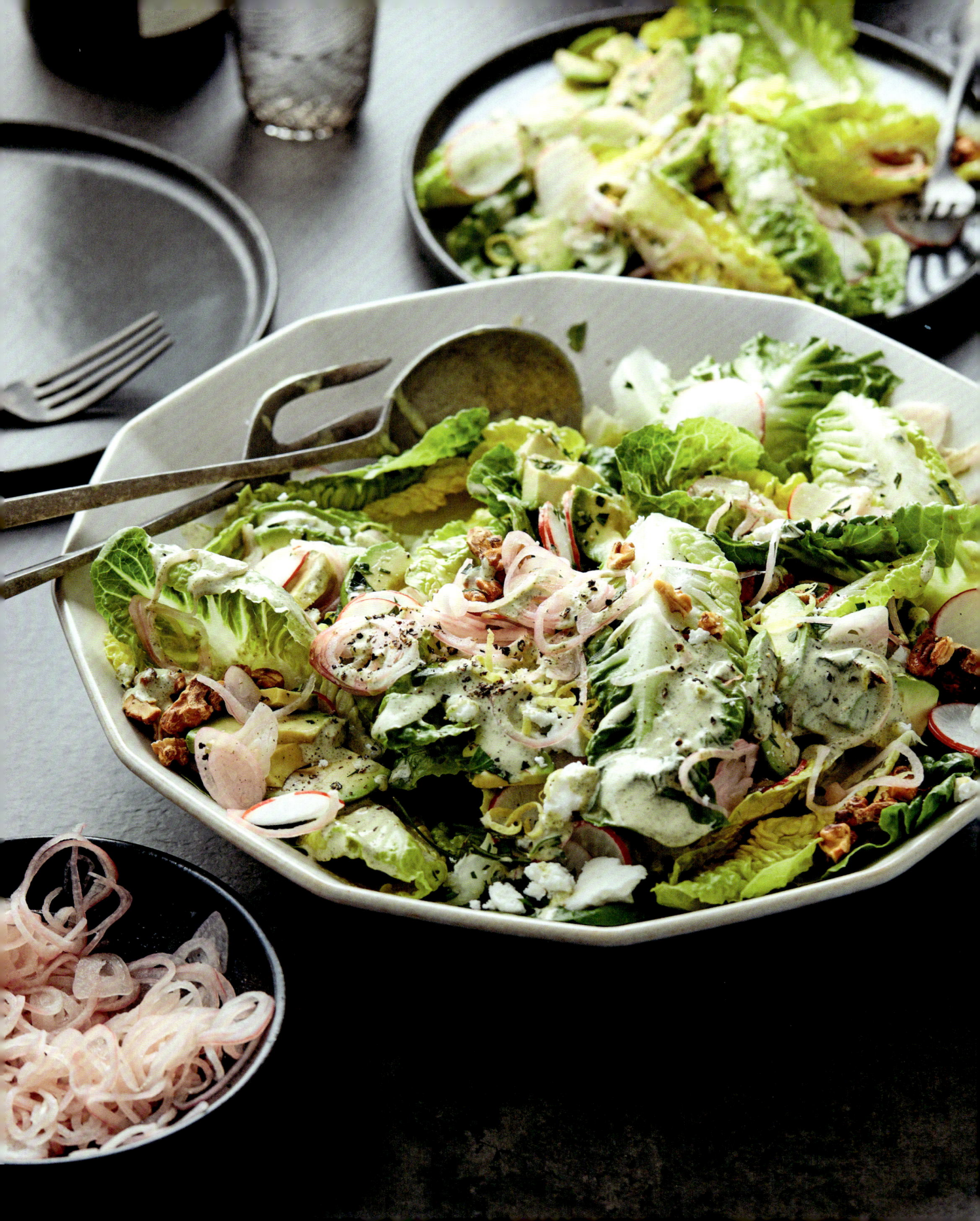

Gem Lettuce Salad

WITH QUICK-PICKLED SHALLOTS

I love when salads can be all the things: nutritious, delicious, and simple to prepare. This crispy gem lettuce salad gets tossed together in just 15 minutes and features quick homemade pickled shallots for a tangy, savory kick. Their zesty flavor is perfect with the creamy, lemony Dijon dressing. Top with avocado, radishes, and toasted walnuts, and you've got a hearty main meal or an elegant side dish to accompany your favorite protein dishes.

1. **For the quick-pickled shallots:** Thinly slice the shallots and add them to a mason jar. Cover with the apple cider vinegar, lemon juice, sweetener of choice, and 2 pinches of salt. Close the lid, shake, and set aside for 15 to 20 minutes.

2. In a small skillet over medium-low heat, toast the walnuts for about 2 minutes, stirring to avoid burning. Set aside to cool and then chop.

3. In a large salad bowl, combine the lettuce, avocado, radishes, toasted walnuts, parsley, and tarragon.

4. **For the dressing:** In a food processor, combine the mayo, olive oil, mustard, lemon juice, mint, and tarragon and blend for a minute. Add salt and pepper to taste.

5. Pour the dressing over the salad. Top with the lemon zest, feta, and as many pickled shallots as desired.

PREP TIME: 15 MINUTES
SERVINGS: 4 TO 6

FOR THE QUICK-PICKLED SHALLOTS

2 small shallots

¼ cup cider vinegar

2 tablespoons freshly squeezed lemon juice

1 teaspoon sweetener of choice (I use allulose)

Salt

¼ cup raw walnuts

6 ounces gem lettuce, washed and dried

1 large avocado, diced

6 medium radishes, thinly sliced

3 tablespoons finely chopped fresh parsley

1 tablespoon finely chopped fresh tarragon leaves

FOR THE DRESSING

3 tablespoons mayonnaise

2 tablespoons olive oil

1 teaspoon Dijon mustard

2 tablespoons freshly squeezed lemon juice

½ cup fresh mint leaves

½ cup fresh tarragon leaves

Salt and freshly ground black pepper

Zest of 1 medium lemon

3 ounces feta cheese, crumbled

Watermelon Feta Salad

Crunchy, creamy, salty, sweet—this watermelon feta salad is true bliss in salad form. The combination of feta cheese, watermelon, and walnuts will forever change the way you look at watermelon. Toss in the blackberries, mint, and lime, and you've really got yourself a party! I love this recipe because the ingredients are so simple and fresh. It takes only minutes to make and brings the wow factor to any gathering or special occasion.

1. In a small skillet over medium-low heat, toast the walnuts for about 2 minutes, stirring to avoid burning. Set aside to cool.

2. In a large bowl, combine the watermelon and cucumbers. Add the blackberries and cooled walnuts. Sprinkle in the feta, lime juice, olive oil, chili lime seasoning, and a pinch of salt.

3. Toss gently and serve immediately.

PREP TIME: 30 MINUTES
SERVINGS: 4 TO 6

⅓ cup raw walnuts

5 cups bite-sized watermelon chunks

2 Persian or mini cucumbers, sliced into thin rounds

6 ounces blackberries or blueberries

4 ounces feta cheese, crumbled

¼ cup freshly squeezed lime juice

2 tablespoons olive oil

1 tablespoon chili lime seasoning, such as Tajín

Salt

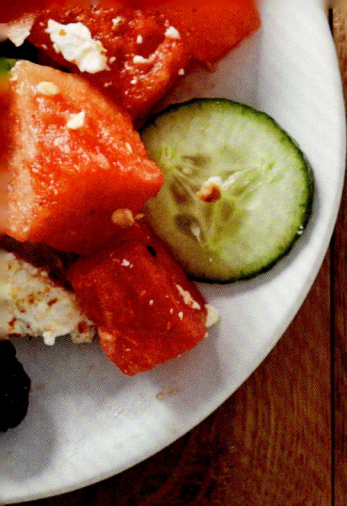

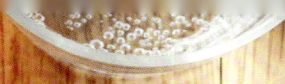

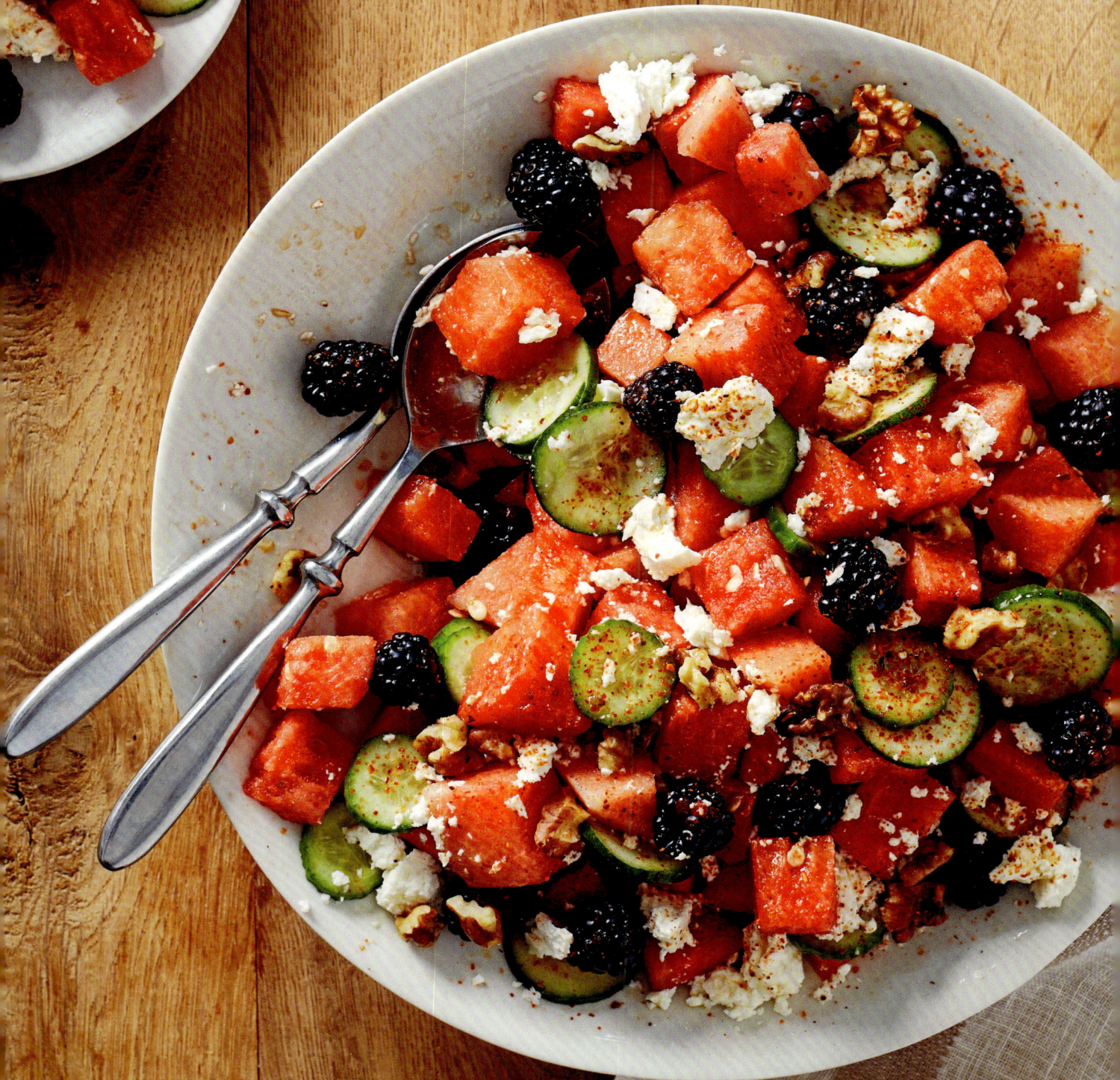

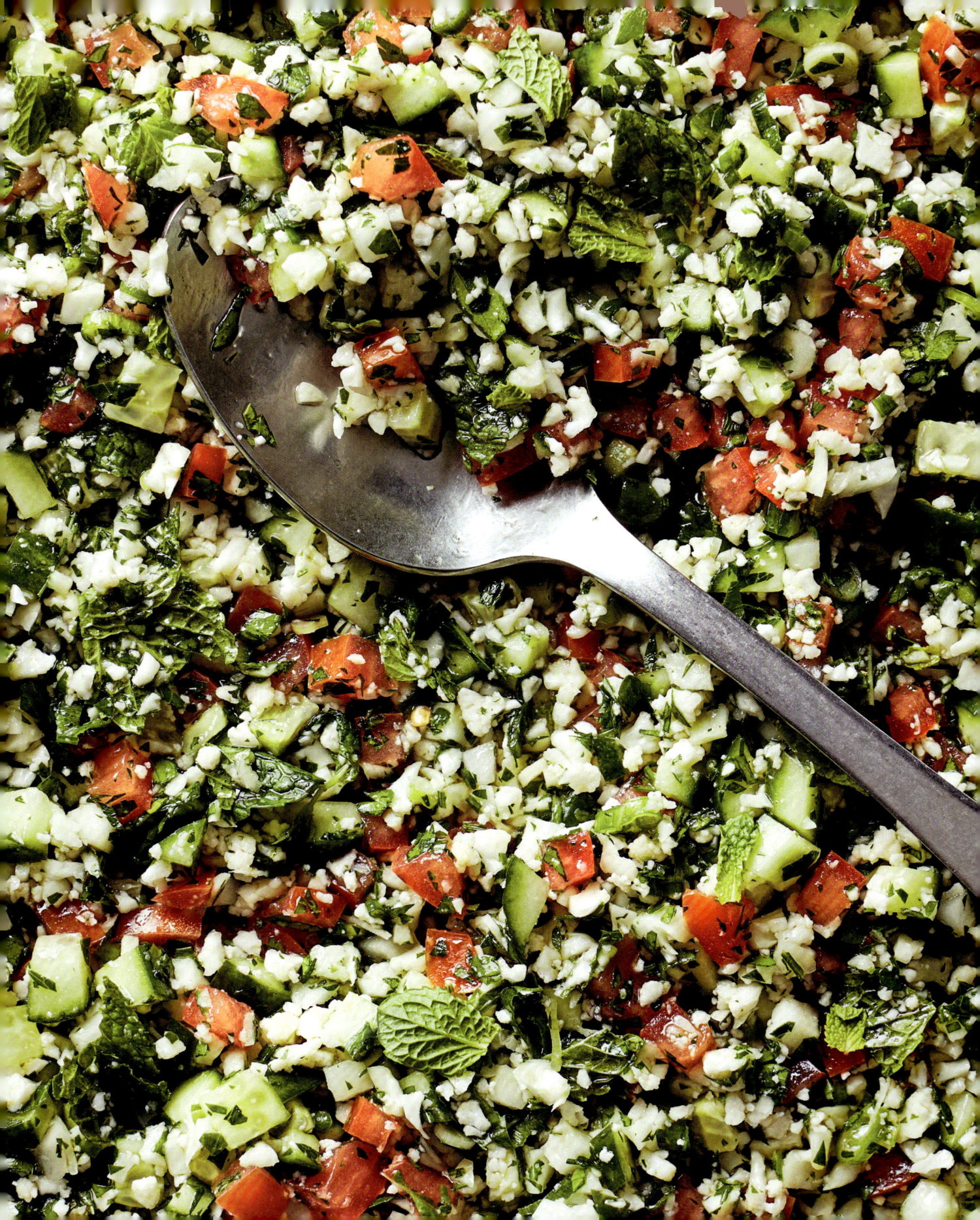

Low-Carb Tabbouleh

Low-carb tabbouleh is my riff on the classic Mediterranean salad I grew up eating with my family. I added finely blended cauliflower into the mix to mimic the texture of bulgur wheat, which, by the way, you won't even miss because the cauliflower soaks up all the good flavor! The lemon juice, garlic, and scallions really helps brighten up each bite. It's fresh, flavorful, and easy to whip up. You can pair it with other shareables such as hummus, baba ghanoush, and matbucha for a family spread or serve as a side dish with Saffron Lemon Grilled Chicken (page 120) or Lamb Koftas (page 112).

1. Thoroughly wash and dry the cauliflower. Cut off the florets and process in a food processor until they are superfine riced (the size of couscous) but be careful not to overprocess. (I don't recommend using pre-packaged cauliflower rice for this recipe.)

2. In a large bowl, combine the cauliflower, cucumbers, tomatoes, scallions, parsley, and mint. (Parsley is the star of the show here. Let it shine!)

3. Add the lemon zest, lemon juice, garlic, olive oil, and salt and pepper to taste and toss well. A good amount of salt is key.

4. This is best served immediately, as is or with your favorite grilled protein.

PREP TIME: 20 MINUTES
SERVINGS: 4 TO 6

½ head cauliflower

3 to 4 Persian or mini cucumbers, finely chopped

2 tomatoes, finely chopped

4 to 5 scallions, white and green parts, finely chopped

1 to 2 bunches fresh parsley, finely chopped

½ handful of fresh mint leaves

1½ teaspoons lemon zest

8 to 9 tablespoons freshly squeezed lemon juice

2 or 3 garlic cloves, minced

⅓ to ½ cup olive oil

Salt and freshly ground black pepper

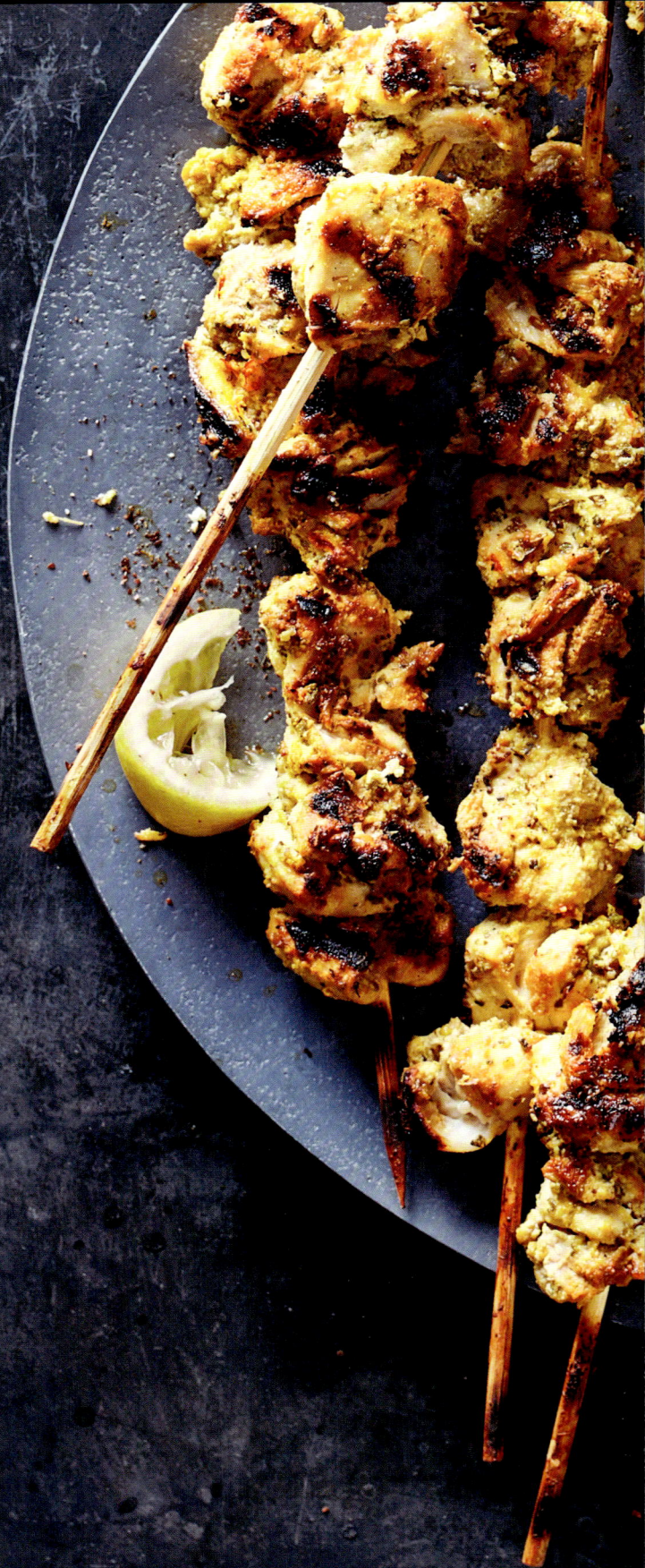

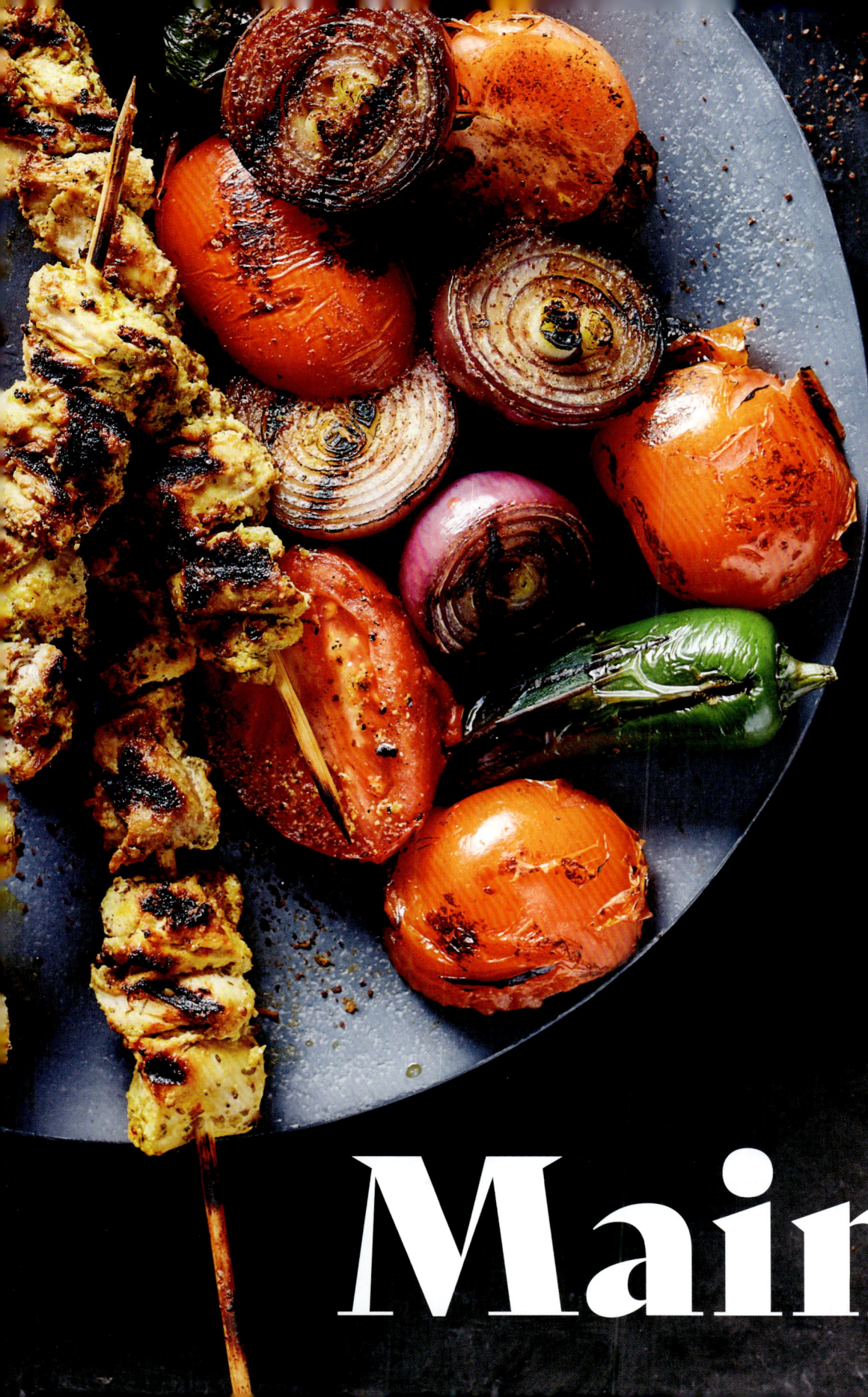

Mains

Do you want dinner on the table faster than ordering takeout, with minimal prep yet maximum flavor? That's what these mains are: sustainable, healthy meals that'll nourish your body *and* make you feel good.

With inspiration from my favorite international cuisines from the Mediterranean, the Middle East, and my own Persian roots, I've included a mix of different meats and fish as well as a few vegetarian options to keep things interesting (but still high in satiating protein). The key is in the marinades and sauces, which are packed with fragrant spices, fresh herbs, healthy fats, and acidity to make your proteins super tender and flavorful. From Persian kabobs to walnut-topped jumbo scallops to hearty vegetable-forward dishes to crave-worthy chicken and lamb, you'll have plenty of options to keep your dinner rotation exciting, satiating, and so good.

These meals should give you a diverse baseline of delicious meals to enjoy on your own or with good company.

Beef Pica Pau

I enjoyed this Portuguese classic in Lisbon and instantly fell in love. I just knew I had to make my own version. The beef is marinated and then cooked in the remaining marinade liquid, along with mustard and butter to make it super flavorful and juicy. Top it with the freshly pickled veggies, olives, and parsley, and serve with toothpicks to enjoy it the traditional way. Or try it with my Kaizen low-carb rice (or the real thing!) and a side salad for a complete and satisfying meal.

PREP TIME: 30 MINUTES,
  PLUS 1 HOUR MARINATING
COOK TIME: 30 MINUTES
SERVINGS: 4 TO 6

20 ounces rib-eye steak or filet mignon

¾ cup white wine or beer

5 garlic cloves, minced

1 teaspoon Tabasco sauce

Salt and freshly ground black pepper

2 tablespoons olive oil

2 tablespoons Dijon mustard

2 ounces unsalted butter, sliced

7 ounces pickled carrots and cauliflower, homemade (recipe follows) or store-bought

2 ounces pitted black olives

1 tablespoon chopped fresh parsley

1. Cut the beef into 1-inch cubes and add them to a medium bowl with the wine, garlic, and Tabasco. Season with salt and pepper. Let marinate for at least 1 hour in the refrigerator.

2. Remove the beef from the marinade and set it in a strainer over a bowl for 2 minutes to drain. Reserve the excess marinade for the sauce.

3. Place a large frying pan over high heat and add the olive oil. Add the beef to the hot oil and sear for 2 to 3 minutes, turning to ensure that it is browned on all sides.

4. Using a slotted spoon or strainer ladle, transfer the beef onto a plate and set aside.

5. Reduce the heat to medium-low and add the mustard and reserved marinade. Whisk for a few minutes to help dissolve the mustard and avoid any clumps.

6. Bring to a boil and let the sauce reduce by half (3 to 4 minutes). Check for salt and adjust if needed.

7. Over low heat, gradually whisk in the slices of cold butter.

8. Once all the butter is melted, add the beef back to the pan and cook for another 1 to 2 minutes.

9. Serve the beef on a large deep platter and top it with the pickled veggies, olives, and fresh parsley. Eat right away!

(recipe continues)

FOR THE PICKLED VEGETABLES

(prepare at least 3 days in advance; makes 1 quart jar)

1. Cut the carrots and cauliflower into ½-inch cubes and place them in a quart mason jar with the garlic.

2. In a small pot over medium-high heat, combine 1 cup water with the vinegar, salt, and monk fruit sweetener. Stir until the mixture comes to a boil and the salt and sweetener are dissolved.

3. Pour the mixture over the vegetables in the jar and seal immediately with the lid. As the liquid cools, it will create a vacuum and seal the jar.

4. Let the vegetables pickle for 4 to 6 hours at room temperature, then refrigerate for 3 days. Store in the fridge after opening.

8 ounces carrots

8 ounces cauliflower

4 garlic cloves, coarsely chopped

2 cups white vinegar

1 tablespoon salt

½ tablespoon monk fruit sweetener or regular sugar

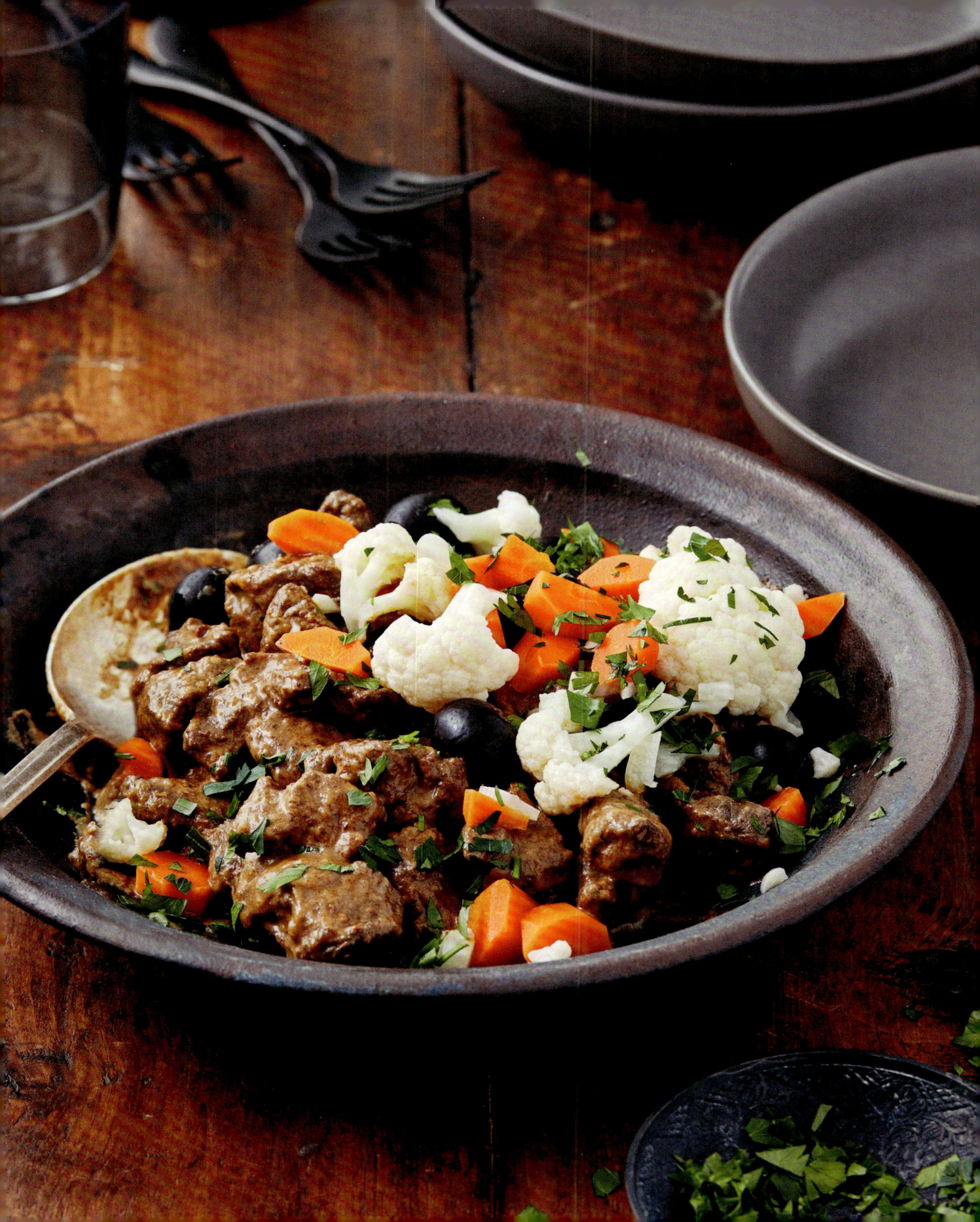

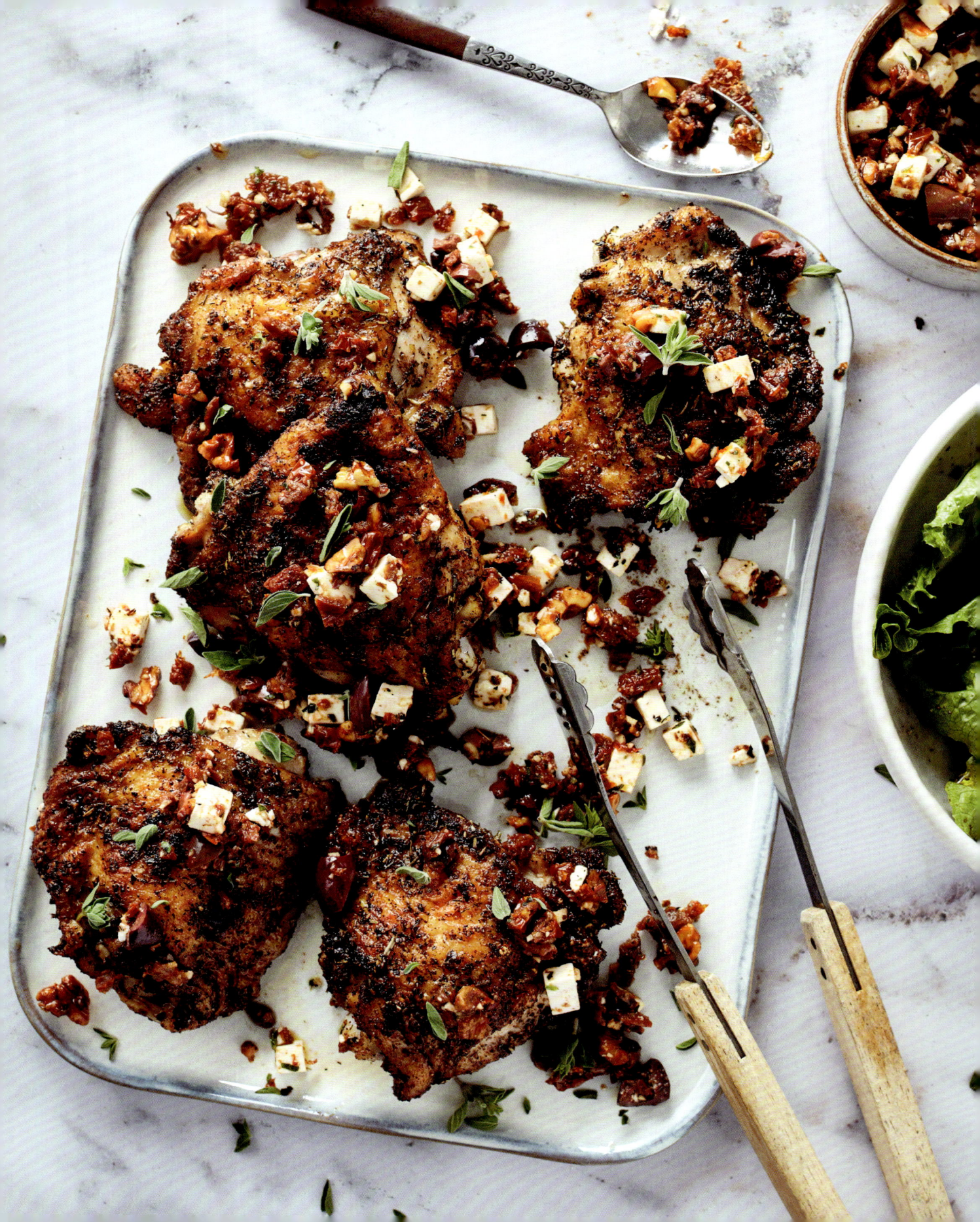

Mediterranean Chicken

WITH OLIVE FETA SALSA

With this Mediterranean chicken, your weeknight dinners are sure to taste fresh and flavorful. It's a simple recipe that covers all the bases: protein, vegetables, and healthy fats. My homemade Greek spice blend provides the chicken a rich depth of flavor, while the olive feta salsa brings in a burst of invigorating Mediterranean flavor. Whether you serve it with a side of your favorite vegetables, with a fresh green salad, or on its own, this dish is sure to become a staple in your meal rotation.

PREP TIME: 30 MINUTES
COOK TIME: 45 MINUTES
SERVINGS: 4 TO 6

6 bone-in, skin-on chicken thighs, about 5 ounces each

3 tablespoons avocado oil

3 tablespoons Greek Spice Blend (page 221)

Salt

FOR THE OLIVE FETA SALSA

¼ cup chopped raw or toasted walnuts

2 ounces feta cheese, cut into small cubes

¼ cup pitted and chopped kalamata olives

8 to 10 halves roasted tomatoes in oil, drained and finely chopped

1 garlic clove, minced

1 tablespoon finely chopped fresh oregano, leaves only, plus extra for garnish

1 tablespoon olive oil

Salt

1. Preheat the oven to 400°F.

2. Pat the chicken thighs with a paper towel to remove the excess moisture.

3. Evenly massage the thighs with 1 tablespoon of the avocado oil and the spice blend and season with salt.

4. Heat the remaining 2 tablespoons of avocado oil in a large pan over medium heat. Sear the chicken for 2 to 3 minutes on each side to lock in the flavors.

5. Transfer the seared chicken onto a rack on a baking sheet and evenly pour the remaining drippings from the pan over the chicken.

6. Bake for 40 to 45 minutes, until the chicken skin is brown and crispy and the chicken is cooked through. Once it is out of the oven, let it rest for a couple of minutes to lock in the juices.

7. For the olive feta salsa: If your walnuts are raw, toast them in a small pan over medium heat for about 2 minutes, tossing continuously to prevent burning. Cool before using.

8. In a small bowl, mix the walnuts, feta, olives, tomatoes, garlic, oregano, and olive oil. Given that both feta and olives are already salty, this salsa does not typically need extra salt, but taste and adjust the salt at the end if needed.

9. Place the chicken on a serving platter and top with the salsa and garnish with more fresh chopped oregano.

10. Serve right away.

Lamb Koftas

WITH CUCUMBER DILL YOGURT SAUCE

If you are looking for maximum flavor to effort ratio, you've found the recipe! These lamb koftas are first marinated in a mix of ingredients like sumac, shallot, garlic, toasted walnuts, and feta before getting cooked on your choice of grill or skillet. To take these to the top, I made a cucumber dill yogurt sauce that pairs perfectly with the bold flavors of the lamb koftas.

1. In a large bowl, combine the ground lamb and beef with a couple of pinches of salt and pepper, the sumac, and the shallot, garlic, parsley, walnuts, and feta. Mix well, cover, and let the meat soak up the flavors for at least 30 minutes.

2. For the cucumber dill yogurt sauce: While the meat is marinating, grab a medium bowl and combine the yogurt, lemon juice, 1 clove of the minced garlic (or 2 cloves for a more garlicky taste), dill, cucumbers, and salt and pepper to taste. Mix them together, give it a taste, and adjust if needed. Set aside in the fridge.

3. When you are ready to make the koftas, dip your fingers in water, then use your fingers to roll the meat into patties, logs, or whatever shape you prefer.

4. If cooking on a charcoal grill: Heat the grill. Once the grill is hot and the flame is gone (a flame will burn the meat), add the koftas. Depending on how well done you prefer them and how hot the grill is, cook them on each side for 3 to 5 minutes, turning them every minute.

5. If cooking in a skillet: Set a large skillet over medium heat. Once the pan is hot, add the koftas and cook until they develop a nice brown crust on all sides. Time depends on the thickness of the koftas; small koftas usually take 2 to 3 minutes per side.

6. Plate the koftas and sprinkle them with 1 teaspoon of the sumac and fresh parsley. Serve with the cucumber dill yogurt sauce.

PREP TIME: 30 MINUTES, PLUS 30 MINUTES MARINATING
COOK TIME: 30 MINUTES
SERVINGS: 4 TO 6

½ pound ground lamb

½ pound 80/20 ground beef

Salt and freshly ground black pepper

1 to 1½ tablespoons sumac, plus extra for garnish

1 small shallot, minced

3 garlic cloves, minced

½ cup finely chopped fresh parsley, plus extra for garnish

⅓ cup toasted walnuts, coarsely chopped

4 ounces feta cheese, crumbled

FOR THE CUCUMBER DILL YOGURT SAUCE

¾ cup thick Greek yogurt

1½ tablespoons freshly squeezed lemon juice

1 to 2 garlic cloves, minced or grated

2 tablespoons fresh dill

2 Persian or mini cucumbers, shredded

Salt and freshly ground black pepper

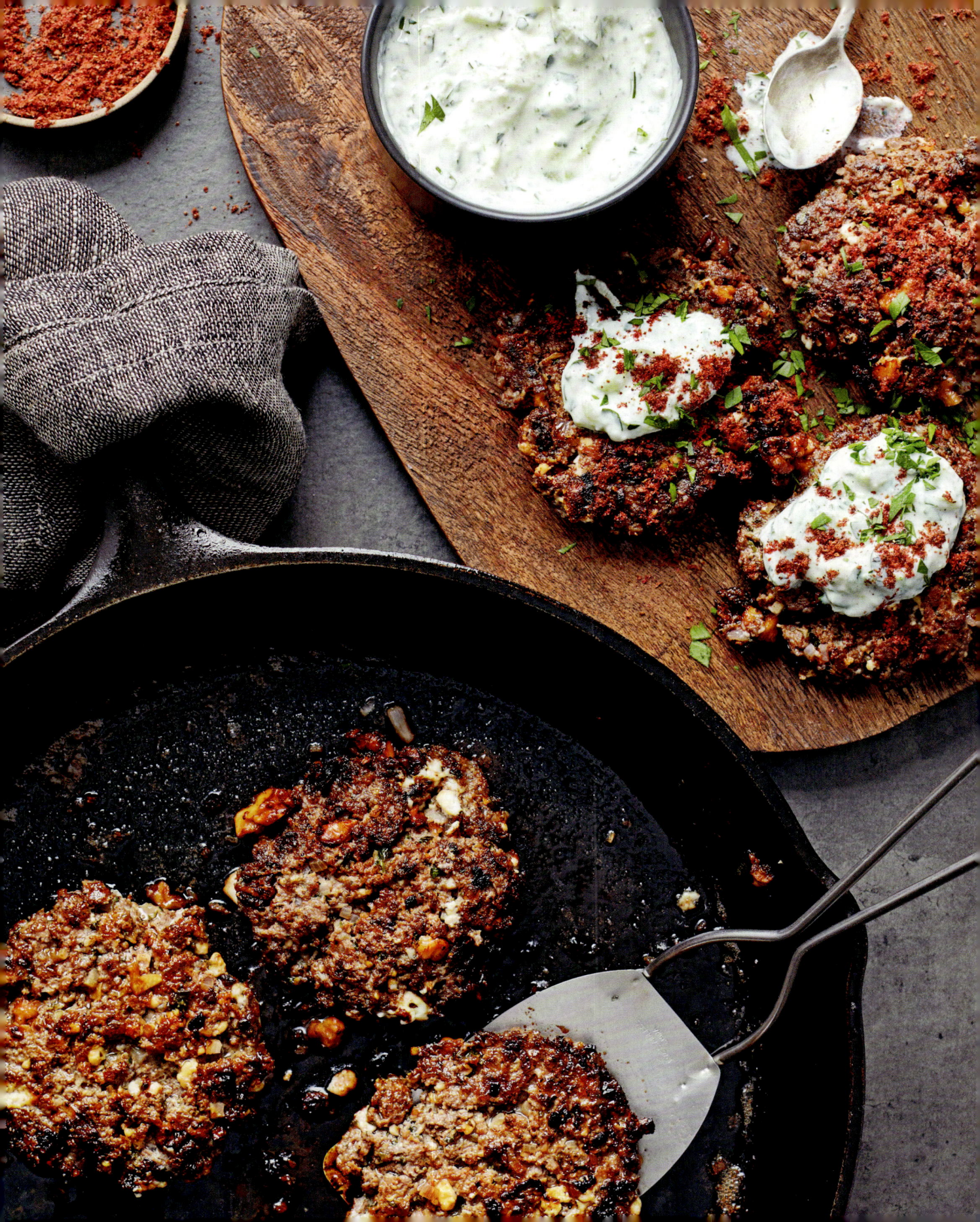

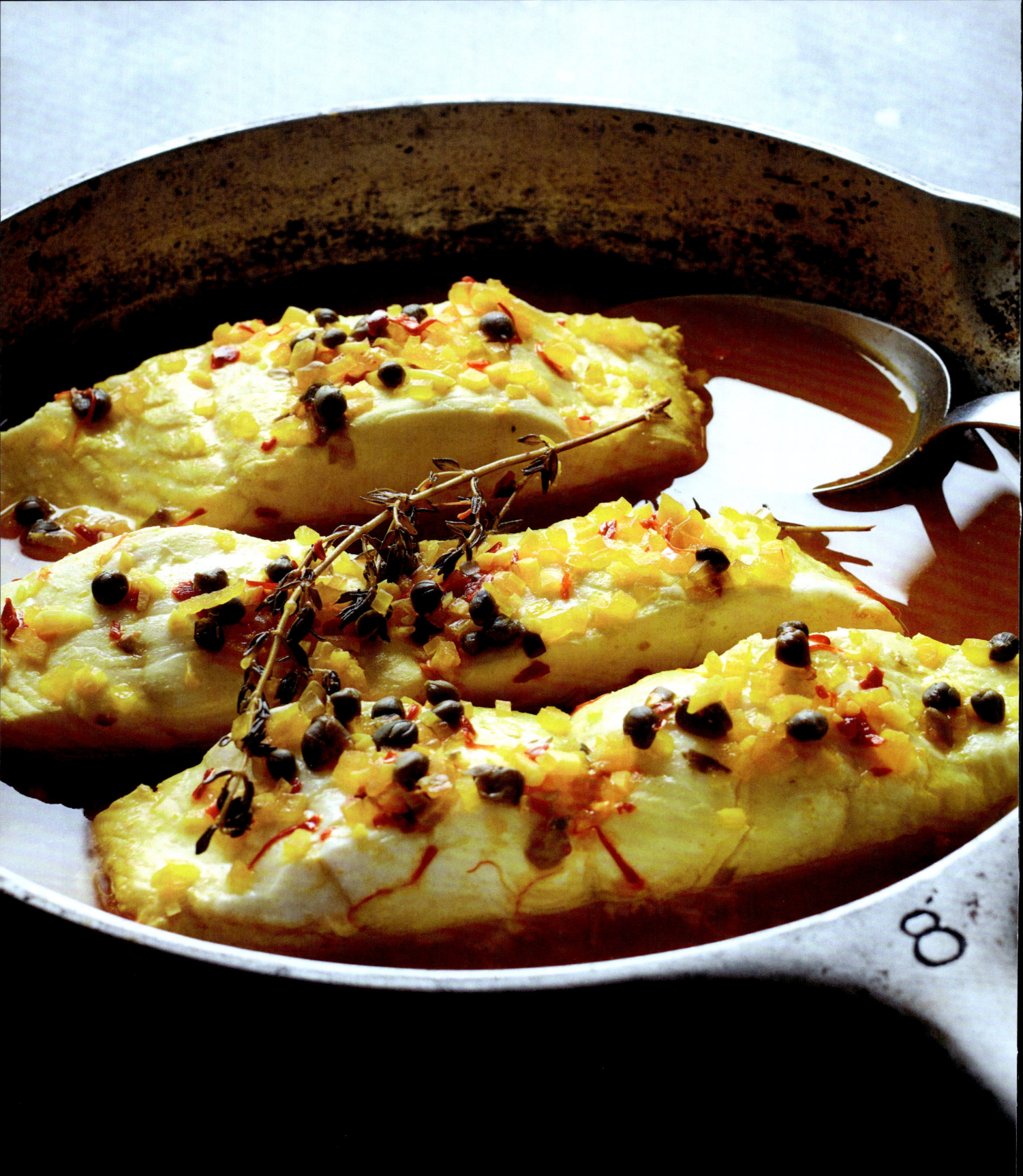

Poached Mediterranean Halibut WITH GARLIC BUTTER

White fish isn't easy to get right, but this poached Mediterranean halibut with garlic butter is sure to be a winner! The fish poaches in a rich broth made with flavorful ingredients like garlic, shallot, wine, lemon juice, capers, and lots of spices. The result is an ultra-moist and juicy halibut packed with Mediterranean flavors that will be the starring act of any dinner.

PREP TIME: 20 MINUTES
COOK TIME: 30 MINUTES
SERVINGS: 2 OR 3

1 pound halibut fillet

Salt and freshly ground black pepper

FOR THE POACHING LIQUID

¾ cup white wine

¾ cup chicken broth

3 tablespoons freshly squeezed lemon juice

1 ounce shallot, minced

3 garlic cloves, minced

2 tablespoons capers

Pinch of saffron threads

1 teaspoon crushed red pepper flakes

2 fresh thyme sprigs

Salt and freshly ground black pepper to taste

1½ ounces unsalted butter, cubed

1 tablespoon chopped fresh chives or parsley, for garnish (optional)

1. Cut the halibut into two or three fillets, depending on how many people you want to serve. Pat them dry with a paper towel and season with salt and pepper to taste. Set aside.

2. **For the poaching liquid:** Choose a shallow pan with a lid that is wide enough to fit all the fillets, but not too wide. Otherwise, the liquid will not cover the fish sufficiently during poaching. Place the pan over medium heat and add the white wine, chicken broth, lemon juice, shallot, garlic, capers, saffron, red pepper flakes, thyme sprigs, and salt and pepper.

3. Bring to a boil and simmer without the lid for a couple of minutes so the liquid is seasoned well and the alcohol from the wine evaporates.

4. Turn the heat down to low, gently place the fish fillets into the poaching liquid, and cover.

5. Poach the fish until the flesh turns opaque, 5 to 8 minutes. Halibut cooks rather fast, so keep an eye on it.

6. Remove the fish from the pan gently (the halibut breaks easily), place it on a deep plate, and let it rest.

7. Bring the heat back up to medium-high and reduce the poaching liquid down to about one third to one half its original volume.

8. Remove the pan from the heat and remove the thyme sprigs from the liquid. Add the butter cubes one by one, whisking to emulsify the sauce.

9. Spoon the sauce over the fish and garnish with fresh chives or parsley (if using).

Ricotta-Stuffed Eggplant Rolls

Vegetables don't have to be boring and flavorless. In fact, these ricotta-stuffed eggplant rolls are quite the opposite! Italian eggplants are sliced thin lengthwise, rolled and filled with three kinds of cheese, covered in a rich marinara sauce, and baked to bubbly perfection. These rolls become a filling meal when placed over a bed of rice, pasta, or any low-carb alternative.

1. Preheat the oven to 450°F.

2. Using a sharp knife, slice the eggplants lengthwise into ¼-inch-thick slices. Sprinkle with salt and let them sit between paper towels for 30 minutes to absorb moisture.

3. Line a large baking sheet with parchment paper and drizzle with some of the olive oil.

4. Brush the eggplant slices on both sides with the remaining olive oil and arrange them in a single layer on the baking sheet.

5. Bake the slices for about 8 minutes, until lightly brown on one side, then flip and bake for another 5 minutes on the other side. Remove from the oven and immediately lower the oven temperature to 350°F. Transfer the eggplant to a plate and set aside.

6. For the marinara sauce: Heat the olive oil in a pan over medium heat and sauté the onion and garlic for 4 to 5 minutes, until the onion is golden brown. Add the thyme and sauté for another minute.

7. Add the tomato puree, red pepper flakes, basil, and balsamic vinegar. Add salt and pepper to taste. Cook until some of the water has evaporated and the sauce is thick and silky.

8. For the cheese filling: In a bowl, combine the ricotta, mozzarella, pecorino, basil, and salt and pepper to taste and mix well.

9. Pour two-thirds of the marinara sauce into a deep oven-safe pan.

10. To make the eggplant rolls, place 2 tablespoons of the cheese filling near one end of an eggplant slice and roll it up. As each roll is formed, place it in the pan. The sauce should partially submerge the rolls.

11. Pour the remaining one-third of the marinara sauce over the rolls and sprinkle with grated pecorino. Bake for 15 to 20 minutes, until the sauce bubbles.

12. Garnish with some more fresh basil and serve hot.

PREP TIME: 45 MINUTES
COOK TIME: 30 MINUTES
SERVINGS: 4 TO 6

2 medium Italian eggplants

Salt

3 tablespoons olive oil

FOR THE MARINARA SAUCE

1 tablespoon olive oil

½ medium onion, minced

4 garlic cloves, minced

2 teaspoons dried thyme

1 (10.75-ounce) can tomato puree

½ teaspoon crushed red pepper flakes

¼ bunch of fresh basil, finely chopped, plus extra for garnish

1 teaspoon balsamic vinegar

Salt and freshly ground black pepper

FOR THE CHEESE FILLING

1 cup ricotta cheese

⅓ cup shredded mozzarella

⅓ cup grated pecorino cheese, plus extra for garnish

¼ bunch of fresh basil, finely chopped

Salt and freshly ground black pepper

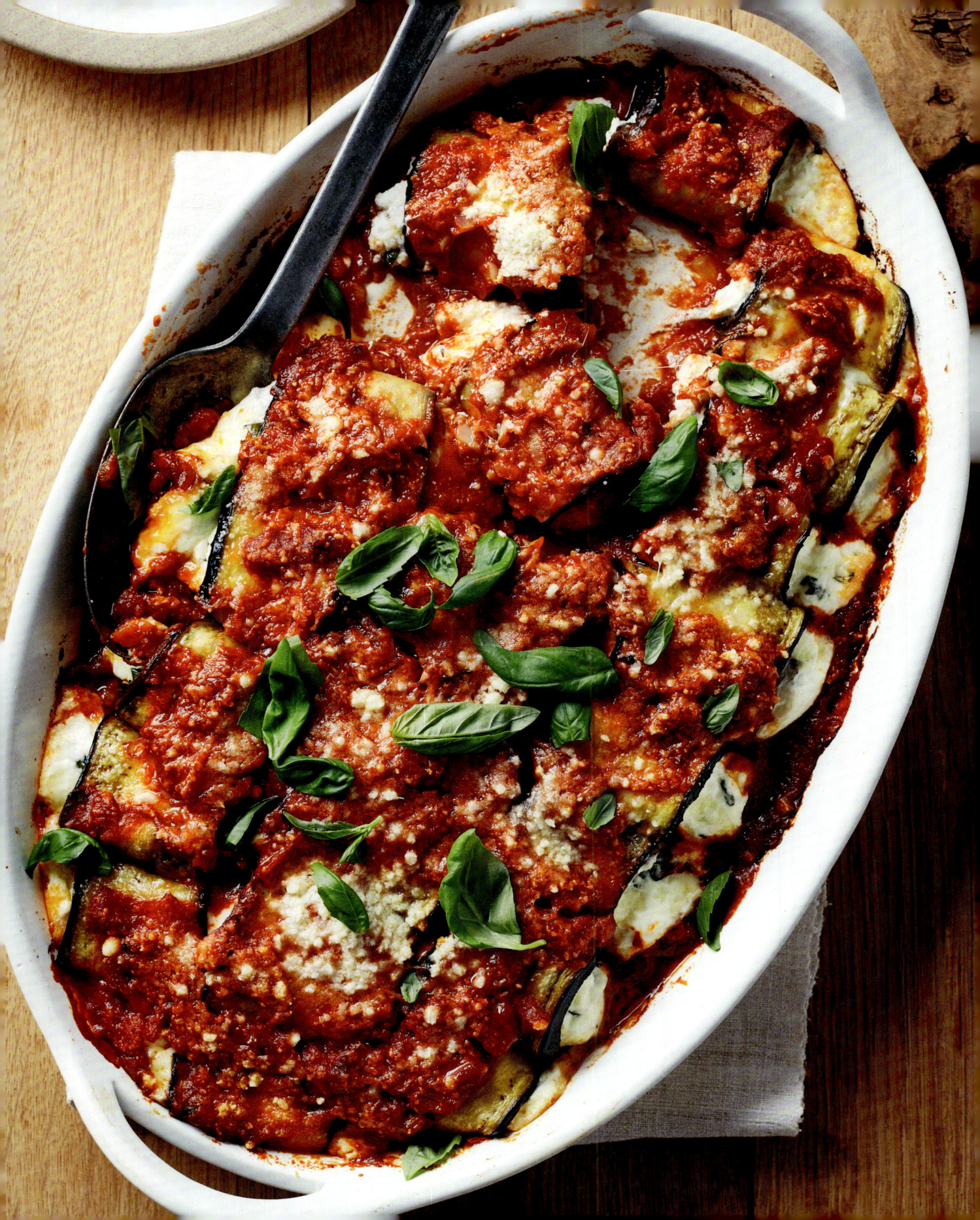

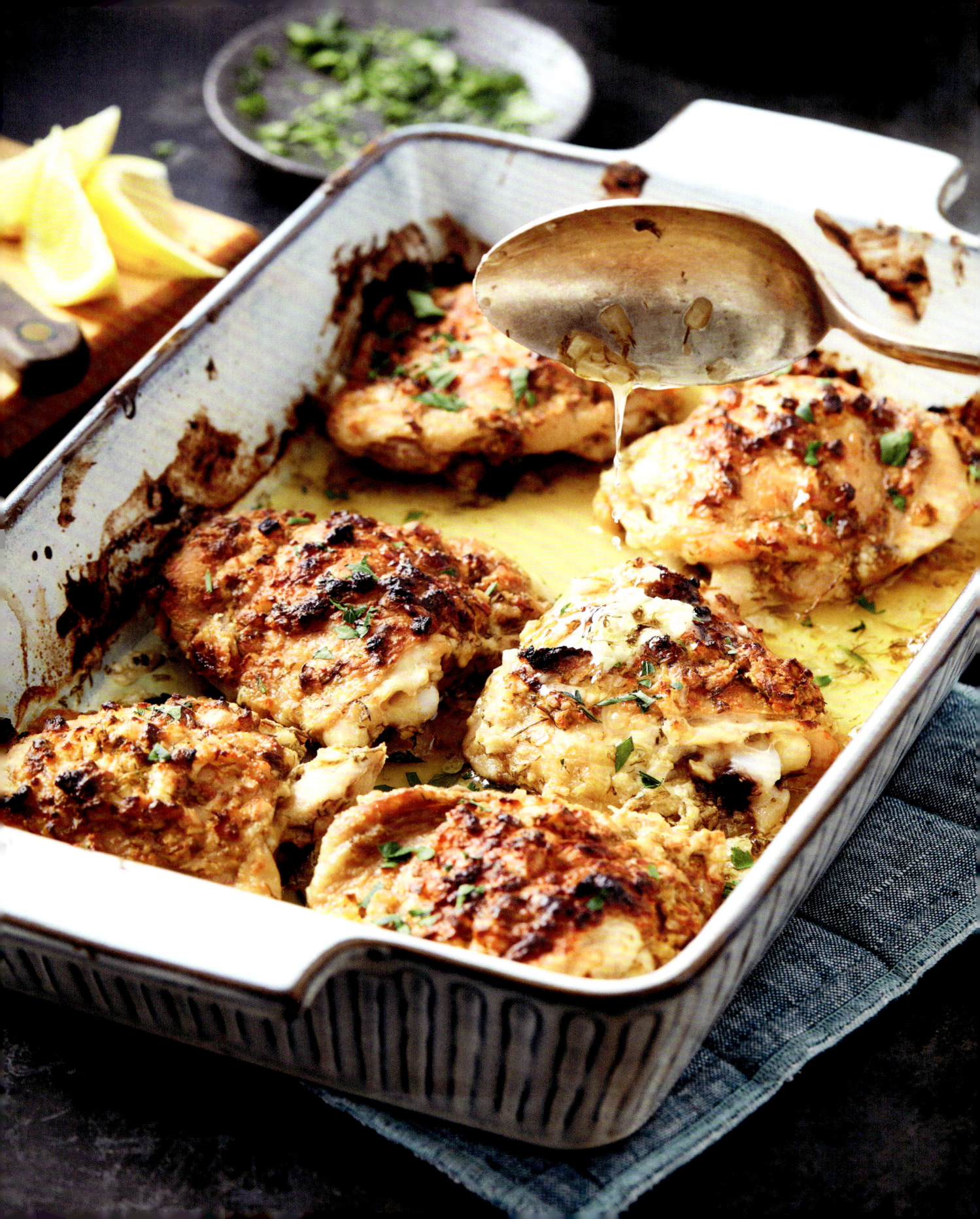

One-Dish Lemony Chicken Bake

There's nothing like a one-pan meal to make you feel like a superstar in the kitchen. This one-dish lemony chicken bake is no exception! It's simple, delicious, and easy to clean up. Plus, it'll make your house smell amazing. The flavor combo of shallot, dill, garlic, lemon, Dijon, and pecorino cheese should really be illegal—it's that dangerously good. Whether you need something nourishing and undemanding on a busy weeknight or a quick Sunday meal prep, this tasty bake will be your right hand. It's always there to save the day when you need some quality protein!

PREP TIME: 15 MINUTES
COOK TIME: 40 MINUTES
SERVINGS: 4 TO 5

2 pounds bone-in, skin-on chicken thighs

3 tablespoons olive oil

Salt and freshly ground black pepper

1 shallot, minced

3 tablespoons finely chopped fresh dill

5 garlic cloves, minced

1 teaspoon lemon zest

2 tablespoons Dijon mustard

¼ cup grated pecorino cheese

6 tablespoons freshly squeezed lemon juice

2 tablespoons finely chopped fresh parsley, for garnish

4 lemon wedges, for garnish

1. Preheat the oven to 425°F.

2. Pat the chicken thighs with a paper towel and place into a large baking dish.

3. Massage the chicken with 2 tablespoons of the olive oil and season with a couple of generous pinches of salt and pepper.

4. Top the chicken with the shallot, dill, garlic, lemon zest, mustard, pecorino, and 4 tablespoons of the lemon juice.

5. Massage all the ingredients thoroughly into the chicken. Space out the thighs so they do not overlap.

6. Pour the remaining 2 tablespoons of lemon juice over the chicken and drizzle with the remaining tablespoon of olive oil.

7. Bake for 30 minutes. Then baste the chicken with the drippings in the pan and return to the oven for an additional 10 minutes, until the chicken skin looks golden brown and the chicken is cooked through.

8. Spoon the drippings over the chicken, garnish with the parsley and lemon wedges, and serve right away.

Saffron Lemon Grilled Chicken

Better known as *joojeh kabob*, this saffron lemon grilled chicken is a traditional Persian dish that brings me back to the fondest memories of my childhood. Every time I get the chance to eat one, it feels like home! The chicken is marinated in a blend of saffron, lemon juice, onion juice, and Greek yogurt to come out super flavorful and tender. These kabobs are best grilled over charcoal, but they'll still taste amazing with what you got. I like to serve them over a bed of Persian rice or my low-carb Kaizen rice, with grilled veggies and a sprinkle of sumac for a finishing touch.

1. Cut the chicken thighs into 1½-inch cubes.

2. In a food processor, process the onion down to a pulp. Pour the pulp into a sieve set over a bowl, letting it strain for a few minutes, until the onion juices have separated into the bowl.

3. In a large bowl, combine just the onion juice, oregano, garlic powder, yogurt, lemon juice, saffron, and a couple generous pinches of salt and pepper.

4. Give the marinade a good mix, then add the chicken. Mix well, ensuring that the chicken is evenly coated.

5. Cover the chicken and let marinate in the fridge for at least 6 hours, or ideally overnight.

6. Remove the chicken from the fridge 30 minutes before grilling and let it come up to room temperature. The chicken is best cooked on a charcoal grill—ideally wood lump charcoal. If using a charcoal grill, preheat it so that the charcoal is evenly glowing and partially ash-covered. You can also use a gas grill or cook these in a large cast-iron pan on your stove. Skewer the marinated chicken onto flat metal skewers to prevent the cubes from rolling. Place the skewers on the charcoal grill or in a skillet on the stovetop and cook for few minutes on each side before rotating on the other side. Switch between sides until the edges are slightly charred and the internal temperature reaches 165°F.

7. This chicken is best served with rice of your choosing, grilled tomato and onion, and fresh herbs. Don't forget to top with a dusting of sumac.

PREP TIME: 30 MINUTES, PLUS 6 HOURS TO OVERNIGHT MARINATING
COOK TIME: 20 MINUTES
SERVINGS: 6 TO 8

2 pounds boneless, skinless chicken thighs, cubed

1 medium yellow onion

2 tablespoons dried oregano

2 tablespoons garlic powder

3 tablespoons plain yogurt

¼ cup freshly squeezed lemon juice

¼ teaspoon saffron threads soaked in 3 tablespoons hot water

Salt and freshly ground black pepper

OPTIONAL SIDE AND TOPPINGS

8 ounces basmati rice or Kaizen rice, cooked

6 medium tomatoes, grilled, for serving

3 medium red onions, grilled, for serving

Fresh herbs, for garnish

Sumac, for garnish

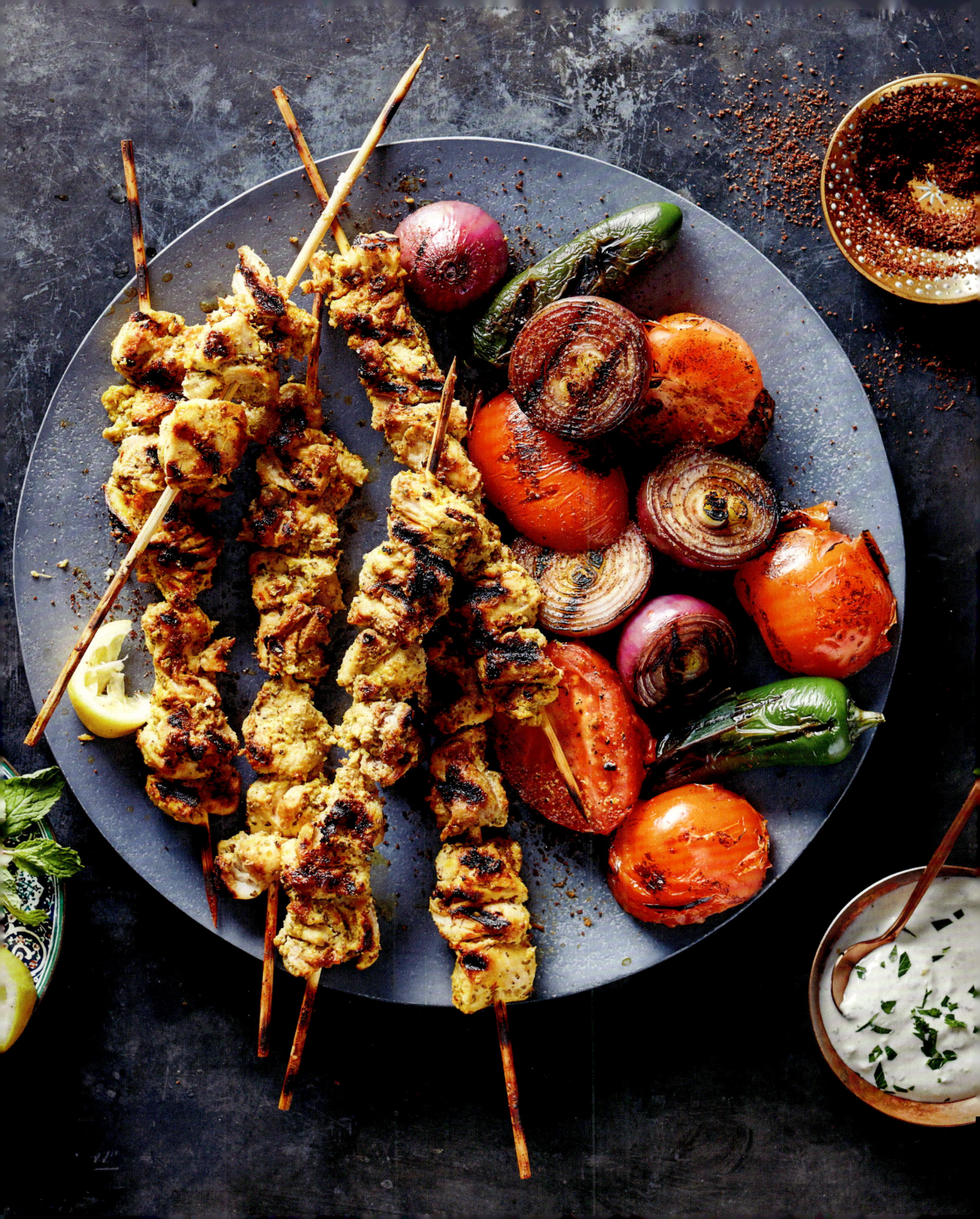

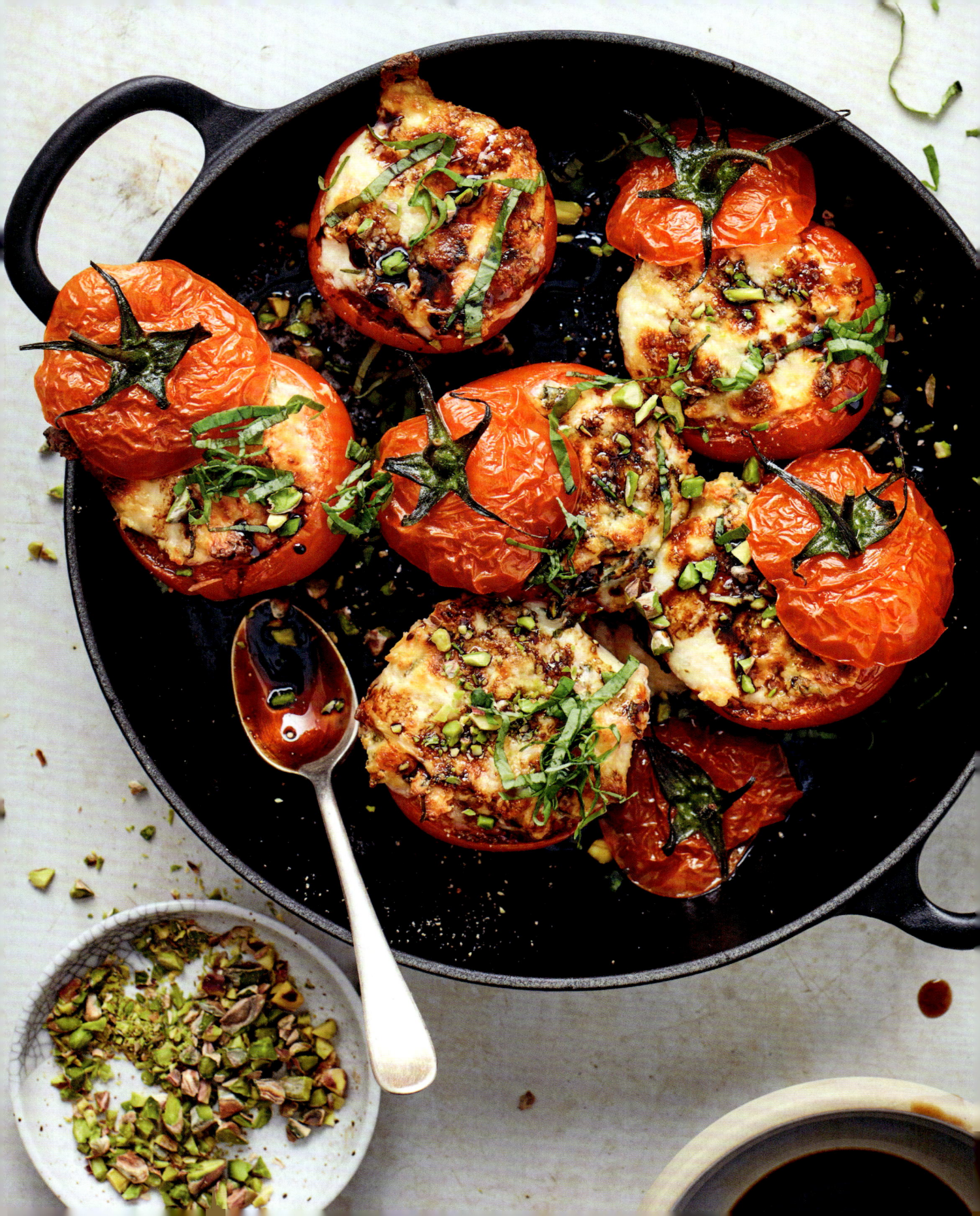

Easy Cheesy Stuffed Tomatoes

I love it when a fruit or vegetable can be a vessel for cheesy deliciousness. This easy cheesy stuffed tomato dish is just that, and then some. The tomatoes come out so juicy and tender, and the mozzarella, ricotta, and Parmesan filling is the perfect creamy, salty, and tangy combination. I add chopped pistachios and basil into the cheese blend and drizzle on some balsamic for an even more robust flavor profile. This dish can be enjoyed in so many ways—as a snack, a meal, or an app! It's like your favorite Margherita pizza but in a little tomato package, no carbs included.

1. Preheat the oven to 400°F.

2. Slice the top off each tomato and scoop out the flesh using a spoon. Do it in small increments to avoid puncturing the walls of the tomatoes. Keep the scooped-out flesh, but discard the seeds and excess tomato water. Keep the tomato tops.

3. Grab a deep oven-safe pan and drizzle in the olive oil. Place the hollowed tomatoes in the pan and season with salt and pepper to taste.

4. Chop the reserved tomato flesh and place it in a mixing bowl. Add the mozzarella, ricotta, pistachios, basil, garlic, and half the Parmesan. Mix well and season with salt and pepper to taste.

5. Using a spoon, stuff the tomatoes with the cheese mixture and top with the remaining Parmesan. Cover the filled tomatoes with the tops.

6. Bake for 15 to 17 minutes, then change the setting to broil, move the tomato tops aside, and let roast another 5 minutes, until the cheese filling is browned and bubbling.

7. Remove from the oven and drizzle with the balsamic vinegar. Garnish with extra fresh basil and crushed pistachios and serve right away.

PREP TIME: 20 MINUTES
COOK TIME: 20 MINUTES
SERVINGS: 4 TO 6

———

6 medium tomatoes

1 tablespoon olive oil

Salt and freshly ground black pepper

3 ounces shredded mozzarella

3 ounces ricotta cheese

1 ounce toasted pistachios, chopped, plus extra for garnish

1 ounce fresh basil, finely chopped, plus extra for garnish

3 garlic cloves, minced

⅓ cup grated Parmesan cheese

1 tablespoon balsamic vinegar

Spatchcock Chicken

WITH ROASTED VEGGIES

Spatchcocking chicken is a cooking technique that involves removing the backbone of a chicken and flattening it out for easier cooking. It may seem intimidating at first, but if you have a sturdy pair of poultry shears, it's actually a straightforward job. The chicken is marinated in a flavorful herby spice blend and roasted with hearty vegetables like bell peppers, cherry tomatoes, red onion, and broccoli. It's an epic meal that'll have the whole fam chowing down, whether it's the holidays, a special occasion, or just a regular weeknight dinner.

1. **For the marinade:** In a food processor, combine the onion, garlic, olive oil, lemon juice, sweet paprika, herbes de Provence, sumac, smoked paprika, and salt and pepper to taste and blend into a smooth paste.

2. Pat the chicken with a paper towel to absorb as much moisture as possible. Turn the chicken breast-side down on a clean cutting board. Using sharp kitchen scissors or a knife, cut along both sides of the backbone and remove it. Turn the chicken over and open the back so the legs are facing down. Place your palms on the center of the breastbone and firmly press down until it cracks (this will allow the chicken to lay flat).

3. Place the chicken on a sheet pan and rub half of the marinade onto both sides of the chicken. You can do this with a kitchen brush or by hand. Make sure to rub it under the skin as well, to the extent possible.

4. Ideally, let the chicken marinate for at least a couple of hours in the refrigerator, but in a hurry, you can cook it right away.

5. Preheat the oven to 350°F. Once the oven is heated, roast the chicken until the skin is brown and crispy and the chicken is cooked through (about 2 hours).

6. While the chicken is roasting, cut the green pepper, yellow pepper, onion, and broccoli into wedges, place them in a large bowl and toss them with the remaining half of the marinade.

7. When the chicken has 30 to 40 minutes to go, add the veggies to the pan beside the chicken and cook together for the remainder of the time.

8. Plate and garnish with fresh parsley, if using.

PREP TIME: 30 MINUTES, PLUS 2 HOURS MARINATING (OPTIONAL)

COOK TIME: 2 HOURS

SERVINGS: 6

FOR THE MARINADE

½ medium onion

4 garlic cloves

3 tablespoons olive oil

5 tablespoons freshly squeezed lemon juice

1 tablespoon sweet paprika

2 tablespoons herbes de Provence

1 teaspoon sumac

1 teaspoon smoked paprika

Salt and freshly ground black pepper

1 whole chicken (about 5 pounds)

1 green bell pepper

1 yellow bell pepper

1 red onion

2 or 3 stalks of broccoli

Fresh parsley, for garnish (optional)

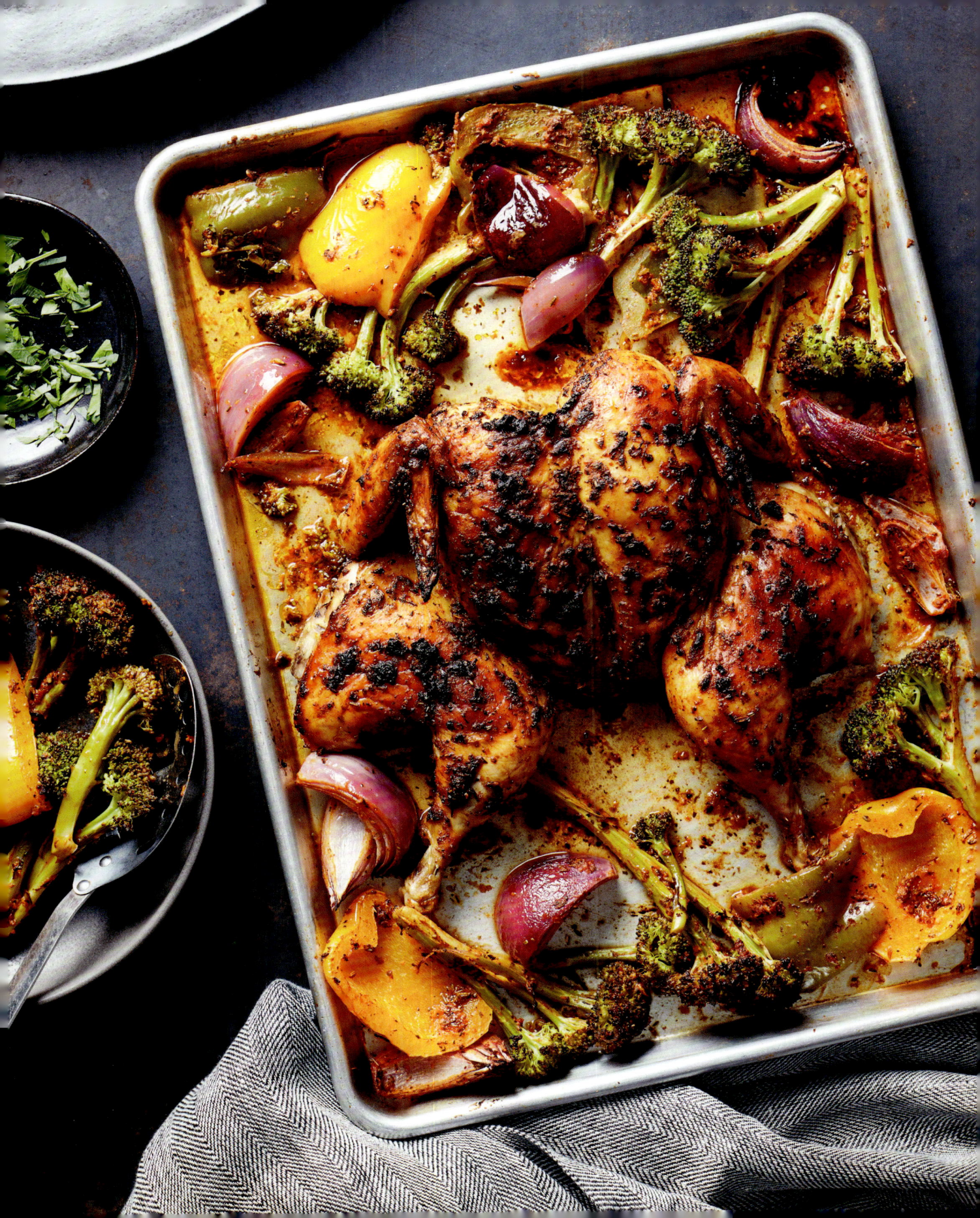

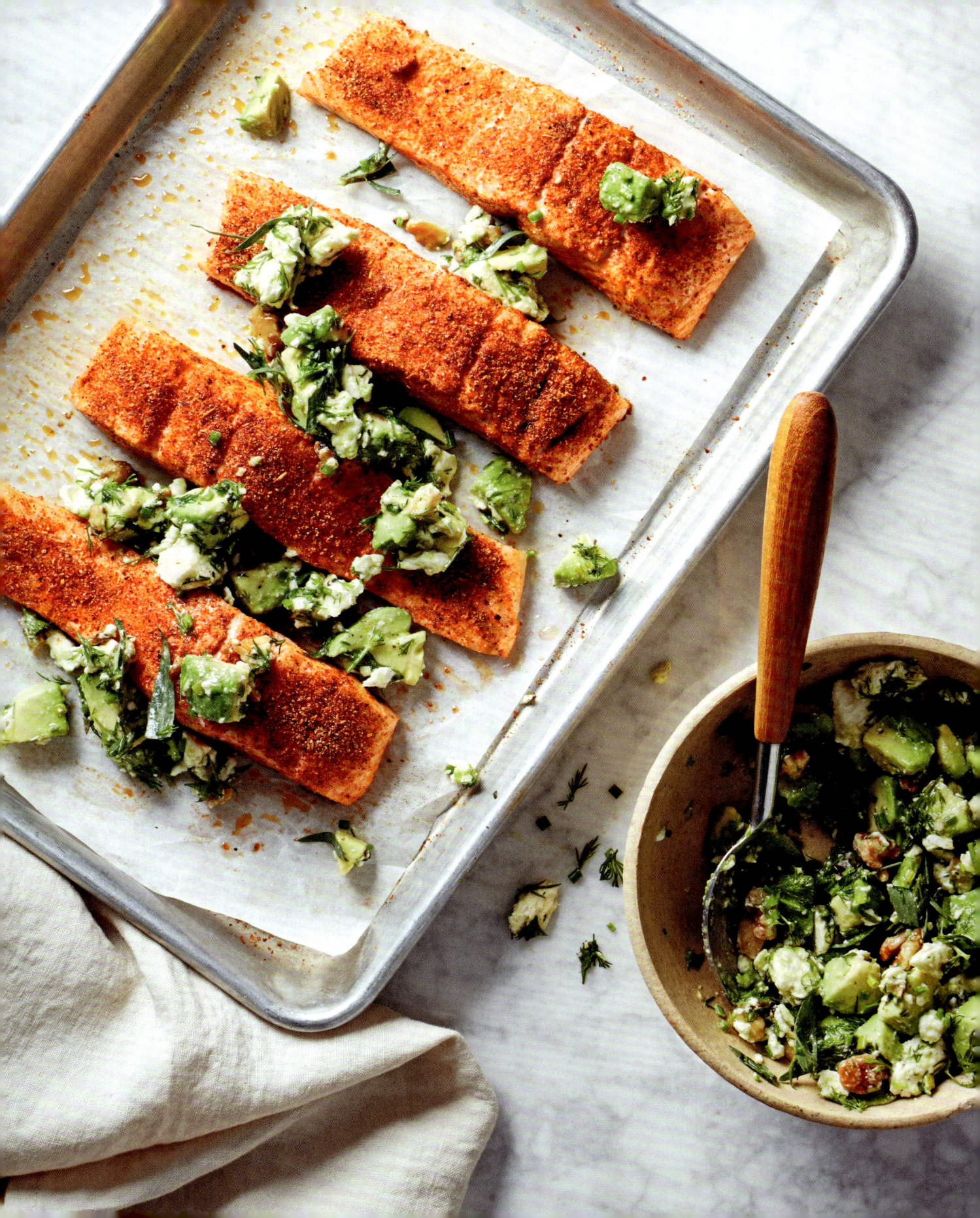

Chili Lime Salmon

WITH BANGIN' AVOCADO SALSA

This salmon with avocado feta walnut salsa is basically a medley of all my favorite foods to create a flavor experience that'll have you hooked after the first bite. The rich and buttery avocado pairs perfectly with the salty feta cheese and crunchy walnuts. Add chili lime–seasoned salmon into the mix and you've got a delicious meal packed with vibrant flavor! And don't worry—if you'd rather cook up the salmon on the stove or in an air fryer, I've included instructions for that too.

1. Cut the salmon into whatever portions you like, then rub with the olive oil. Season with the garlic powder, chili lime seasoning, fennel, smoked paprika, and salt. If you can, let the salmon sit for 15 to 30 minutes to really soak up the flavors.

2. For the bangin' avocado salsa: Cut the avocado into chunks and add to a medium bowl with the dill, tarragon, chives, lemon zest, lemon juice, olive oil, feta, walnuts, and salt and pepper to taste. Give it a mix and add whatever else you like. If you like a little spice, add some fresh chiles or red pepper flakes.

3. If baking the salmon: Preheat the oven to 400°F. Transfer the salmon to a sheet pan. Once the oven reaches temperature, cook for 10 to 15 minutes, depending on the thickness of the fillets, until the flesh turns opaque.

4. If pan-frying the salmon: Place the salmon in a cast-iron or large pan and set over medium heat. Cook for 4 to 5 minutes on each side, until the salmon has a nice sear.

5. If air-frying the salmon: Preheat the air fryer to 400°F. Once the air fryer reaches temperature, add the salmon and cook for 12 to 15 minutes. Time varies by air fryer and the thickness of your salmon, so you may need to play around to find what works best for you. When gently pressed with a fork, the salmon should easily flake apart.

6. Once your salmon is ready, plate it up and top liberally with salsa.

PREP TIME: 30 MINUTES
COOK TIME: 20 MINUTES
SERVINGS: 4 TO 6

---

1 pound wild salmon fillet

1 tablespoon olive oil or avocado oil

1 teaspoon garlic powder

1 teaspoon chili lime seasoning, such as Tajín

Pinch of ground fennel

1 teaspoon smoked paprika or chipotle powder

Salt

FOR THE BANGIN' AVOCADO SALSA

1 avocado

1 tablespoon roughly chopped fresh dill

1 tablespoon roughly chopped fresh tarragon leaves

1 tablespoon roughly chopped fresh chives

Zest of 1 medium lemon

3 tablespoons freshly squeezed lemon juice

1 to 2 tablespoons olive oil

1 ounce feta cheese, crumbled

¼ cup toasted walnuts, chopped

Salt and freshly ground black pepper

Finely chopped fresh chiles or crushed red pepper flakes (optional)

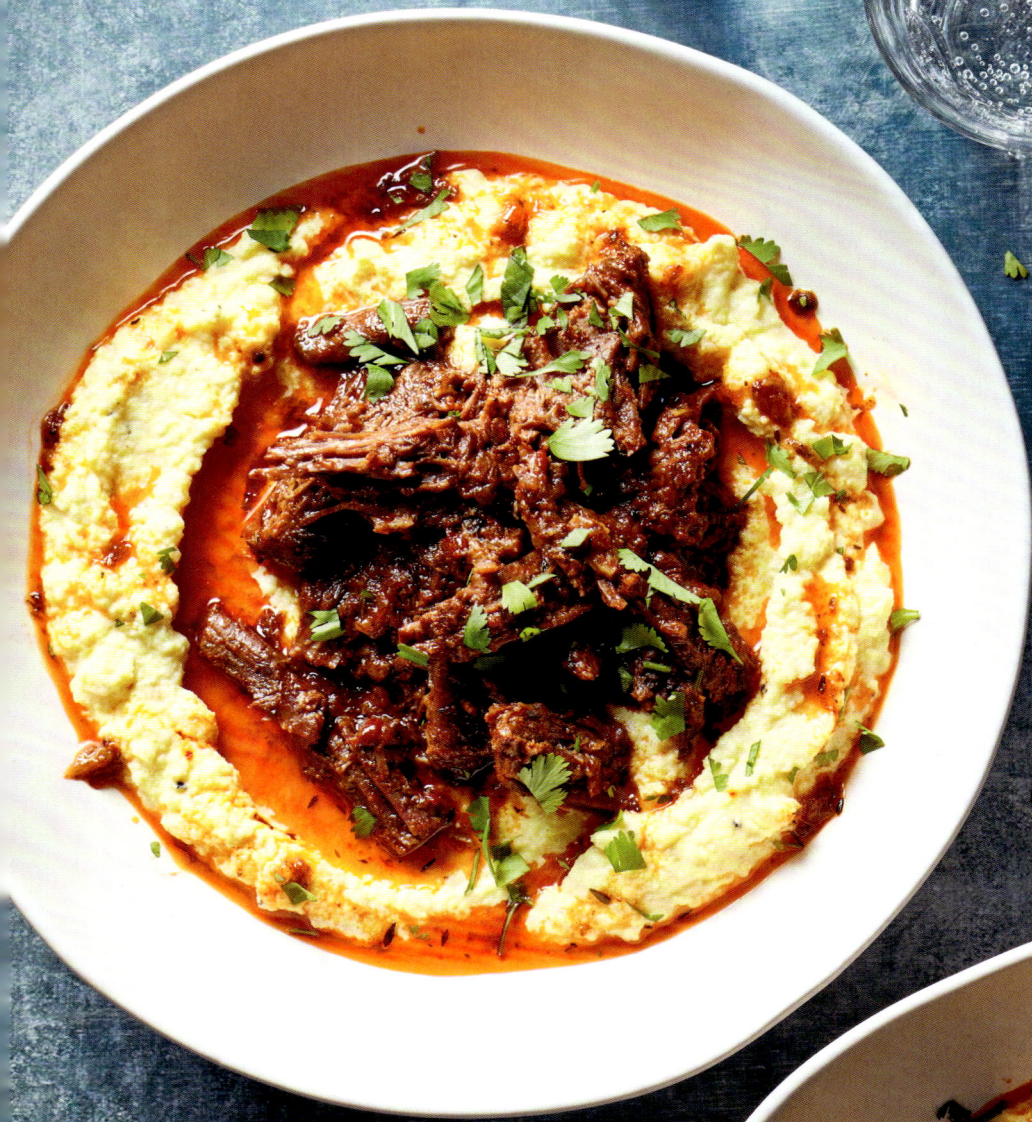

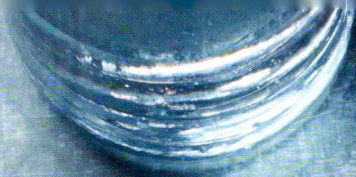

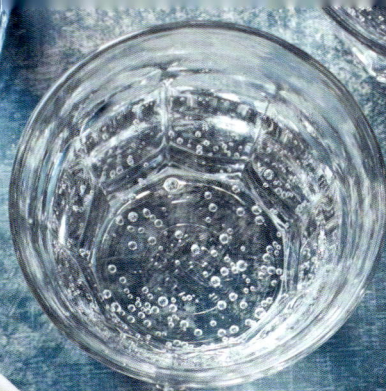

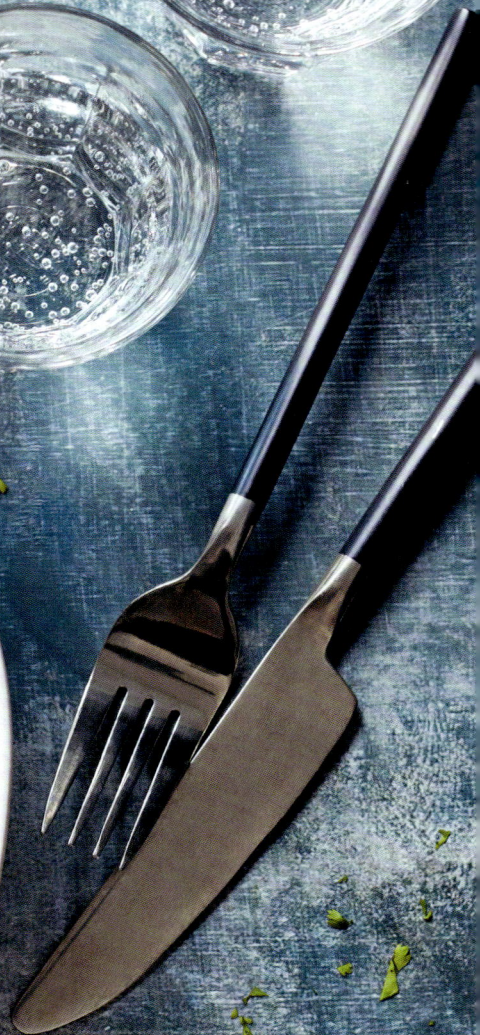

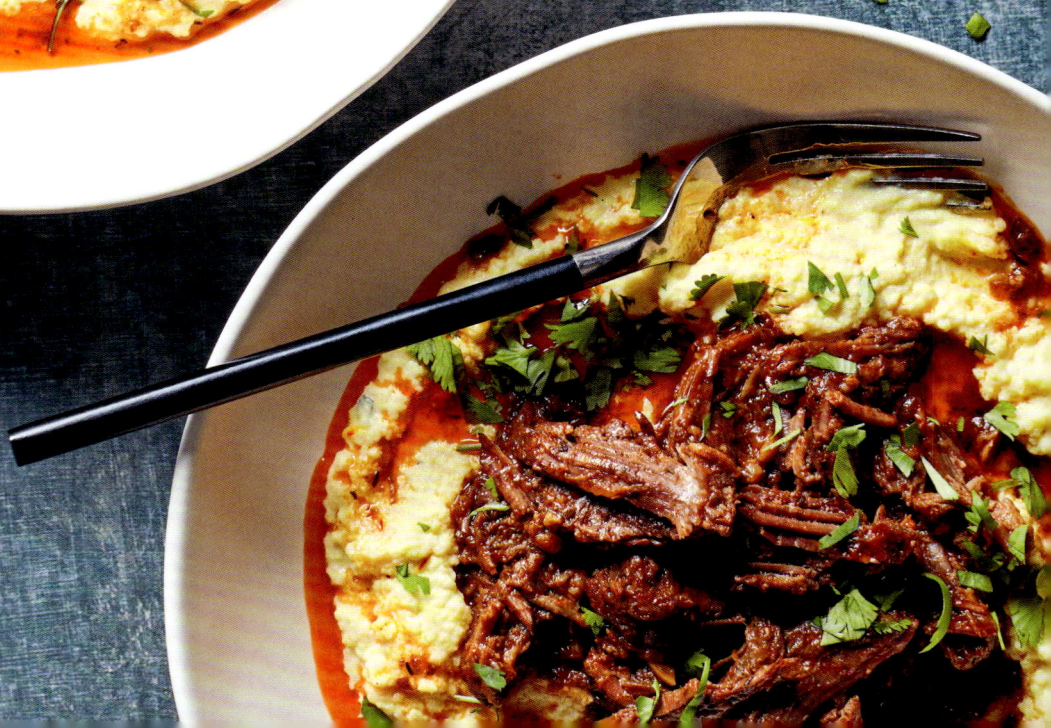

Barbacoa Chuck Roast

OVER SAFFRON CAULIFLOWER MASH

Nothing goes together quite like meat and potatoes. But eating low-carb doesn't mean the days of enjoying those amazing flavors are over. With this barbacoa chuck roast over saffron cauliflower mash, you can still indulge in this classic comfort food combo, without all the carbs. The cauliflower comes out super creamy, and the saffron adds a depth of flavor that takes this dish to the next level. Top the mash with the chuck roast and a drizzle of a delicious tomato adobo sauce to reap all the rewards of this low-carb, high-flavor meal.

1. Preheat the oven to 350°F.

2. **For the chuck roast rub:** In a small bowl, combine the smoked paprika, onion powder, cumin, thyme, and salt and pepper to taste and mix.

3. Using two-thirds of the rub, thoroughly season all sides of the chuck roast.

4. Heat 1 tablespoon of the olive oil in a large cast-iron or stainless-steel pan over medium-high heat. Add the beef and sear for about 2 minutes on each side, until the meat browns.

5. Set the beef in a deep oven-safe dish with a lid.

6. In the same pan used to sear the beef, combine the onion, garlic, and remaining 1 tablespoon of olive oil. Sauté until the onion turns golden. Add the chipotles in adobo and tomato paste and continue to sauté for another 1 to 2 minutes.

7. Add the beef broth and stir to fully dissolve the tomato paste. Bring the sauce to a boil and then remove from the heat. (Optional: For a smooth texture, blend the sauce with an immersion blender or, after cooling, a food processor.)

8. Pour the mixture over the meat. The roast should be submerged at least halfway. Cover the dish with the lid and roast the beef in the oven for 2 hours first. At the 2-hour mark, add the white wine (if using). Cover again to continue cooking for another 30 minutes. At the 2½-hour mark, remove from the oven and lightly break the meat into smaller chunks or shreds with a fork. With the lid back on, return the pot to the oven for another 20 to 30 minutes. In total, the meat should cook for about 3 hours for a 2-pound roast—aim for about 1½ hours per pound, depending on how large your chuck roast is.

PREP TIME: 30 MINUTES
COOK TIME: 3 HOURS
SERVINGS: 6 TO 8

FOR THE CHUCK ROAST RUB

1 tablespoon smoked paprika (or chipotle powder for extra heat)

1 tablespoon onion powder

1 tablespoon ground cumin

2 tablespoons dried thyme

Salt and freshly ground black pepper

2-pound beef chuck roast

2 tablespoons olive oil

1 medium yellow onion, minced

8 garlic cloves, minced

2 chipotle peppers in adobo sauce, chopped

2 tablespoons tomato paste

2 cups beef broth

⅓ cup white wine (optional)

FOR THE SAFFRON CAULIFLOWER MASH

2 pounds cauliflower florets

1 ounce unsalted butter in ½-inch cubes

Pinch of saffron threads

3 tablespoons heavy cream

Salt and freshly ground black pepper

1 tablespoon chopped fresh cilantro, for garnish

(recipe continues)

9. **For the saffron cauliflower mash:** While the meat is cooking, bring a large pot of salted water to a boil and cook the cauliflower florets until they are soft but not mushy, about 20 minutes.

10. Remove from the water and allow to drain for 5 minutes.

11. In a medium bowl, mash the florets into a paste with a potato masher or immersion blender. Add the butter cubes and whisk the paste until the cubes melt.

12. Add the saffron and heavy cream gradually while continuing to whisk. Whisk for a couple of minutes more, until the saffron is fully incorporated into the mash. Add salt and pepper to taste.

13. Transfer the cauliflower mash to a serving platter, then set the chuck roast chunks on top and pour a few tablespoons of the sauce on top.

14. Garnish with the cilantro and serve right away.

Miso-Marinated Chilean Sea Bass

Melt-in-your-mouth good, this miso-marinated sea bass is a dream in each bite. The key here is the miso marinade. It's a combination of cooked sake, mirin, and miso paste, with monk fruit sweetener to add just the right amount of sweet. It's a beautiful Japanese-inspired dish. The marinating process takes two to three days, but once the fish has absorbed all the flavorful goodness, the cooking process is super quick and easy. All that's left to do is make your tasty caramelized bok choy, add an optional side like my Kaizen low-carb high-protein rice, and you're golden.

PREP TIME: 40 MINUTES, PLUS 2 TO 3 DAYS MARINATING
COOK TIME: 20 MINUTES
SERVINGS: 3 OR 4

FOR THE MARINADE

⅓ cup sake

⅓ cup mirin

⅓ cup white miso paste

¼ cup monk fruit sweetener or sugar

1 pound sea bass fillets, cut into 4-ounce pieces

2 tablespoons avocado oil

2 heads bok choy, cut in quarters

FOR THE SEASONED RICE (OPTIONAL)

8 ounces Kaizen rice or regular short grain rice

¼ cup rice vinegar

1 tablespoon monk fruit sweetener or regular sugar

1. **For the marinade:** Set a medium saucepan over high heat, add the sake and mirin, and bring to a boil. Boil for 20 seconds to evaporate the alcohol. Reduce the heat to medium and whisk in the miso. When the miso has dissolved completely, increase the heat to high again and add the monk fruit sweetener, whisking constantly to ensure that the sugar doesn't burn on the bottom of the pan. Remove the pan from the heat once the sweetener is fully dissolved. Cool to room temperature.

2. With a paper towel, pat the sea bass fillets dry. In a ceramic or glass dish, add the fillets and cover with three-quarters of the miso glaze. Refrigerate the rest and save to use for the bok choy later. Cover the sea bass with a plastic wrap or a lid and leave it to marinate in the refrigerator for 2 to 3 days.

3. Once the fillets are marinated, you can cook them in the air fryer or the oven. First, drain off any excess miso marinade, but don't rinse.

4. **To cook in the air fryer:** Preheat the air fryer to 400°F. Brush the sea bass with 1 tablespoon avocado oil and cook in the air fryer for 12 to 14 minutes, until the fish has a blackened crust and is opaque and flakes easily.

5. **To cook in the oven:** Preheat the oven to 400°F. Set an oven-safe skillet over medium heat. Film the pan with 1 tablespoon avocado oil, then place the fish skin-side up in the pan and cook until the bottom of the fish blackens, about 2 minutes. Flip and cook the skin side for another 2 minutes, until brown. Set the skillet in the oven and bake for 10 to 15 minutes, until the fish is opaque and flakes easily.

(recipe continues)

6. Heat the remaining 1 tablespoon avocado oil in a skillet over medium-high heat. Once the oil is hot, toss in the bok choy quarters and sauté for 2 to 3 minutes on each side, until the bok choy browns. Add the remaining miso marinade and cook for another 4 to 5 minutes, until the bok choy softens but is still crunchy and caramelized on the side.

7. Once the sea bass is cooked, set on a plate together with the bok choy.

8. **For the seasoned rice (optional):** Cook the rice per the instructions on the packaging. Combine the rice vinegar and monk fruit sweetener and drizzle over the rice. Gently fold the rice—by lifting and folding it on top of itself, rather than stirring and smooshing the rice—until the vinegar is evenly mixed in. Serve with the sea bass and bok choy.

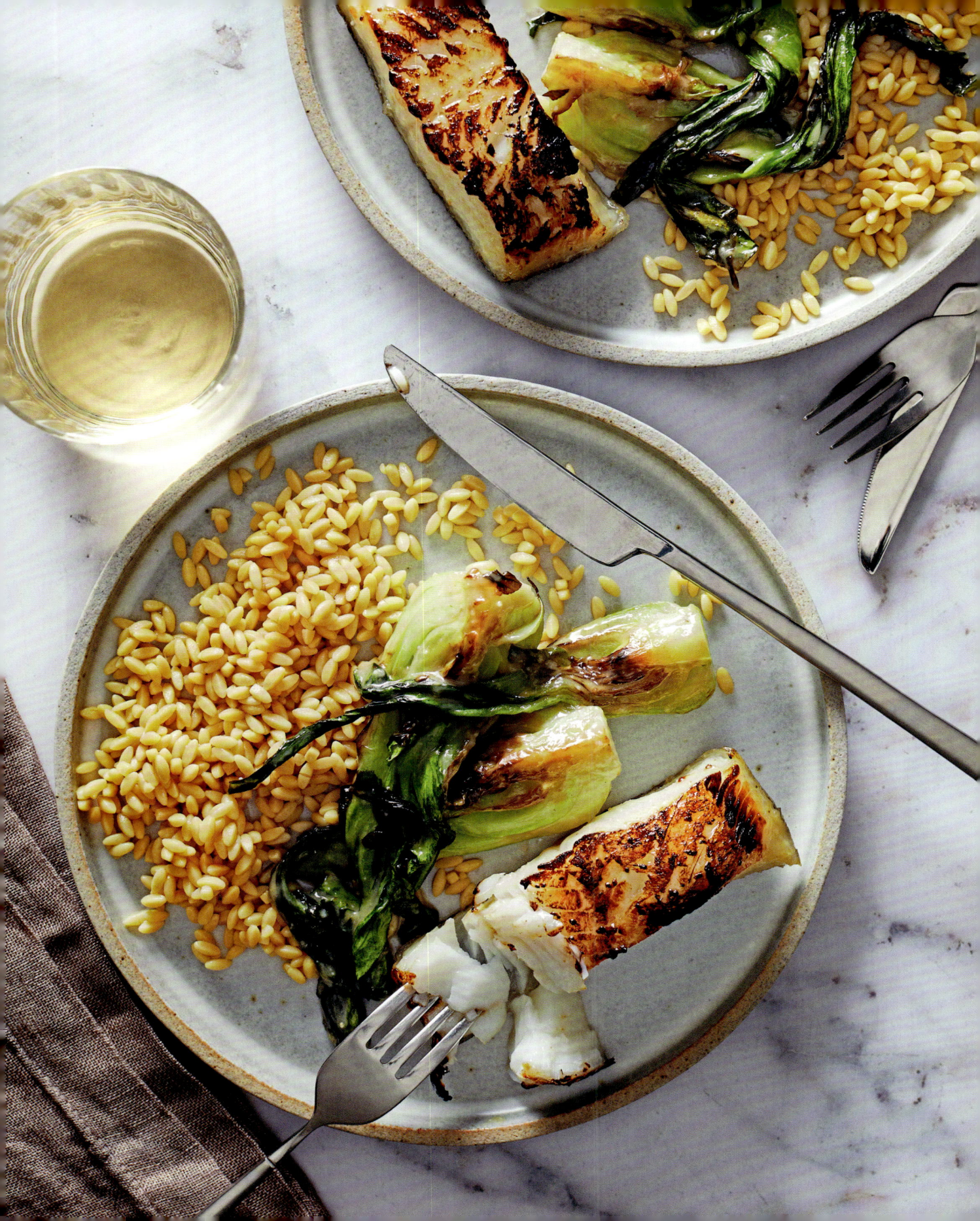

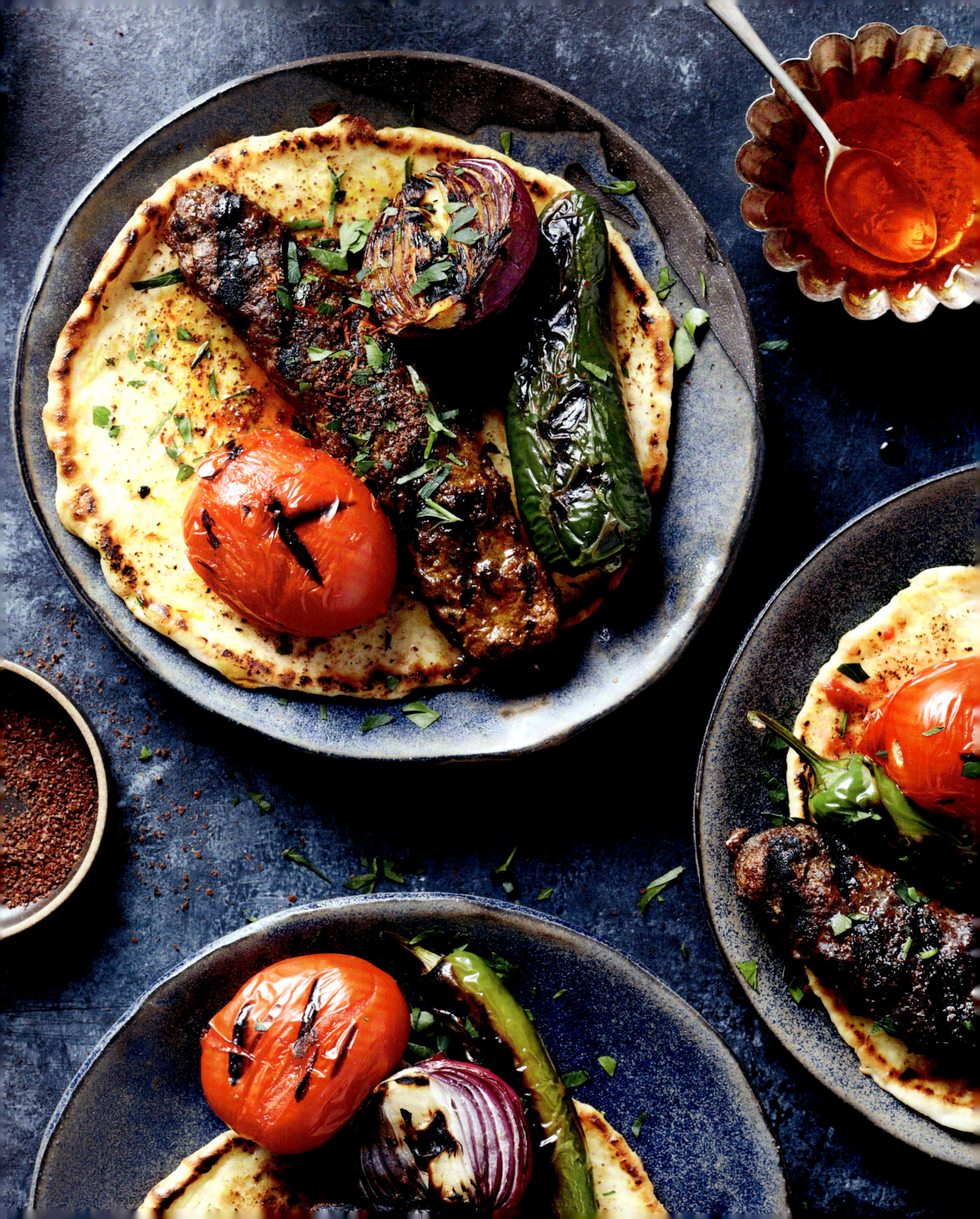

Persian Kabob Koobideh

Alright, it's not easy picking favorites, but you've made it to my absolute favorite meal. This is a Persian classic, and it tastes best grilled to a nice char over charcoal. The beef is flavored with onion and spices, grilled with lots of love and care, and served with a delicious topping of bloomed saffron water and butter. It takes a bit of effort, but it's worth it. This book truly wouldn't be complete without this recipe. If there is one dish to order when dining at any Persian restaurant, this would be it.

Koobideh is barbecued on wide, flat skewers (22 inches long and ¾ inch wide) that are meant to rest on the bowl of the grill so the meat is directly over the fire and won't stick to the grill grates. You can find these at any Middle Eastern store or online by searching for "Persian kabob skewers."

1. In a large food processor, blend the onions until pureed. Transfer to a strainer and let sit for 3 to 4 minutes to drain out the excess liquid.

2. Add just the drained onion pulp back to the food processor with the ground beef, turmeric, garlic powder, sumac, and salt and pepper to taste. Pulse until everything is blended.

3. Transfer the meat mixture into a bowl and knead it a few more times with your hands. Cover and refrigerate for at least 2 hours. The meat will firm up slightly, which is critical for grilling.

4. While the meat is resting in the fridge, bloom the saffron by mixing it with 4 tablespoons hot water. Stir, let it sit, and stir again in about 5 minutes. Set this aside.

5. **For the optional grilled veggies:** Cut the tomatoes and onions in half and place them on skewers along with the jalapeños.

6. Remove the grates from the grill and start the fire about 20 minutes before cooking. The grill is ready when the charcoal is evenly glowing and partially ash-covered. Preheating is essential for the kabobs to grill properly.

7. Before you assemble the kabobs and vegetables for grilling, prepare the rice (if using) per the instructions on the packaging.

8. Remove the meat from the fridge and divide into 4½-ounce balls. This will make 8 to 9 skewers.

PREP TIME: 30 MINUTES, PLUS 2 HOURS CHILLING
COOK TIME: 15 MINUTES
SERVINGS: 4 TO 8

2 medium yellow onions

2 pounds 80/20 ground beef

1 teaspoon ground turmeric

1 teaspoon garlic powder

2 teaspoons sumac

Salt and freshly ground black pepper

¼ teaspoon saffron threads

FOR THE GRILLED VEGGIES (OPTIONAL)

6 medium tomatoes

3 medium red onions

2 jalapeño peppers

FOR THE RICE (OPTIONAL)

8 ounces basmati rice (or Kaizen rice)

5 low-carb pitas or other flatbreads

2 tablespoons unsalted butter, sliced

OPTIONAL GARNISHES

1 to 2 tablespoons sumac

Fresh herbs such as lemon basil, mint, tarragon, or flat-leaf parsley

(recipe continues)

9. Place one portion of meat onto each skewer, using your fingers to evenly distribute the meat along the middle of the skewer, shaping it into a kabob 7 to 8 inches long and ½ inch thick on each side of the skewer. Use your fingers to press small indentations at bite-sized intervals for the classic koobideh look.

10. Place the skewers across a rimmed baking sheet as they are assembled, so the meat doesn't touch the surface and fall apart.

11. **For the grilled veggies (optional):** Grill the vegetable skewers for 6 to 8 minutes, rotating between sides every 2 to 3 minutes.

12. Grill the kabobs for 3 to 3½ minutes, flipping them every 10 to 15 seconds to prevent the meat from falling off.

13. Layer the bottom of a large serving dish with a couple of the low-carb pita breads. Remove the grilled kabobs from the grill one by one, and, using another piece of bread, loosen the kabob meat from the skewer and transfer onto the pita bread. Keep the dish covered using the remaining pita breads.

14. Once all kabobs are grilled, drizzle with the bloomed saffron water. Add the butter slices and let them melt onto the finished kabobs. The juice from the cooked meat, saffron, and melted butter will infuse the bread, making it the perfect side once the kabob is ready to serve.

15. This dish is traditionally served with basmati rice (optional) along with the grilled veggies, fresh herbs, and sumac.

Green Herb–Crusted Salmon

This herb-crusted salmon is inspired by the Persian dish *hashoo*. It's one of my all-time favorite recipes my mom made for us growing up. The sweet and sour flavors of the tamarind paste and the burst of freshness from the cilantro are what truly make this dish unforgettable. This gets sautéed with other tasty additions like red onion, garlic, ginger, tomato paste, turmeric, and curry powder to create a heavenly combination of flavors. From there, all that's left to do is spread it over the salmon and bake until a beautiful crust forms on top. It's simple, elegant, and delicious—the perfect dish for any occasion! PHOTO ON PAGES 138–139

PREP TIME: 20 MINUTES
COOK TIME: 30 MINUTES
SERVINGS: 6 TO 8

4 tablespoons olive oil

1 large red onion, minced

Salt

1 teaspoon ground turmeric

8 garlic cloves, minced

1 tablespoon freshly grated ginger

1 tablespoon tomato paste

1 tablespoon curry powder

4 cups fresh cilantro (about 3 large bunches), finely chopped

1 tablespoon dried fenugreek leaves (optional)

½ tablespoon crushed red pepper flakes (optional)

3 tablespoons tamarind paste

2-pound wild salmon fillet

1. Preheat the oven to 400°F.

2. Heat 3 tablespoons of the olive oil in a skillet over medium heat. Add the red onion and sauté until translucent. Add 2 to 3 generous pinches of salt and the turmeric and mix.

3. Add the garlic, ginger, tomato paste, and curry powder. Mix well.

4. Add the cilantro and, if using, the fenugreek and red pepper flakes and continuously stir over medium heat until the water from the cilantro evaporates, 4 to 5 minutes.

5. Add the tamarind paste and mix again. Set aside.

6. Pat the salmon dry, season it with a generous pinch of salt, and make three small slits across the top of the fillet.

7. Top the salmon with a ¼-inch layer of the cooked cilantro mixture and drizzle with the remaining 1 tablespoon of olive oil.

8. Pop into the oven for 15 to 18 minutes, until the herb crust is brown and the salmon is evenly pink on the inside.

9. Plate the salmon and serve with your favorite base. I like it with a cauliflower mash, like the one with my Barbacoa Chuck Roast (page 129), but without the saffron, and Gem Lettuce Salad with Quick-Pickled Shallots (page 99).

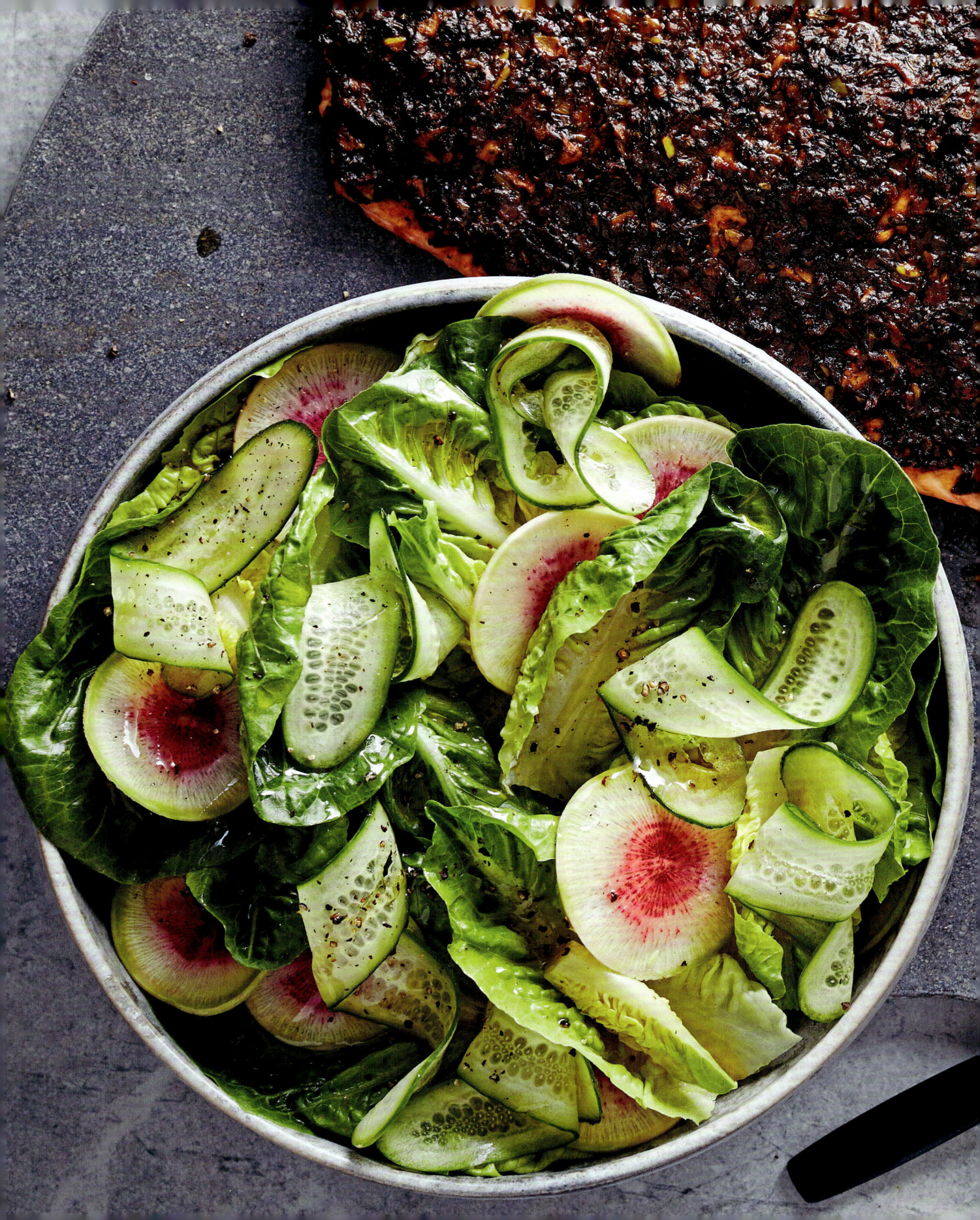

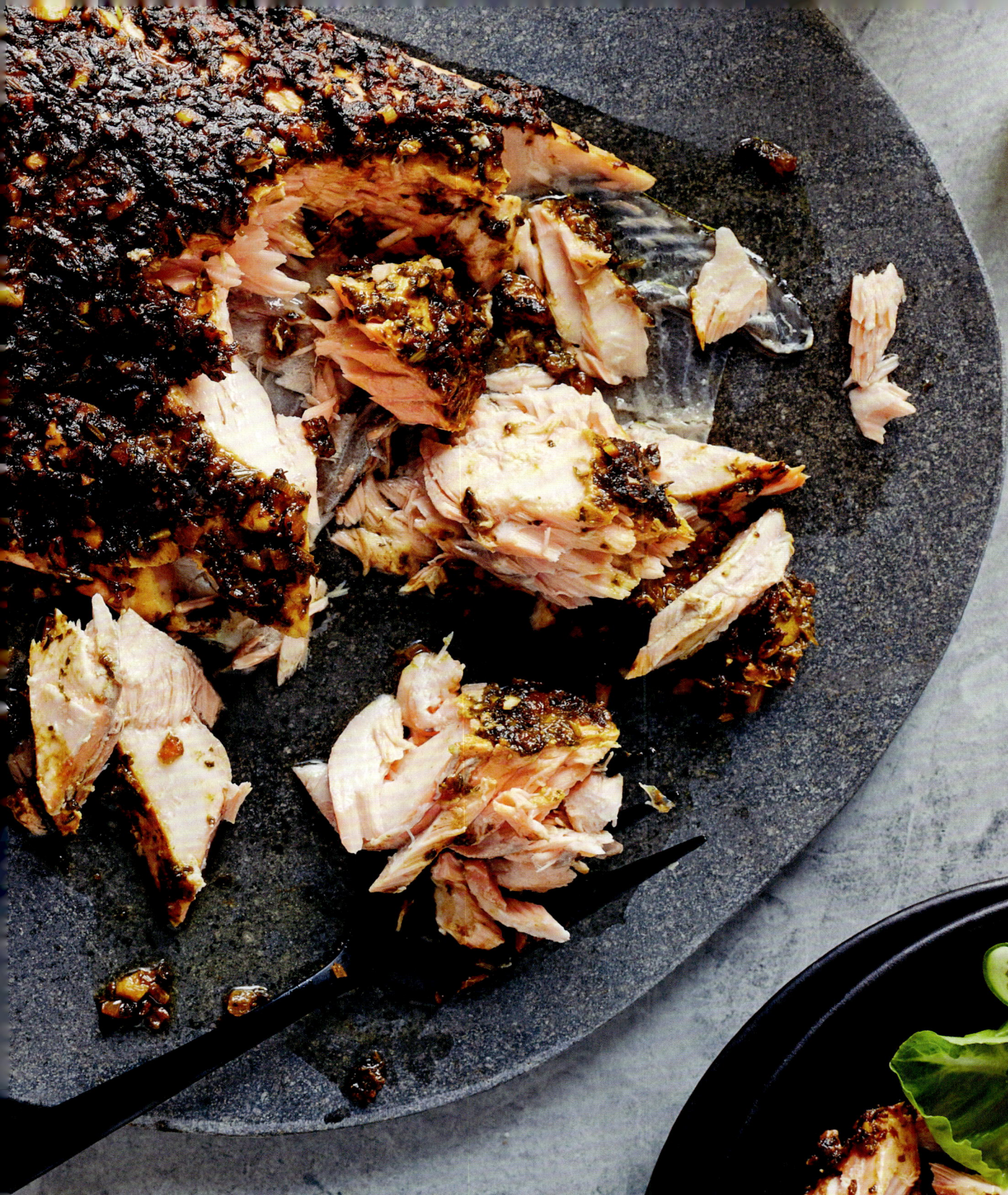

Sun-Dried Tomato Chicken

WITH PISTACHIOS & ARTICHOKES

Pistachio artichoke sun-dried tomato chicken is my personal antidote when I'm bored with the same ol' chicken dishes in my rotation. It's a perfect combination of sweet and savory, with the crunch of pistachios and the tanginess of sun-dried tomatoes. Pistachios are an excellent low-carb alternative to breadcrumbs, and blended with sun-dried tomatoes, marinated artichokes, and other flavorful ingredients, they create a unique spin on a classic dish.

1. In a food processor, combine the artichokes, sun-dried tomatoes, 2 to 3 tablespoons of the olive oil from the sundried tomatoes, pistachios, garlic, lemon juice, white wine vinegar, basil, and a couple of pinches of salt and pepper to taste. Blend well, but keep a slight chunkiness. Set aside.

2. Coat the chicken thighs with the olive oil and season with smoked paprika, baking powder, and salt and pepper. Massage well, ensuring that all the chicken is coated. Let sit for 30 minutes to 2 hours in the refrigerator for optimal flavor. Bring it back to room temperature before cooking.

3. Preheat the oven to 425°F.

4. Place the seasoned chicken thighs into a cast-iron pan. Top each chicken thigh with a big spoonful of the artichoke and sun-dried tomato mixture, spreading it as thin or thick as you'd like.

5. Bake for 35 to 40 minutes.

6. Remove from the oven. Roughly chop the reserved pistachios. Garnish with the pistachios, fresh basil, and red pepper flakes and serve.

PREP TIME: 20 MINUTES, PLUS 30 MINUTES TO 2 HOURS MARINATING
COOK TIME: 40 MINUTES
SERVINGS: 4 TO 6

_____

1 cup artichokes marinated in olive oil

12 to 14 sun-dried tomato halves in olive oil, plus the oil

¾ cup toasted pistachios, plus extra for garnish

2 or 3 garlic cloves

5 to 6 tablespoons freshly squeezed lemon juice

1½ tablespoons white wine vinegar

4 to 5 fresh basil leaves, plus extra for garnish

Salt and freshly ground black pepper

2 pounds bone-in, skin-on chicken thighs

2 tablespoons olive oil

1 tablespoon smoked paprika

1 teaspoon baking powder

Crushed red pepper flakes, for garnish

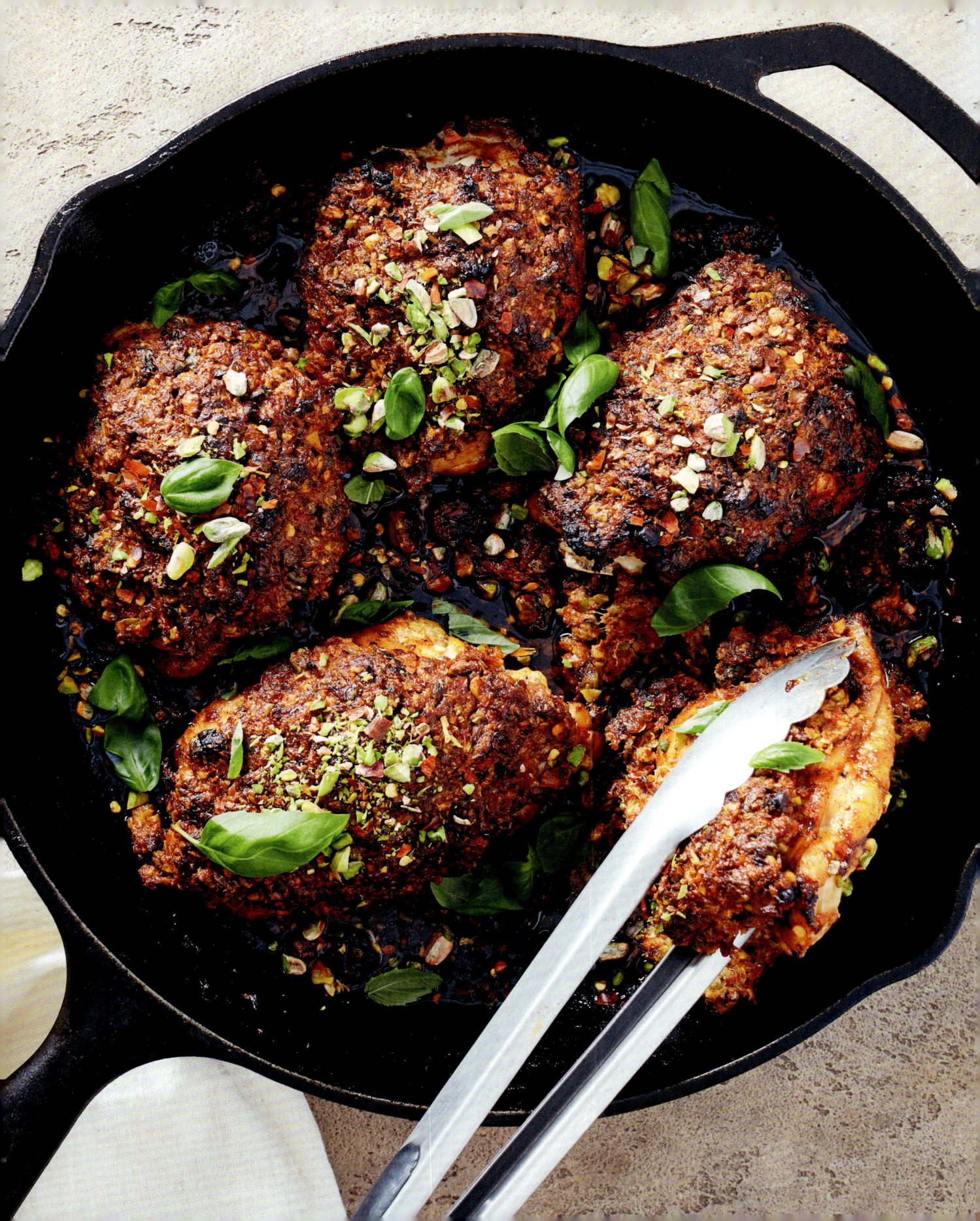

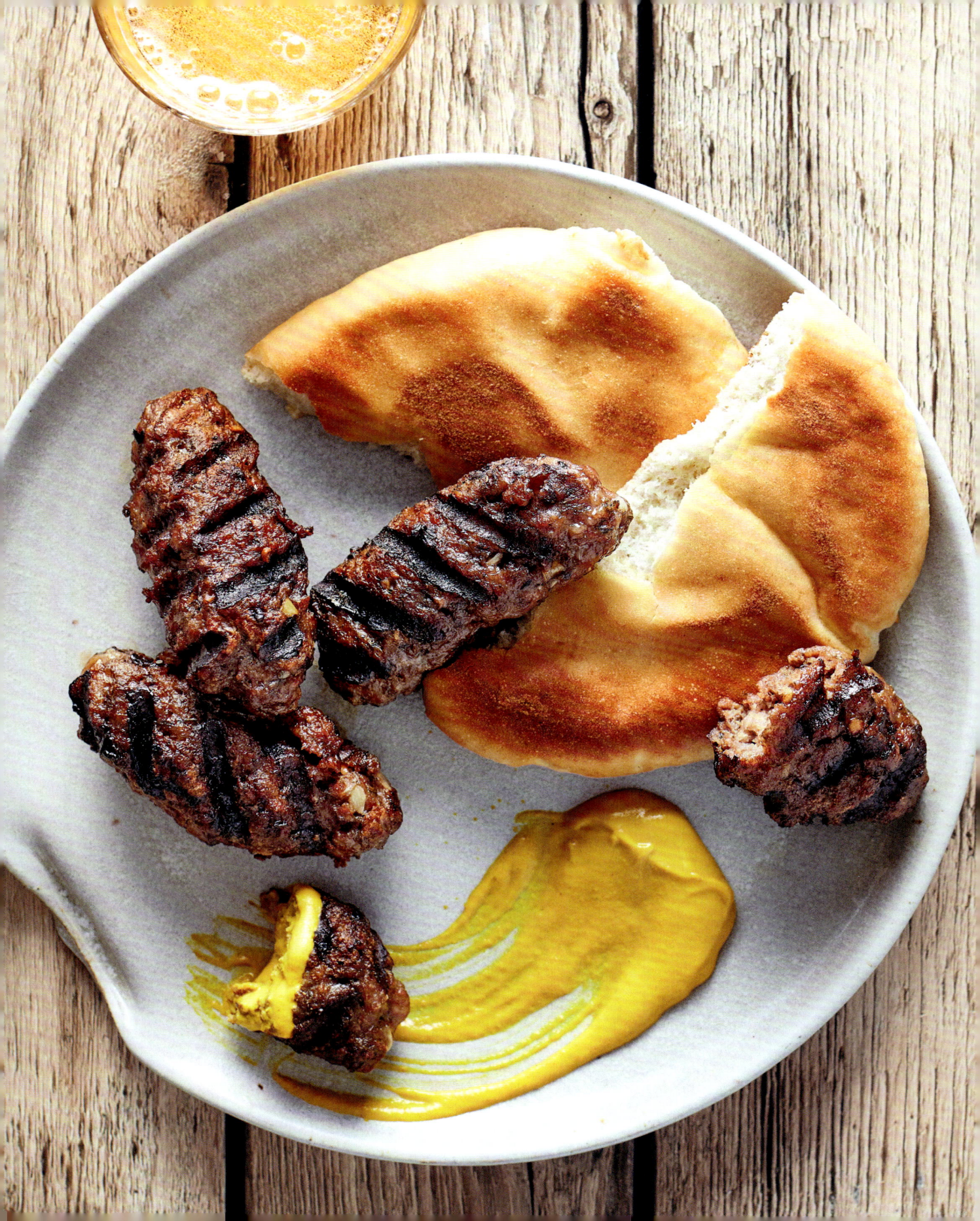

Charcoal Grilled Mici

These incredible (and garlicky!) little bites are called *mici* (pronounced meech) or *mititei* (me-tee-tay), a must have every time I visit Romania! I just had to put my own spin on them. No worries if you don't have a grill. I've got a stovetop version using a cast-iron pan that will do the trick. These flavorful sausages are super simple to make and are perfect dipped in mustard. Once you have them, you'll understand why I always look forward to making the real thing every time we visit Madalina's home country in the summer. These are traditionally eaten with yellow mustard and bread, but use your imagination and serve them up however you want. They are so good, you will probably eat a few straight up without anything!

PREP TIME: 30 MINUTES, PLUS 4 HOURS TO OVERNIGHT MARINATING
COOK TIME: 30 MINUTES
SERVINGS: 6 TO 8

1¼ pounds 80/20 ground beef, or 85/15 or 90/10 if preferred

¾ pound ground lamb

2 tablespoons dried thyme

2 teaspoons baking soda

6 garlic cloves, minced

Salt and freshly ground black pepper

¾ cup bone broth

Neutral cooking oil or grease (optional)

OPTIONAL, FOR SERVING

Yellow mustard

Bread

1. In a large bowl, combine the ground beef, lamb, thyme, baking soda, and garlic. Season with salt and pepper. Give everything a good mix (get those hands in there), add the bone broth, and mix well until the seasonings and liquid are well incorporated.

2. Cover the mixture and let it sit in the fridge for at least 4 hours, or ideally overnight.

3. When you're ready to make the mici, remove the mixture from the fridge and shape the meat into approximately 16 little cylinders about 3½ inches long.

4. Traditionally, mici are grilled on an outdoor charcoal grill for maximum flavor, but you can also do it on a gas grill. If outdoor grilling is not an option, a cast-iron pan on the stovetop will do as well.

5. If using an outdoor grill (gas or charcoal), cook the mici until the meat has been cooked through, using tongs to turn them every 30 to 40 seconds until they have grill marks with a nice crust on all sides.

6. If using a cast-iron pan, set the stove to medium heat. Coat a large cast-iron pan with the cooking oil and cook the mici until the meat has been cooked through, using tongs to turn them until they have a nice crust on all sides.

7. Serve immediately. Don't forget the yellow mustard!

Spicy Walnut Jumbo Scallops

These scallops combine unique, vibrant flavors to create a ridiculously tasty appetizer, lunch, or dinner option. The scallops are topped with a spicy, garlicky, and crunchy sauce made with crushed toasted walnuts, chili garlic crunch (oil infused with garlic and red pepper flakes), and South African smoke seasoning (a blend of dried garlic, onion, basil, and smoked paprika). This dish may taste gourmet, but it's surprisingly easy to make. Serve these scallops on their own, or pair them with a light salad or cauliflower mash for a satisfying meal.

PREP TIME: 30 MINUTES
COOK TIME: 15 MINUTES
SERVINGS: 4 TO 6

1 pound raw wild scallops

⅓ cup raw walnuts

1 tablespoon soy sauce or tamari

½ tablespoon sesame oil

1 tablespoon chili garlic crunch

1 teaspoon crispy fried garlic, homemade (see instructions) or store-bought

½ teaspoon South African smoke seasoning

2 tablespoons avocado oil

Finely chopped fresh chives, for garnish

1. Peel off the side muscle on the scallops and discard, then place the scallops in one layer on top of a paper towel. Cover with another paper towel and gently press down to remove excess moisture. Let sit for 15 to 30 minutes.

2. In a small dry skillet over medium heat, toast the walnuts for 3 to 5 minutes, stirring occasionally. Remove from the stove and let cool.

3. Add the cooled walnuts to a mortar and crush. (You don't want to crush them too finely. Keep the pieces fairly coarse.)

4. **For the crispy fried garlic:** You can find it in stores ready-made, but if you want to make your own, just peel and mince a few garlic cloves and fry them in a medium pan on low heat in a few tablespoons of olive oil or avocado oil until golden brown. It should only take 10 to 15 minutes. Strain and either use right away or store in the fridge for up to a week to use for other dishes.

5. Transfer the crushed walnuts to a mixing bowl and add the soy sauce, sesame oil, chili garlic crunch, crispy fried garlic, and South African smoke seasoning. Mix well. Taste and adjust to your liking.

6. Heat the oil over medium-high heat. Arrange the scallops in the skillet so they are not crowding one another (cook in batches, if needed). Cook for 1½ to 2 minutes, then use tongs to flip once the bottom is golden brown and no longer sticks to the pan.

7. Top each scallop with a small spoonful of the walnut mixture and cook for another 1 to 2 minutes, until the second side is golden brown and no longer sticks.

8. Plate the scallops, garnish with the chives, and serve right away.

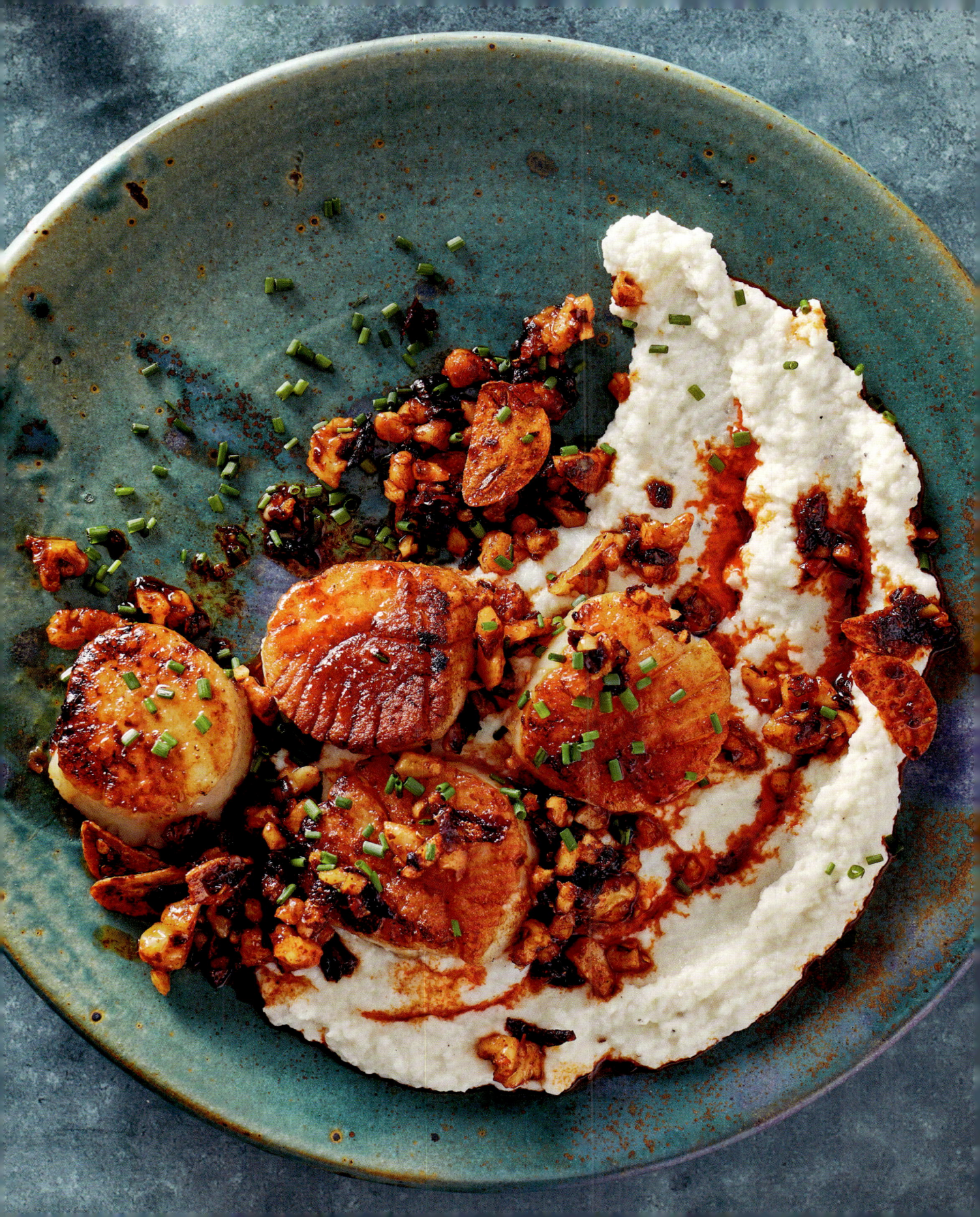

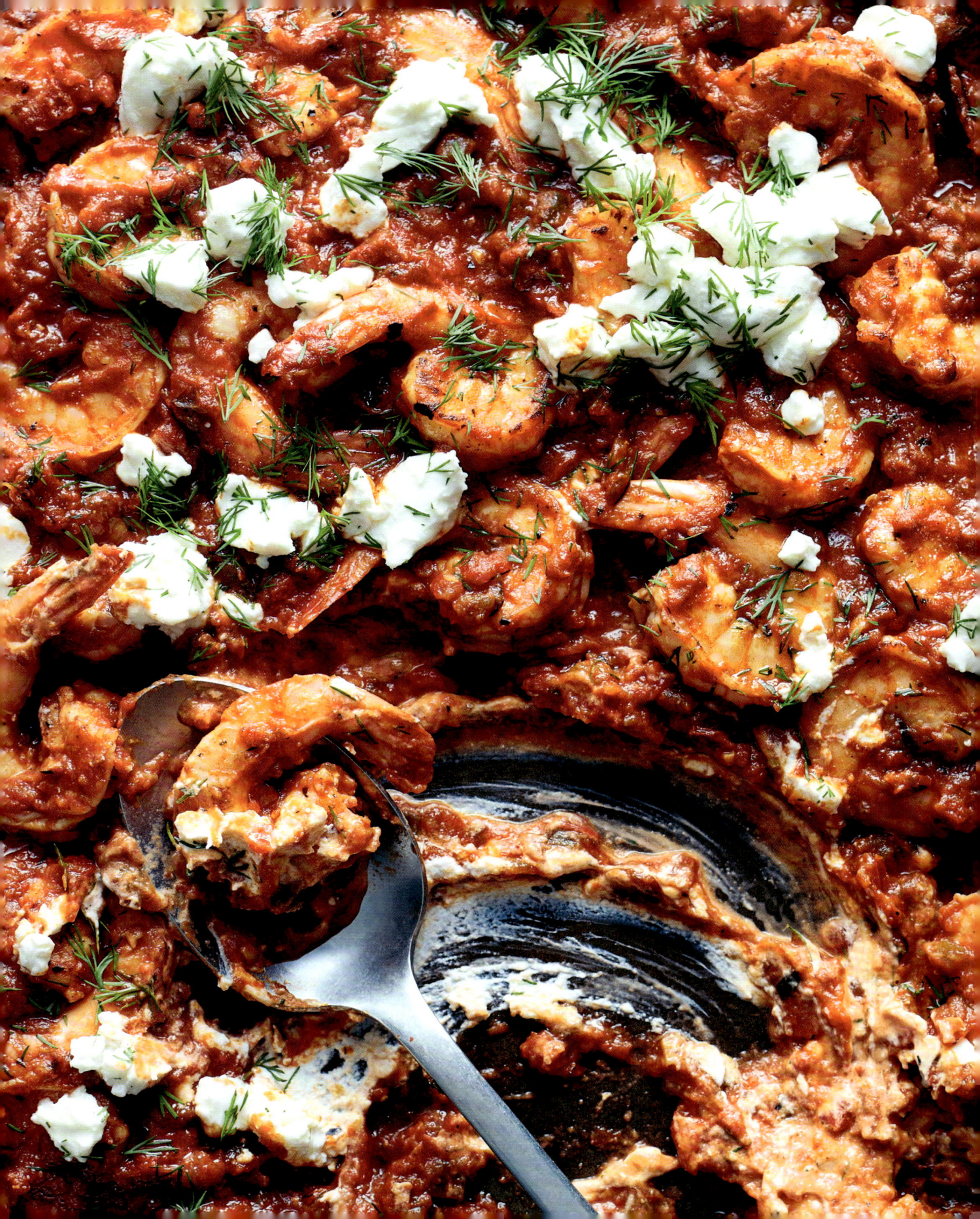

Shrimp Matbucha

WITH GOAT CHEESE

This shrimp matbucha with goat cheese is one of the most incredible ways to serve friends and guests shrimp. It's the combination of spicy matbucha and creamy goat cheese that makes this stand out as something truly special. Matbucha is a spicy Moroccan tomato and pepper dish often featured as a dip or condiment, but it works wonders here alongside the succulent shrimp and tangy goat cheese. Serve it as an appetizer or light meal for a get-together, and watch it disappear in seconds.

PREP TIME: 40 MINUTES
COOK TIME: 1½ HOURS
SERVINGS: 4 TO 6

1 pound raw shrimp, peeled and deveined

Salt and freshly ground black pepper

1 tablespoon olive oil

4 cups Moroccan Tomato Spread (page 65)

5 ounces goat cheese, crumbled

1 tablespoon chopped fresh dill, for garnish

1. Pat the shrimp dry and season with salt and pepper. Drizzle with the olive oil and mix well.

2. In a large shallow skillet over medium heat, sear the shrimp for 1 minute on each side. The shrimp should have a nice pink sear on each side but should not be fully cooked. Remove from the skillet and set aside.

3. In the same skillet, heat the matbucha. Once the sauce starts to bubble, return the shrimp to the pan and cook for another 2 minutes.

4. Place on a serving platter and sprinkle with the crumbled goat cheese. Garnish with the dill and serve hot.

Za'atar Chicken

If you're looking for something convenient and flavorful, this za'atar chicken is exactly what you need. Made all in one dish, this recipe requires little prep and saves you from washing a bunch of dishes. The chicken thighs are seasoned with a blend of tangy za'atar and sweet and spicy Aleppo pepper to create an aromatic and succulent dish perfect for busy weeknights or hosting guests. To make it even more mouthwatering, serve it with a homemade za'atar dipping oil for the ultimate Mediterranean-inspired meal. You can eat it as is or pair it with a salad or your favorite low-carb base. I like to have it with my Rustic Walnut Tomato Salad (page 92) and my Kaizen low-carb rice.

PREP TIME: 15 MINUTES
COOK TIME: 40 MINUTES
SERVINGS: 4 TO 6

---

3 shallots, thinly sliced

2 pounds bone-in, skin-on chicken thighs

2 tablespoons olive oil

1 tablespoon za'atar, homemade (page 222) or store-bought

½ tablespoon Aleppo pepper

½ tablespoon baking powder

Salt and freshly ground black pepper

FOR THE ZA'ATAR OIL

2 tablespoons olive oil

1 tablespoon za'atar

1 tablespoon toasted sesame seeds, for garnish

1. Preheat the oven to 425°F.

2. Grab an oven-safe dish and place the shallots on the bottom.

3. Pat the chicken thighs dry and drizzle with the olive oil. In a small bowl, combine the za'atar, Aleppo pepper, baking powder, salt and pepper to taste and mix the spices well. Add the spice mixture to the chicken and massage well to ensure that the thighs are coated evenly.

4. Place the chicken thighs over the shallots and bake for 35 to 40 minutes and the chicken is golden and crispy on the outside.

5. **For the za'atar oil:** While the chicken is baking, mix together the olive oil and za'atar and set aside to infuse.

6. Plate the chicken and top with all the juices and caramelized shallots from the bottom of the baking dish. Garnish with the sesame seeds, and serve right away with the za'atar oil for dipping.

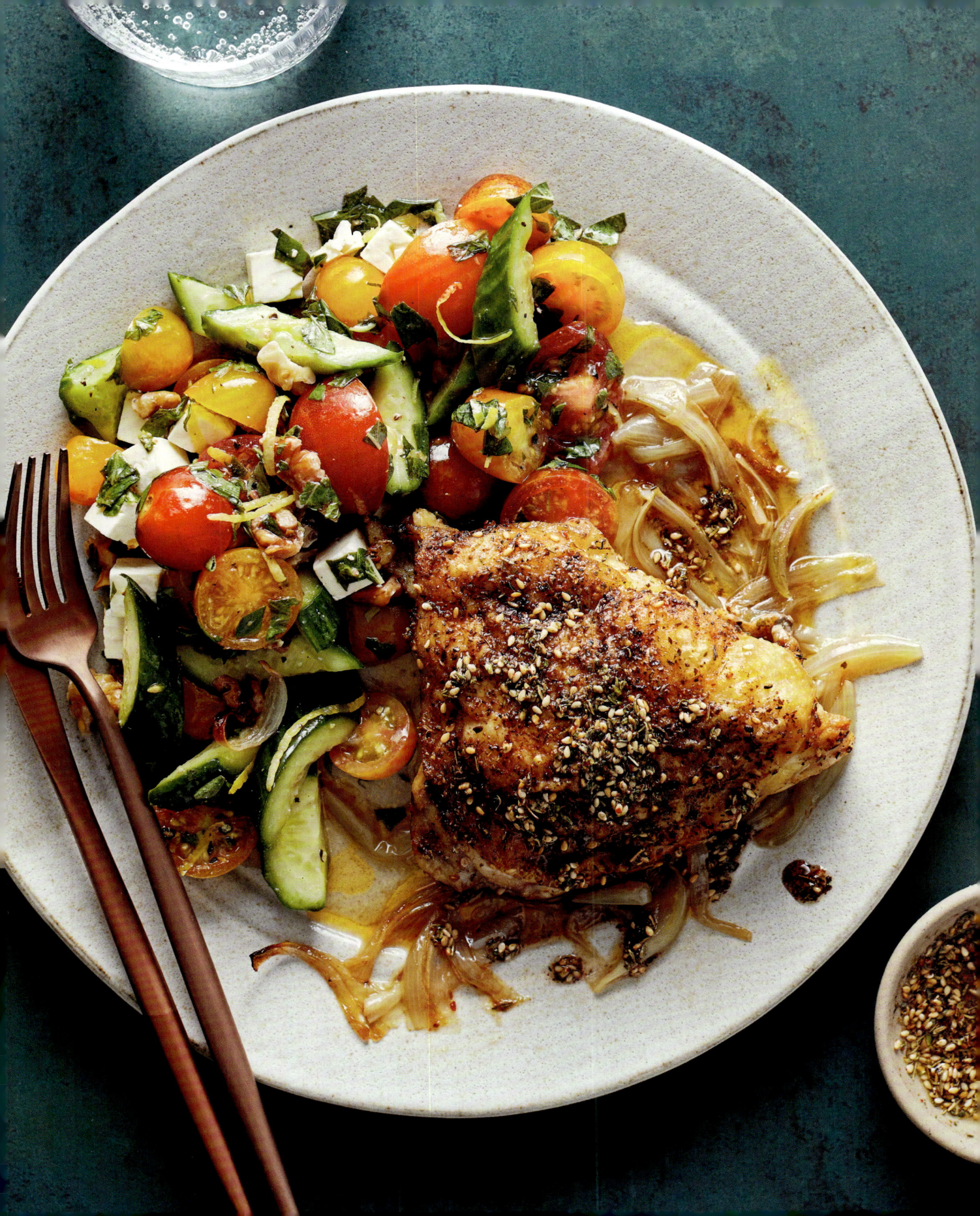

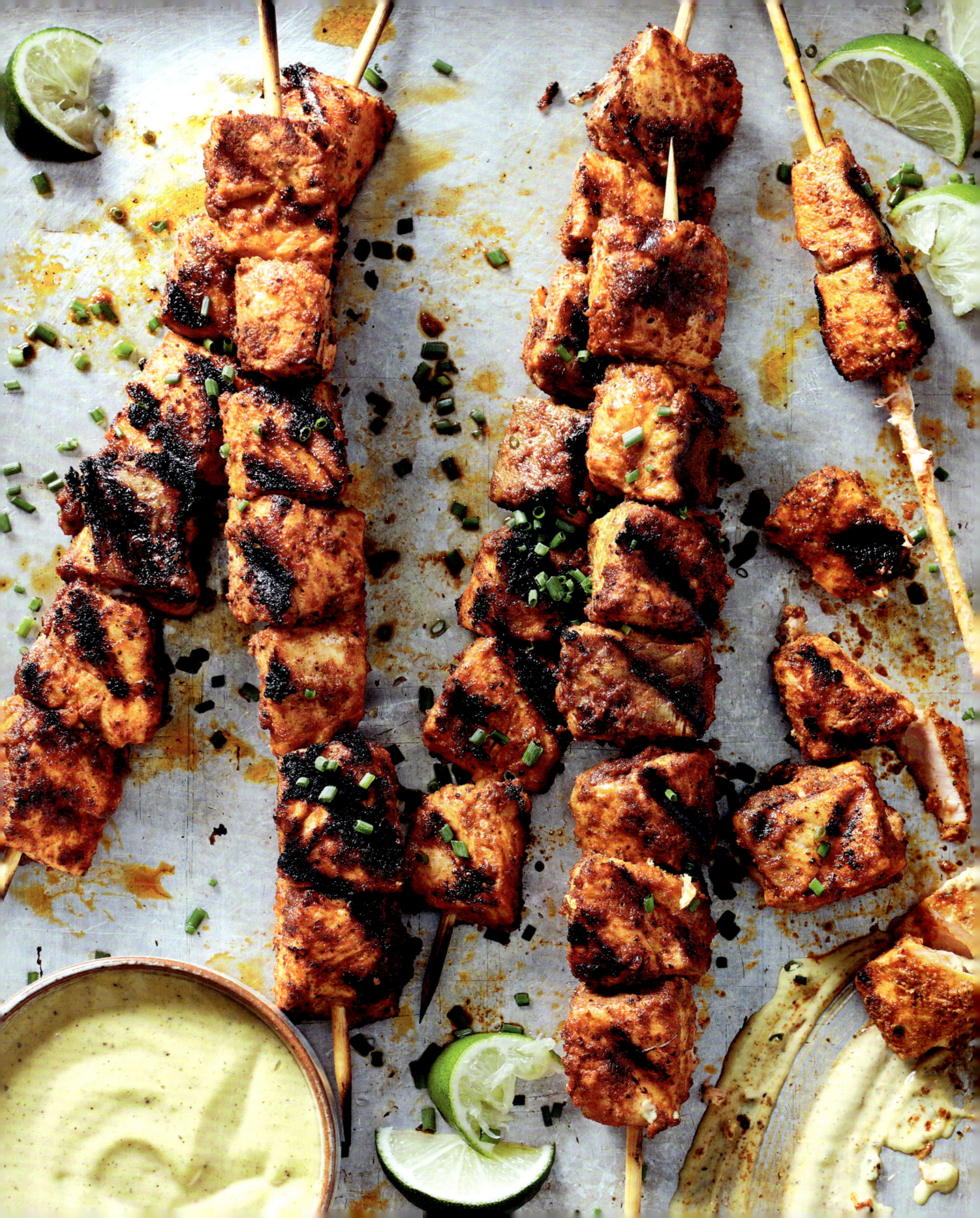

Salmon Skewers

If you need a good addition to your regular grilling routine, this recipe is a treat. These salmon skewers come out perfectly seasoned and bursting with flavor. The key here is the marinade, which consists of simple ingredients that pack a punch, like lemon juice, sumac, Aleppo pepper, turmeric, and more. Just let it marinate for at least 30 minutes before grilling outside or cooking it up on the stove. Whichever method you choose, I've got you covered! Serve with roasted veggies and/or my super tasty Homemade Lime Aioli (page 206) for dipping.

PREP TIME: 15 MINUTES, PLUS 30 MINUTES TO 1 HOUR MARINATING
COOK TIME: 20 MINUTES
SERVINGS: 4 TO 6

———

1 pound skinless wild salmon fillet

2 tablespoons freshly squeezed lemon juice

3 garlic cloves, minced

2 teaspoons sweet paprika

1 teaspoon onion powder

1 teaspoon sumac

2 tablespoons olive oil

½ teaspoon Aleppo pepper or crushed red pepper flakes

⅛ teaspoon ground turmeric

Salt and freshly ground black pepper

1 tablespoon finely chopped fresh chives, for garnish

1. Cut the salmon into 1-inch cubes and set aside.

2. In a medium bowl, combine the lemon juice, garlic, paprika, onion powder, sumac, 2 teaspoons of the olive oil, the Aleppo pepper, turmeric, and salt and pepper to taste. Give it a good mix.

3. Add the salmon cubes and fold them into the marinade until all sides are evenly coated. Let marinate for 30 minutes to 1 hour at room temperature.

4. Place the cubes on wooden skewers. Make sure to measure the skewers first to ensure that they fit on your grill or in your stovetop pan.

5. **If cooking on an outdoor grill:** Grease the grill with the remaining olive oil well to prevent the skewers from sticking, or use a nonstick grill grid. Place the skewers over medium heat and cook for 3 to 4 minutes on each side, until the fish is opaque and flaky.

6. **If cooking on the stove:** Grab a cast-iron grill pan (or a regular pan, if you don't have a grill pan) and set it over medium heat. Coat the pan with the remaining olive oil. (Use a cooking brush to help ensure that the pan is completely coated.) Once the pan is hot, add the skewers and cook for 2 to 3 minutes on each side, until the fish is opaque and flaky.

7. Place on a serving plate and garnish with the chopped chives, and serve.

Tamarind Chicken

Tamarind is a nutrient-rich fruit native to Africa, but it can now be found in many tropical regions around the world. It has a special sweet and tangy taste that I just had to incorporate into a chicken dish! Making this is super easy: Just pop your marinade ingredients in a food processor, marinate your chicken, and cook in a cast-iron skillet until gorgeously seared and juicy. It'll taste great with anything from rice to quinoa or even as a filling for tacos or burritos.

1. **For the tamarind marinade:** In a food processor, combine the tamarind paste, olive oil, chipotle powder, garlic, onion, cilantro, and salt and pepper to taste and blend into a smooth paste.

2. Place the chicken thighs in a medium bowl and pour in the marinade, thoroughly massaging it into the chicken. Marinate in the fridge for at least a couple of hours, ideally overnight.

3. Preheat the oven to 350°F.

4. In a cast-iron skillet, heat the olive oil over medium-high heat. Remove the chicken thighs from the marinade, letting most of the sauce drip off, and add them to the hot skillet. Sear for 3 to 4 minutes on each side.

5. Move the skillet to the oven to finish cooking the chicken, another 10 to 15 minutes, depending on the thickness of the thighs. The chicken is done when it is no longer pink in the center and the juices run clear when pierced with a fork.

6. Serve right away, with additional cilantro if you like. I served these as tacos over tortillas with a touch of sour cream, pickled red onion, fresh cilantro, and more sliced red chile.

PREP TIME: 15 MINUTES, PLUS 2 HOURS TO OVERNIGHT MARINATING
COOK TIME: 20 MINUTES
SERVINGS: 3 TO 5

FOR THE TAMARIND MARINADE

1½ tablespoons tamarind paste

2 tablespoons olive oil

2 teaspoons chipotle powder

4 garlic cloves

½ medium onion, coarsely chopped

½ bunch fresh cilantro, plus more for garnish (optional)

Salt and freshly ground black pepper

1½ pounds boneless, skinless chicken thighs

1 tablespoon olive oil

1 to 2 red chiles, finely sliced (optional)

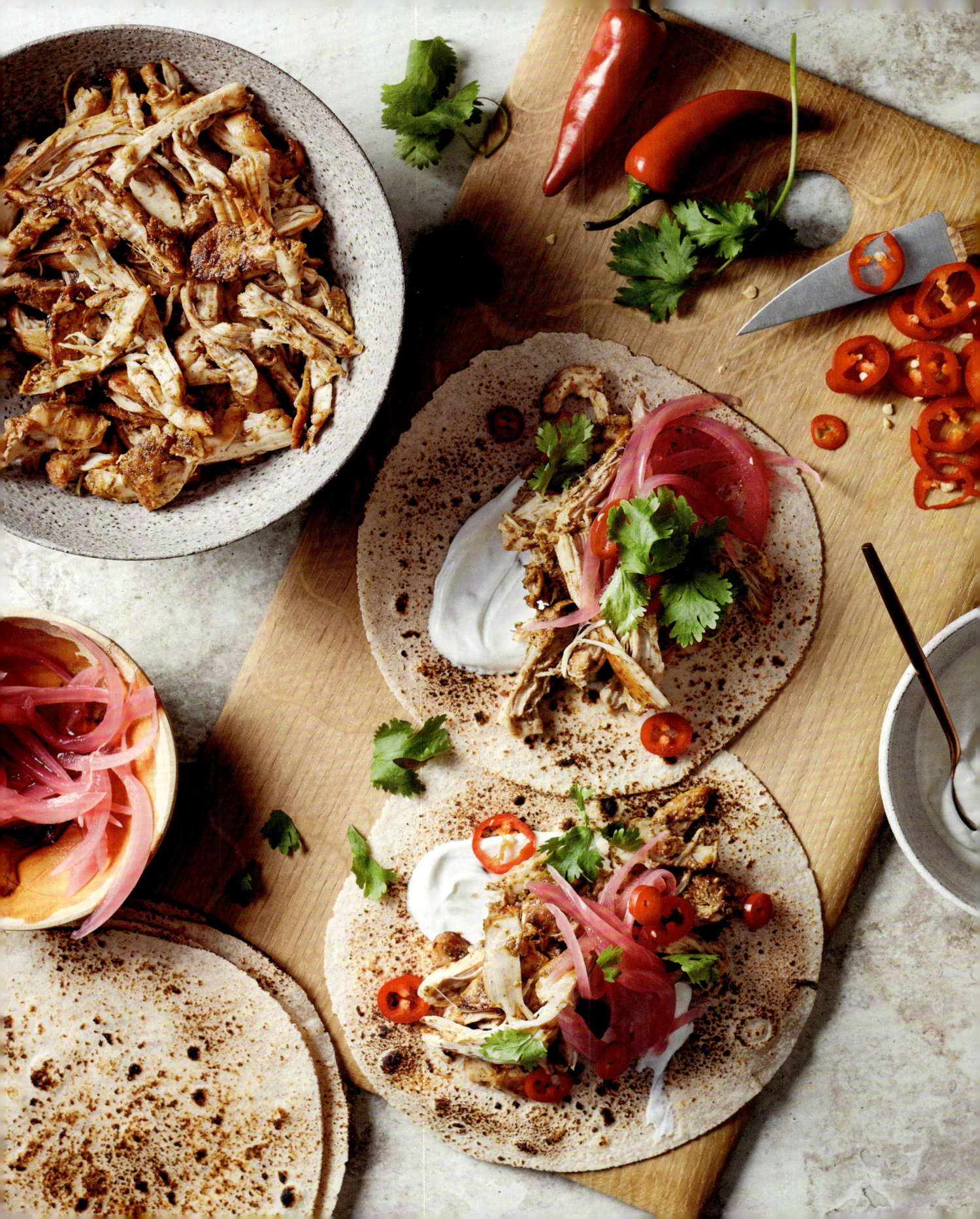

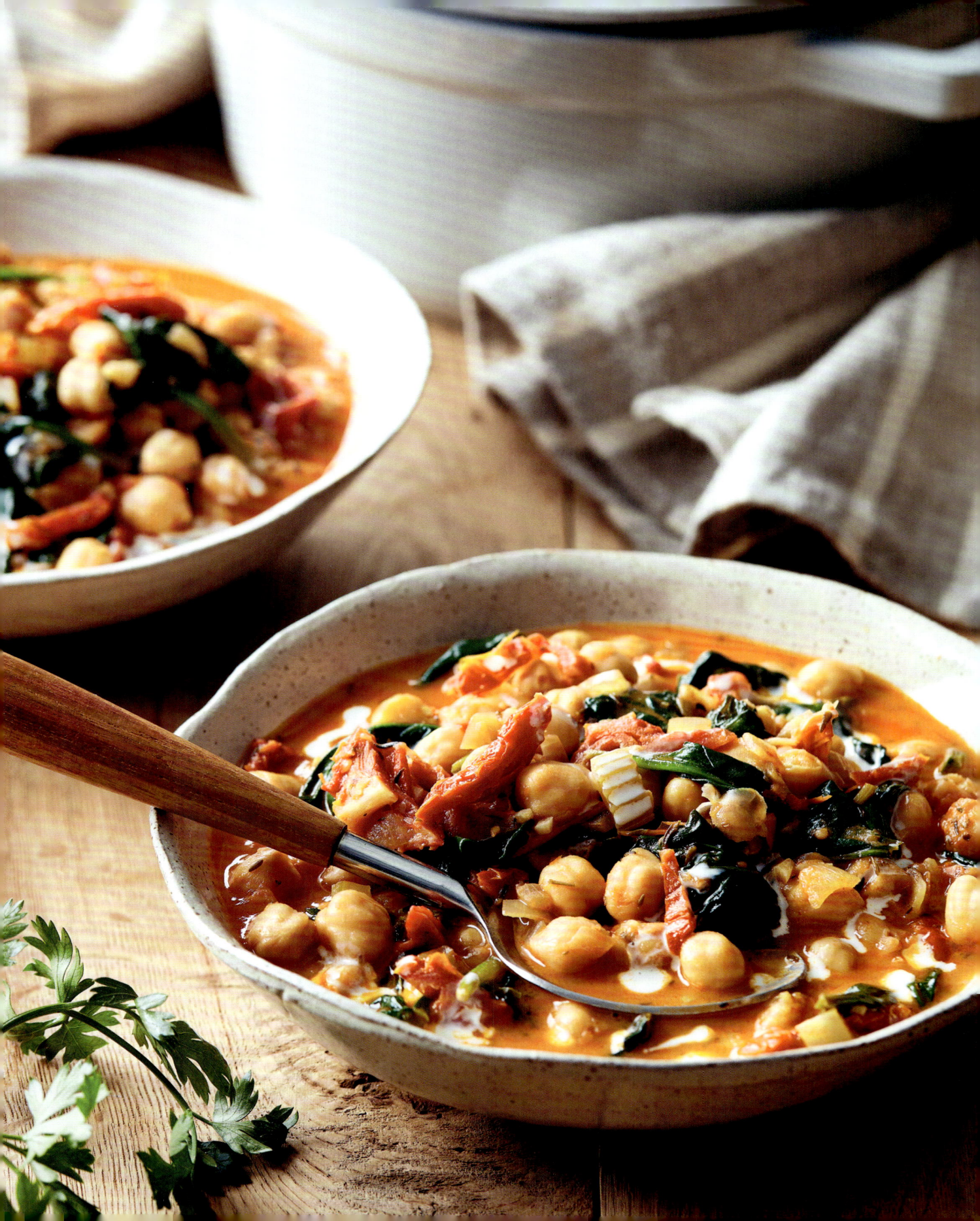

Chickpea & Spinach Stew

When you're in the mood for something hearty and comforting, this chickpea and spinach stew is just what you need. The protein-packed chickpeas, sweet tomatoes, and fresh spinach make this dish delicious, nutritious, and super filling, so you can easily enjoy it as a main course. To make it ultra-creamy, I mash some of the chickpeas in broth. It's perfect for those busy weeknights when you need something quick and easy but oh-so-satisfying.

1. Place a medium-size deep skillet over medium heat and add the olive oil. Once the oil is hot, add the onion, cherry tomatoes, and celery and sauté until the onions are golden brown.

2. Add the thyme and red pepper flakes and stir for another minute.

3. Add the tomato paste, garlic, and sun-dried tomatoes. Cook for another 2 to 3 minutes.

4. Add the chickpeas, lemon juice, and salt and pepper to taste and stir for another 2 minutes. (To thicken the stew, save a couple of spoonfuls of chickpeas and mash them with a fork in a small bowl with a couple of tablespoons of the broth before adding to the pan. Traditionally, a thick and silky texture is achieved by another starch, like bread or potatoes—but using this method, you will get a similar texture without the extra starch.)

5. Add the bone broth and cream to the skillet and stir to help dissolve the paste. Add more salt and pepper to taste.

6. Bring to a boil, reduce the heat, and simmer for 10 minutes.

7. Add the spinach and cook for another couple of minutes, until wilted, and it is ready to serve.

8. Top with fresh parsley and a bit more cream for decoration.

PREP TIME: 15 MINUTES
COOK TIME: 30 MINUTES
SERVINGS: 4 TO 6

---

2 tablespoons olive oil

1 medium onion, minced

10 ounces cherry tomatoes, halved

2 medium celery stalks, chopped

2 tablespoons dried thyme

½ teaspoon crushed red pepper flakes

2 tablespoons tomato paste

4 garlic cloves, minced

1½ ounces sun-dried tomatoes, julienned

1½ (15.5 ounce) cans chickpeas, drained

5 tablespoons freshly squeezed lemon juice

Salt and freshly ground black pepper

2 cups bone broth

⅓ cup heavy cream, plus extra for garnish

4 ounces fresh spinach

Fresh parsley, for garnish

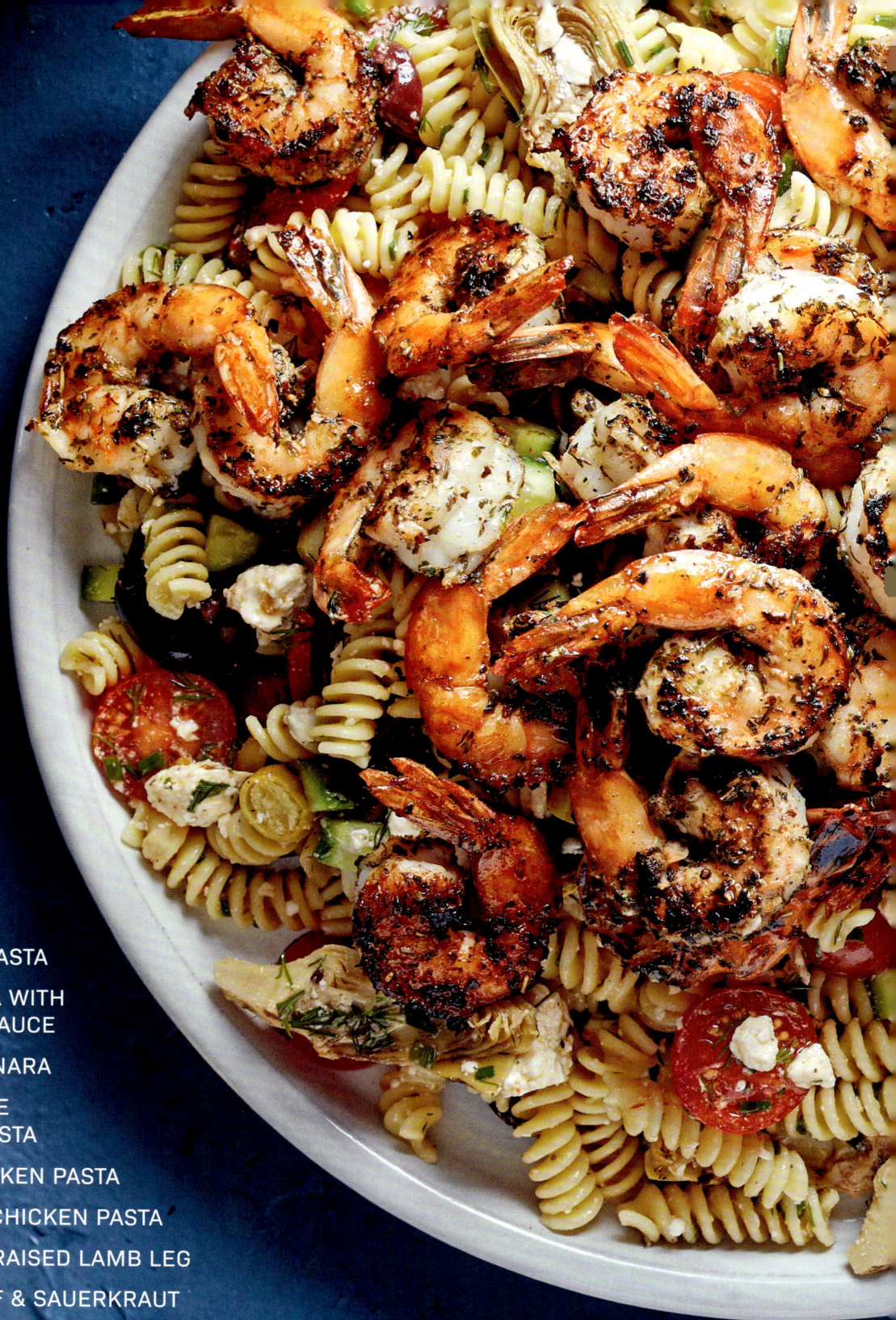

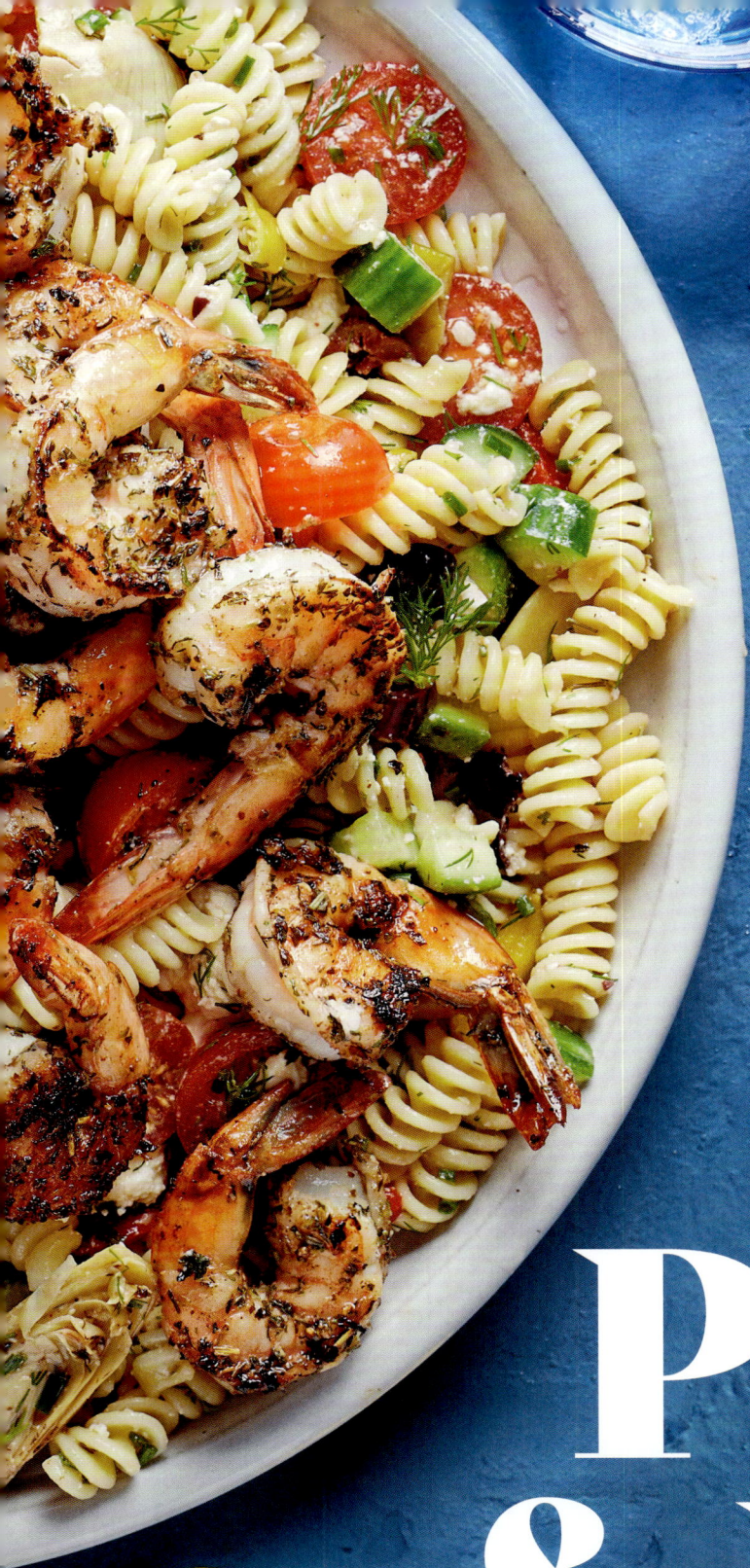
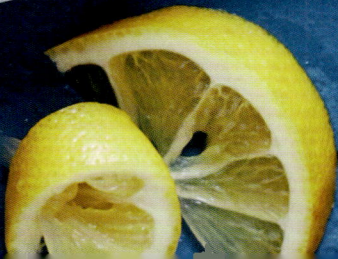

Pasta & Rice

That's right, I wrote a low-carb cookbook with an entire chapter on pasta and rice. And no, I didn't use zucchini noodles, spaghetti squash, or any of those low-carb pasta alternatives that taste like sacrifice. These dishes are made with a special ingredient that is near and dear to my heart, a passion project of mine: my Kaizen lupini pasta!

If you love pasta or rice as much as I do, you'll know that it is not easy to find a low-carb alternative that checks all the boxes when it comes to flavor, texture, and nutritional value. After years of struggling to find the perfect low-carb pasta, I took matters into my own hands and created Kaizen, low-carb pasta and rice made with lupini beans. With only 6 grams of net carbs and a whopping 20 grams of protein, you can finally indulge in a big bowl of pasta or rice without the sleepy carb crash or breaking your macros.

Whether you're craving a creamy pasta salad, a simple yet unique one-pan meal, or a delicious spin on a classic, these recipes will leave you satisfied and nourished. And of course, if you enjoy regular pasta or rice or prefer another alternative, go ahead and substitute whatever you prefer.

Bolognese Pasta

Who said you can't enjoy your favorite pasta dishes while on a low-carb diet? Certainly not me. This Bolognese pasta dish is made with my Kaizen low-carb pasta, which is made with lupini beans. Of course, you can also feel free to use your favorite low-carb pasta or regular pasta. The beefy marinara sauce is packed with flavor and the perfect balance of herbs, aromatics, and spices. Let someone try this dish and then blow their mind by telling them it's low-carb! PHOTO ON PAGES 160–161

PREP TIME: 15 MINUTES
COOK TIME: 40 MINUTES
SERVINGS: 4

1 tablespoon olive oil

½ medium onion, minced

4 garlic cloves, minced

2 celery stalks, minced

1 medium carrot, minced

2 tablespoons dried oregano

1 teaspoon crushed red pepper flakes

1 pound 80/20 ground beef

Salt and freshly ground black pepper

1 (28-ounce) can tomato puree

1 teaspoon balsamic vinegar

2 tablespoons chopped fresh basil, plus extra for garnish

⅓ cup grated Parmesan cheese

8 ounces Kaizen ziti or regular pasta

1. Place a large pan over medium-high heat. Add the olive oil, onion, garlic, celery, and carrot and sauté until the onion is golden brown (5 to 8 minutes). Add the oregano and red pepper flakes. Cook for another minute.

2. Add the ground beef and, using a meat masher or spatula, keep chopping the meat to prevent large clumps from forming. Season with salt and pepper to taste.

3. Once the meat starts to brown and the excess moisture is gone, add the tomato puree, balsamic vinegar, and basil.

4. Reduce the heat to medium-low and simmer for 10 to 15 minutes to further reduce the tomato puree. Add half of the Parmesan and disperse it with a spatula to prevent clumps.

5. While the meat sauce is cooking, bring a large pot of salted water to a boil and cook the pasta per the instructions on the packaging. Drain, rinse, and set aside.

6. Once the meat sauce is cooked, serve it on top of the pasta. Garnish with the remaining half of the Parmesan and more fresh basil. Serve right away or store in the fridge for up to 5 days.

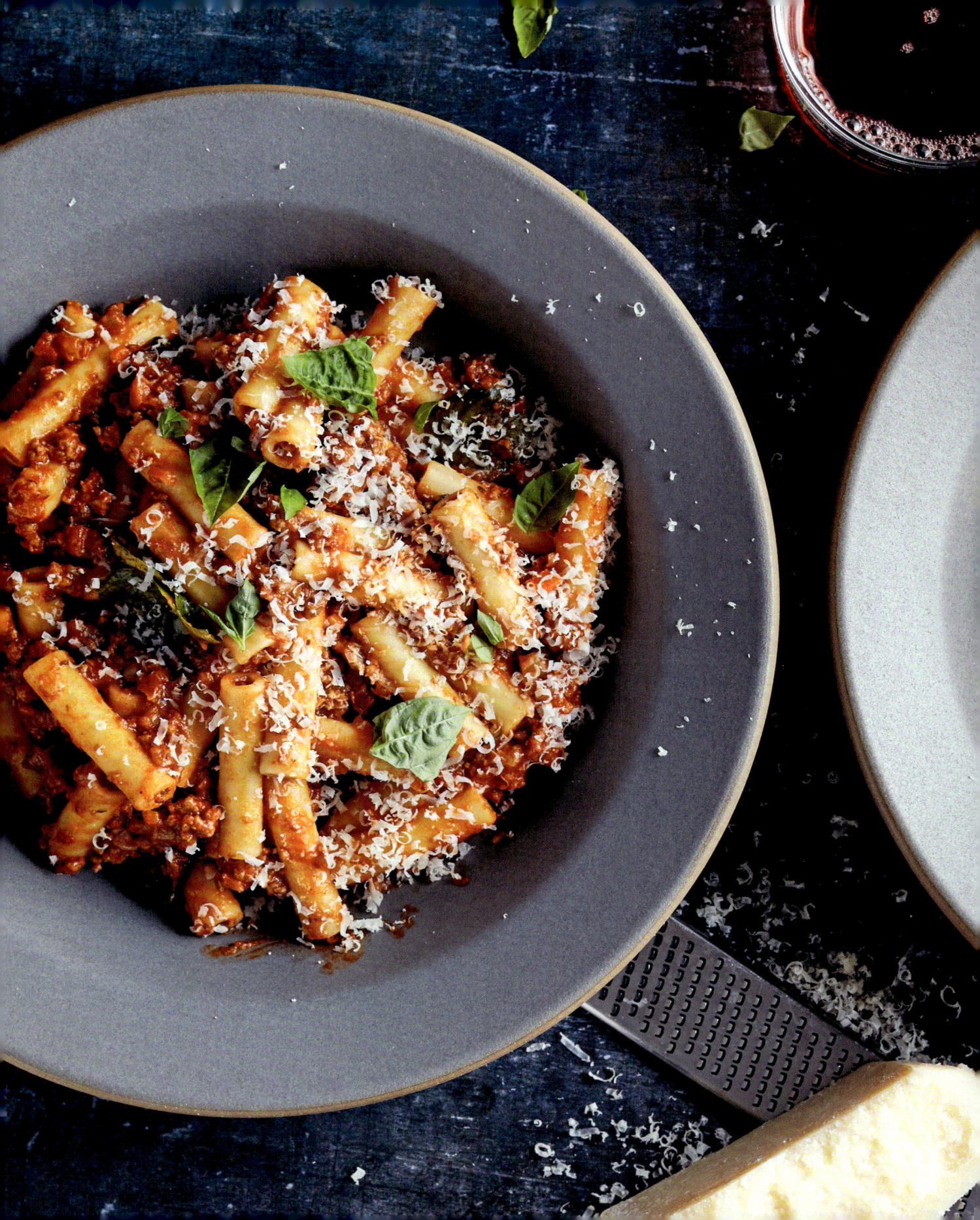

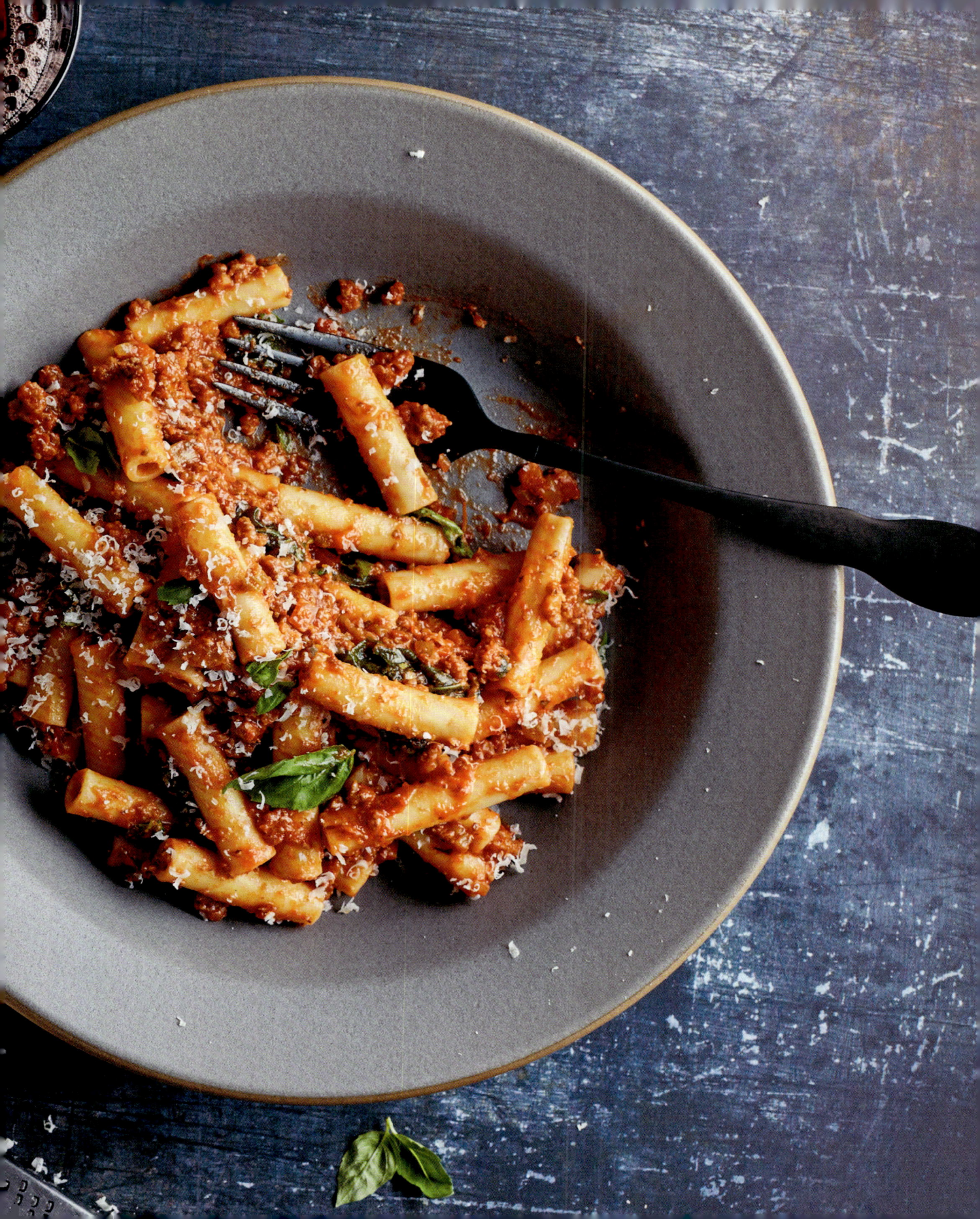

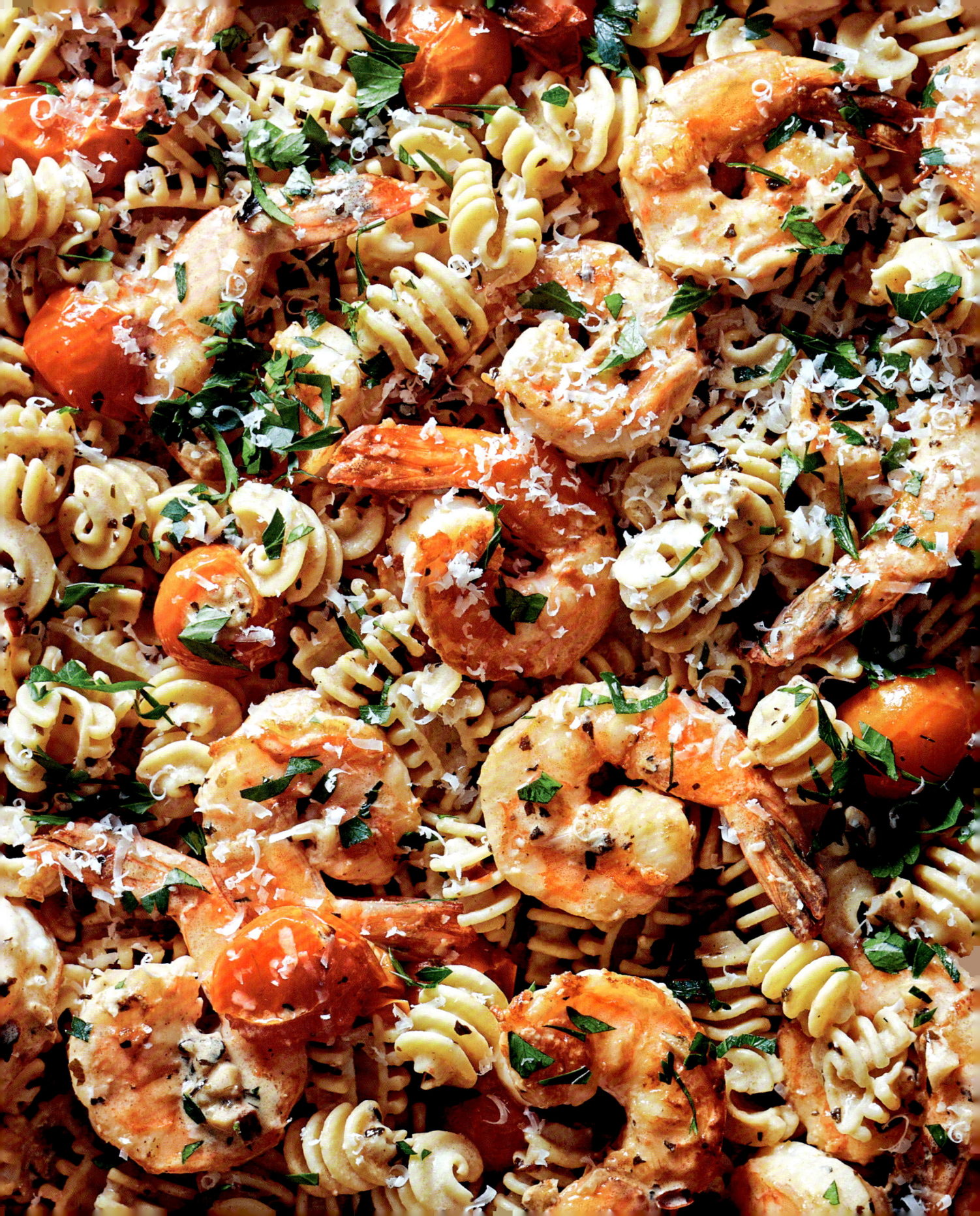

Shrimp Pasta

WITH WHITE WINE SAUCE

I love a good shrimp and pasta dish! This shrimp pasta with white wine sauce is one of my favorite creamy and flavorful low-carb meals. Ready in under an hour, this simple yet satisfying dish is perfect for a weeknight dinner or even a special occasion. The shrimp gives it a touch of luxury, while the white wine and sautéed and seasoned cherry tomatoes add a depth of flavor and richness to the sauce that is just phenomenal. It's fresh, flavorful, and indulgent without being heavy—perfect for my low-carb friends!

PREP TIME: 20 MINUTES
COOK TIME: 20 MINUTES
SERVINGS: 4 TO 6

———

Salt

8 ounces Kaizen fusilli or regular pasta

5 ounces cherry tomatoes

1 pound raw shrimp, peeled and deveined

Freshly ground black pepper

2 tablespoons olive oil

4 garlic cloves, minced

1 teaspoon dried basil

1 teaspoon crushed red pepper flakes

⅓ cup white wine

⅓ cup heavy cream

¼ cup grated Parmesan cheese, for garnish

1 tablespoon chopped fresh parsley, for garnish

1. Bring a large pot of salted water to a boil and cook the pasta per the instructions on the packaging. Drain, rinse, and set aside. While the pasta is cooking, prepare the rest. Poke the cherry tomatoes with the tip of a knife and set aside. This will help prevent the tomatoes from popping and splashing while they cook.

2. Pat the shrimp dry and season with salt and pepper.

3. Grab a wide skillet (this will need to fit all the ingredients at the end) and heat 1 tablespoon of the olive oil over medium heat. Sear the shrimp for 1½ to 2 minutes on each side and set aside.

4. In the same pan, heat the remaining 1 tablespoon of olive oil, add the tomatoes, and sauté for 2 minutes, until the tomatoes are all soft and collapsed. Add the garlic, basil, and red pepper flakes and sauté for another minute.

5. Add the wine and cook for 2 to 3 minutes to eliminate the alcohol, then add the heavy cream.

6. Add the cooked pasta and shrimp back to the skillet and fold them in with the sauce for about 1 minute.

7. Place the pasta and shrimp on a serving plate and garnish with grated Parmesan and fresh parsley.

Pasta Carbonara

Treat yourself to gourmet-level flavor using the most minimal effort with this easy pasta carbonara. It's a low-carb spin on the classic, using my Kaizen pasta, which gets tossed in crispy melted guanciale, an Italian staple for adding flavor to pasta dishes. Don't have guanciale? No problem. This will taste great with bacon too! The sauce is just a mixture of egg yolks and Parmesan cheese, diluted with warm water, making it deliciously creamy and silky. Ready in under 30 minutes, this low-carb pasta dish is as easy and quick as it gets! Whip it up for a quick weeknight dinner, or impress your guests with a fancy yet simple dish.

PREP TIME: 10 MINUTES
COOK TIME: 15 MINUTES
SERVINGS: 4 TO 6

---

4 ounces guanciale or bacon

4 egg yolks

⅓ cup grated Parmesan cheese, plus extra for garnish

Salt

8 ounces Kaizen fusilli or regular pasta

Freshly ground black pepper

1. Cut the guanciale into ⅓-inch cubes and set aside.

2. Place the egg yolks in a small mixing bowl, add the Parmesan, and give it a mix. Gradually add ½ cup warm (not hot) water and set aside.

3. Bring a large pot of salted water to a boil and cook the pasta per the instructions on the packaging. Drain, rinse, and set aside.

4. Place a medium pan over medium heat and add the cubed guanciale. Sear until it starts to crisp up and has a golden brown color.

5. Add the pasta to the pan and toss it a couple of times using a spatula to coat it with the melted guanciale fat (this step is key).

6. Turn off the heat but leave the pan on the stove. Add the egg yolk and Parmesan mixture and continuously fold into the pasta for 1 to 2 minutes, using the remaining heat from the pan to cook the yolks and melt the Parmesan. The mixture will turn into a delicious sauce. Remove the pasta from the stove to prevent it drying out. Check for salt and pepper and adjust as needed.

7. Place in a serving bowl, garnish with extra Parmesan and freshly ground pepper, and serve right away.

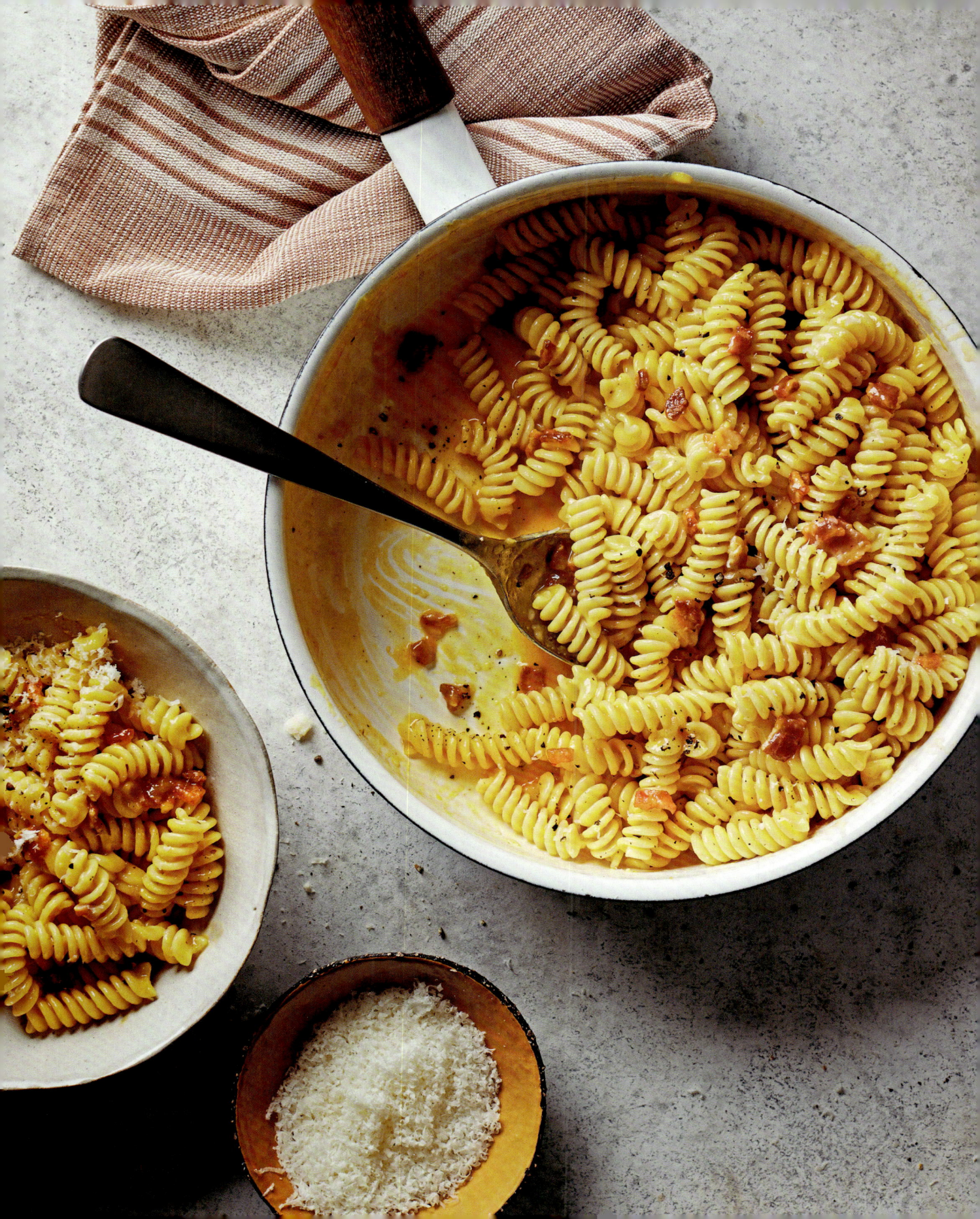

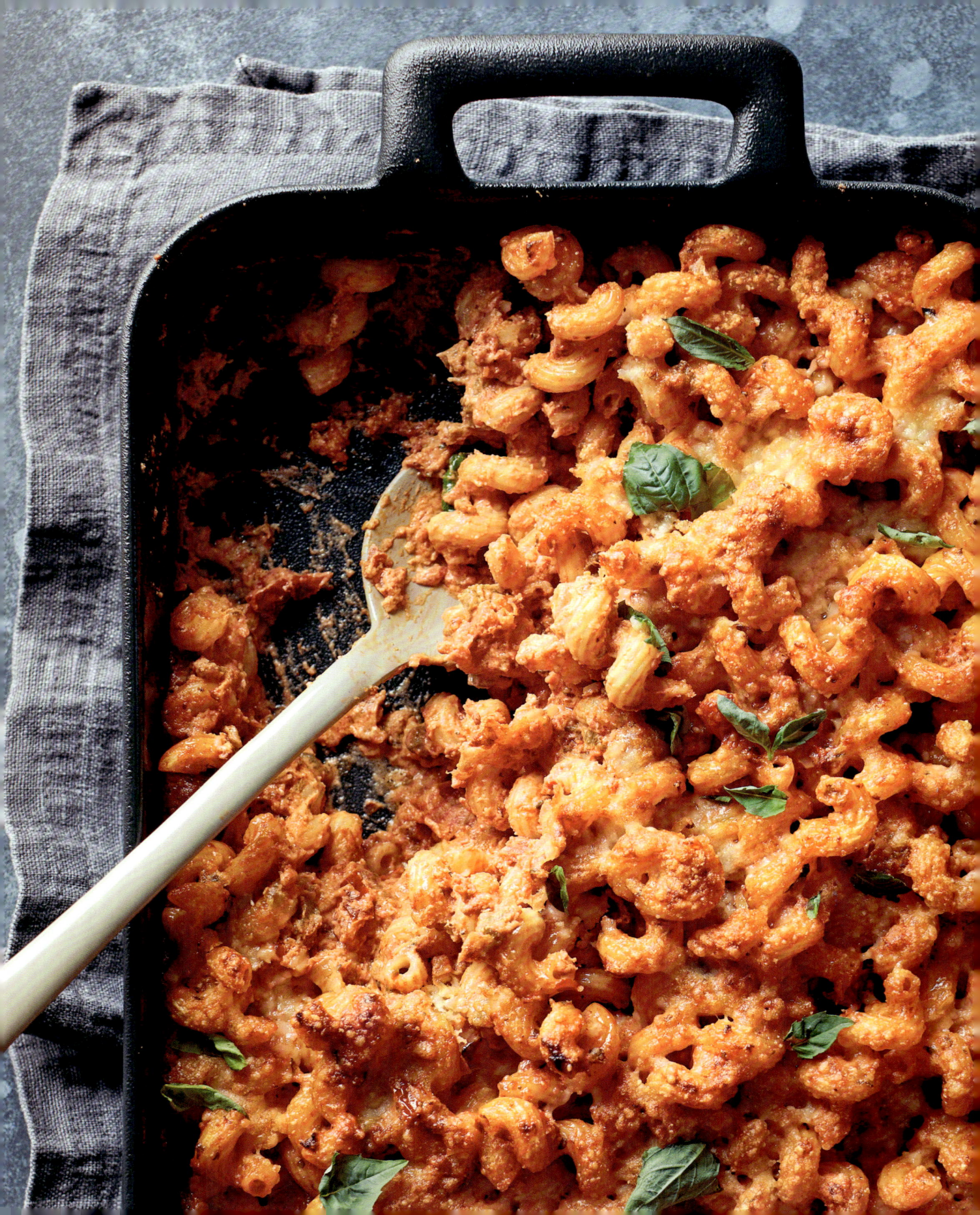

Baked Cheese Matbucha Pasta

I wanted to merge my love for pasta with my love for the Moroccan dish matbucha, so I came up with this delicious baked cheese matbucha pasta to indulge all my comfort food cravings. The matbucha is first baked with some olive oil and your choice of Boursin or feta cheese, to create a dreamy cheese base for the pasta. After that, fold in your favorite low-carb pasta (I use Kaizen pasta) and sprinkle it with Parmesan cheese before broiling it until the top is deliciously crusty and bubbly. Mmm.

1. Preheat the oven to 400°F.

2. Add the matbucha sauce to a medium-size deep oven-safe dish and place the Boursin on top. If using feta, add the oregano, chives, and garlic powder. (Boursin contains herbs already.) Drizzle on the olive oil.

3. Bake the cheese and sauce for 20 minutes, until warmed through and softened.

4. While the cheese and sauce are baking, prepare the pasta. Bring a large pot of salted water to a boil and undercook the pasta by 1 to 2 minutes compared to the instructions on the packaging to keep it al dente, since this will cook further in the oven. Drain, rinse, and set aside.

5. Remove the sauce from the oven and crush the cheese into the sauce with a fork.

6. Add the pasta and gently fold it into the sauce. Top with the grated Parmesan.

7. Set the oven to broil. Place the pasta in the oven for another 5 minutes, until the cheese melts and creates a light crust on top.

8. Garnish with fresh basil and serve right away!

PREP TIME: 1 HOUR
COOK TIME: 2 HOURS
SERVINGS: 4 TO 6

---

4 cups Moroccan Tomato Spread (page 65)

10 ounces Boursin cheese or feta cheese, crumbled

ADDITIONAL INGREDIENTS IF USING FETA

½ tablespoon dried oregano

½ tablespoon dried chives

½ tablespoon garlic powder

1 tablespoon olive oil

Salt

8 ounces Kaizen pasta or regular pasta

½ cup grated Parmesan cheese

2 tablespoons chopped fresh basil, for garnish

Buffalo Chicken Pasta

One of the keys to my 100-pound weight-loss journey has been eating more protein. And this dish delivers that from every angle, as it's loaded with protein from not just the chicken but also my Kaizen low-carb lupini pasta, which boasts a mighty 20 grams of protein per serving (but feel free to use any pasta that you like). And the protein keeps coming—cottage cheese and yogurt make up the rich and creamy base for the buffalo sauce. It strikes the perfect balance between indulgent and filling, without causing a food coma.

1. Preheat the oven to 400°F.

2. In a food processor, combine the cottage cheese, yogurt, ranch seasoning, and buffalo sauce and blend for about a minute, until smooth.

3. In a medium oven-safe dish, combine the chicken and the sauce, mixing until the chicken is evenly coated. Add salt and pepper to taste.

4. Cook the pasta per the instructions on the packaging.

5. Add the cooked pasta to the dish and give it another mix to blend the pasta with the chicken and sauce. Top with the shredded Cheddar.

6. Bake for 12 to 15 minutes, until the cheese is melted.

7. Remove from the oven and top with the scallions and red pepper flakes.

PREP TIME: 15 MINUTES
COOK TIME: 15 MINUTES
SERVINGS: 4 TO 6

½ cup cottage cheese

½ cup plain yogurt

1 packet ranch seasoning

½ cup buffalo sauce

2 cups diced rotisserie chicken or other cooked chicken

Salt and freshly ground black pepper

8 ounces Kaizen ziti or regular pasta

1 cup shredded Cheddar cheese

2 scallions, white and green parts, finely chopped

1 teaspoon crushed red pepper flakes

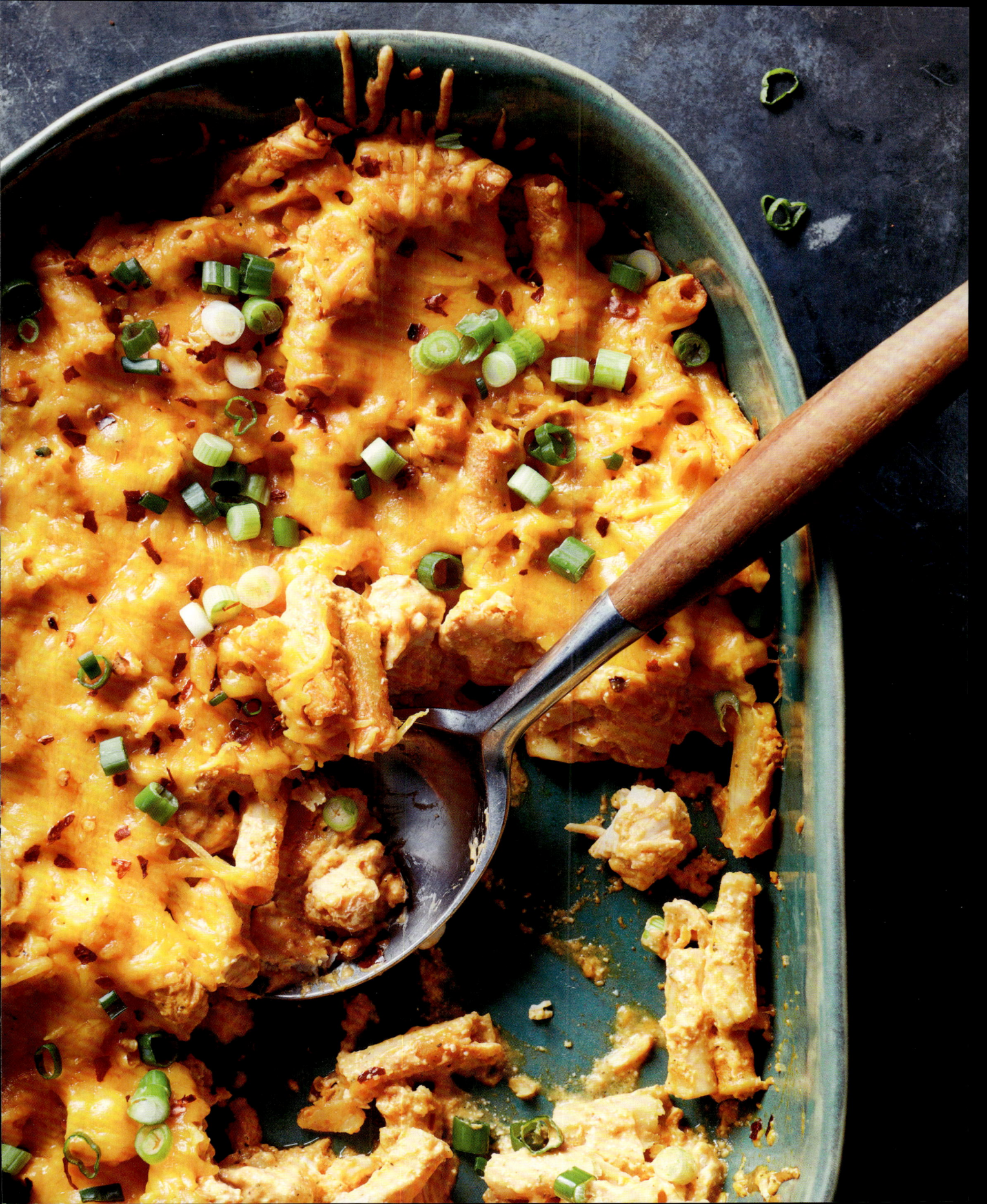

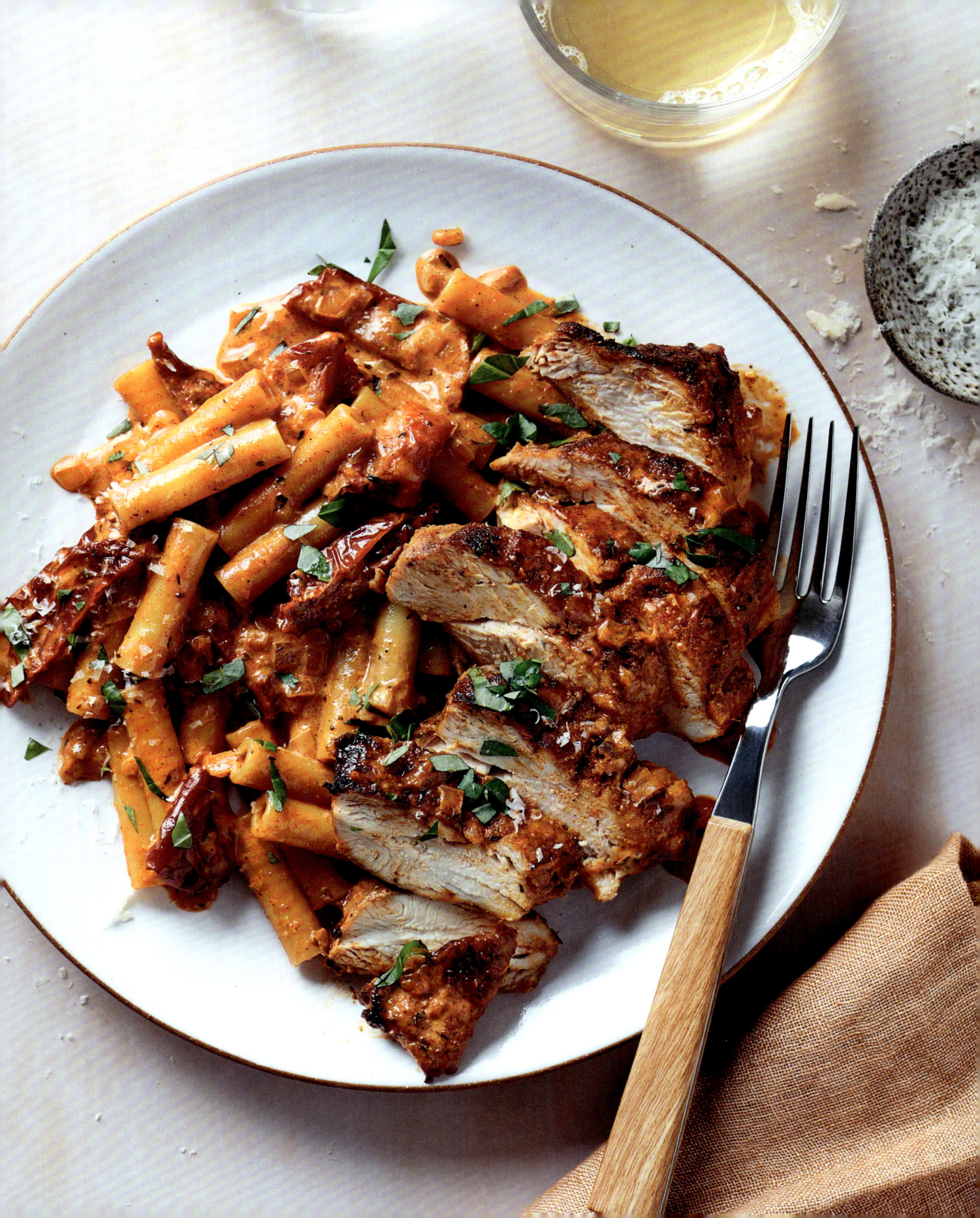

"Marry Me" Chicken Pasta

Prepare yourself for what I call a "mouth party" as you dive right into this delightful chicken and pasta dish. I used my Kaizen low-carb ziti here. Add sun-dried tomatoes, fresh basil, and a creamy, cheesy sauce into the mix, and you'll want to make a marriage proposal to this dish. I do, I do! Serve it on a special occasion for a crowd or as an easy chicken dinner for your family at home (it's faster than delivery!). No matter the time and place, know that you'll have everyone raving—even those who aren't watching their carbs!

PREP TIME: 10 MINUTES
COOK TIME: 25 MINUTES
SERVINGS: 4 TO 6

- 1 tablespoon onion powder
- 1 tablespoon garlic powder
- 1 tablespoon sweet paprika
- 1 tablespoon dried thyme
- ½ teaspoon cayenne pepper
- Salt and freshly ground black pepper
- 4 chicken breasts
- 2 tablespoons olive oil
- ½ large yellow onion, minced
- 1 tablespoon unsalted butter
- 2 tablespoons tomato paste
- ¾ cup heavy cream
- ¾ cup bone broth
- ½ cup sun-dried tomatoes
- 4 to 5 sprigs fresh basil, plus extra for garnish
- 8 ounces Kaizen ziti or regular pasta

- ¼ cup freshly grated pecorino cheese, for garnish

1. In a small bowl, combine the onion powder, garlic powder, paprika, ½ tablespoon of the thyme, the cayenne, and salt and pepper to taste. Rub the seasoning on the chicken, ensuring that all sides are covered thoroughly.

2. Heat the oil in a large pan over medium heat. Place the chicken in the pan and sear for about 3 minutes on each side. Once the chicken is golden brown on both sides, transfer to a plate and set aside.

3. Return the pan to medium heat and add the onion and butter. Mix well. Then season with salt, pepper, and the remaining ½ tablespoon of thyme. When the onion turns translucent, add the tomato paste, cream, and bone broth, mixing well with a spatula.

4. Add the sun-dried tomatoes and basil. Transfer the chicken back to the pan. Spoon the sauce over the chicken and put the lid on for 4 to 5 minutes, or until the chicken is cooked through.

5. While the chicken cooks, bring a large pot of salted water to a boil and cook the pasta per the instructions on the packaging. Drain, rinse, and set aside.

6. When the chicken is cooked, remove it from the pan, slice it, and set aside.

7. Add the pasta to the sauce, turn off the heat, and gently fold it until the pasta is evenly coated.

8. Plate up the pasta and top it with the sliced chicken, fresh basil, and pecorino and serve right away.

Moroccan Braised Lamb Leg

Cooked long and slow (as it should be!), this Moroccan braised lamb is the perfect centerpiece for any dinner party. This flavorful dish features all the best spices the region has to offer, combined with tender lamb meat. It's absolutely delicious and surprisingly easy to make! The oven does most of the cooking for you. It's one of those meals that will taste as good as gourmet, but without all the effort!

1. Rub all sides of the lamb with 2½ tablespoons of the Moroccan spice blend, plus salt and pepper. Let it marinate for at least 1 hour.

2. Preheat the oven to 300°F.

3. Heat 1 tablespoon of the olive oil in a skillet over medium heat. Sear the meat on each side until brown (2 to 3 minutes per side). Set aside on a plate.

4. In a small dry skillet, toast the walnuts until the edges start to brown. Set aside to cool.

5. Using the same skillet as for the meat, add the remaining 1 tablespoon of olive oil, then add the onion, garlic, and carrot and sauté for 3 to 4 minutes, until the onion turns golden brown.

6. Add the remaining ½ tablespoon of Moroccan spice blend to the veggies and sauté for another minute.

7. Pour the veggies into a deep oven-safe dish with a lid. Add the tomato puree, a pinch of saffron, and the bone broth, and give it a quick mix to incorporate the puree and saffron. Add salt and pepper to taste. Place the meat in the liquid, then add the cauliflower florets, apricots, and toasted walnuts.

8. Cover and bake for 3½ hours until the meat is fork tender and you're able to shred it off the bone with two forks.

9. Thirty minutes before the meat is ready, cook the rice per the instructions on the package.

10. Place the rice on a serving platter, then add the lamb and cooked veggies and drizzle the sauce from the baking dish on top. Serve hot!

PREP TIME: 30 MINUTES, PLUS 1 HOUR MARINATING
COOK TIME: 4 HOURS
SERVINGS: 4 TO 6

2 pounds lamb leg steak or shanks

3 tablespoons Moroccan Spice Blend (page 223)

Salt and freshly ground black pepper

2 tablespoons olive oil

1 ounce raw walnuts, chopped

1 medium onion, cut into strips

6 garlic cloves, minced

1 medium carrot, diced

1 (15-ounce) can tomato puree

Pinch of saffron threads

2 cups bone broth

5 cups cauliflower florets (1 medium head cauliflower)

5 to 6 dried apricots, cut in quarters

8 ounces Kaizen rice, couscous, or basmati rice

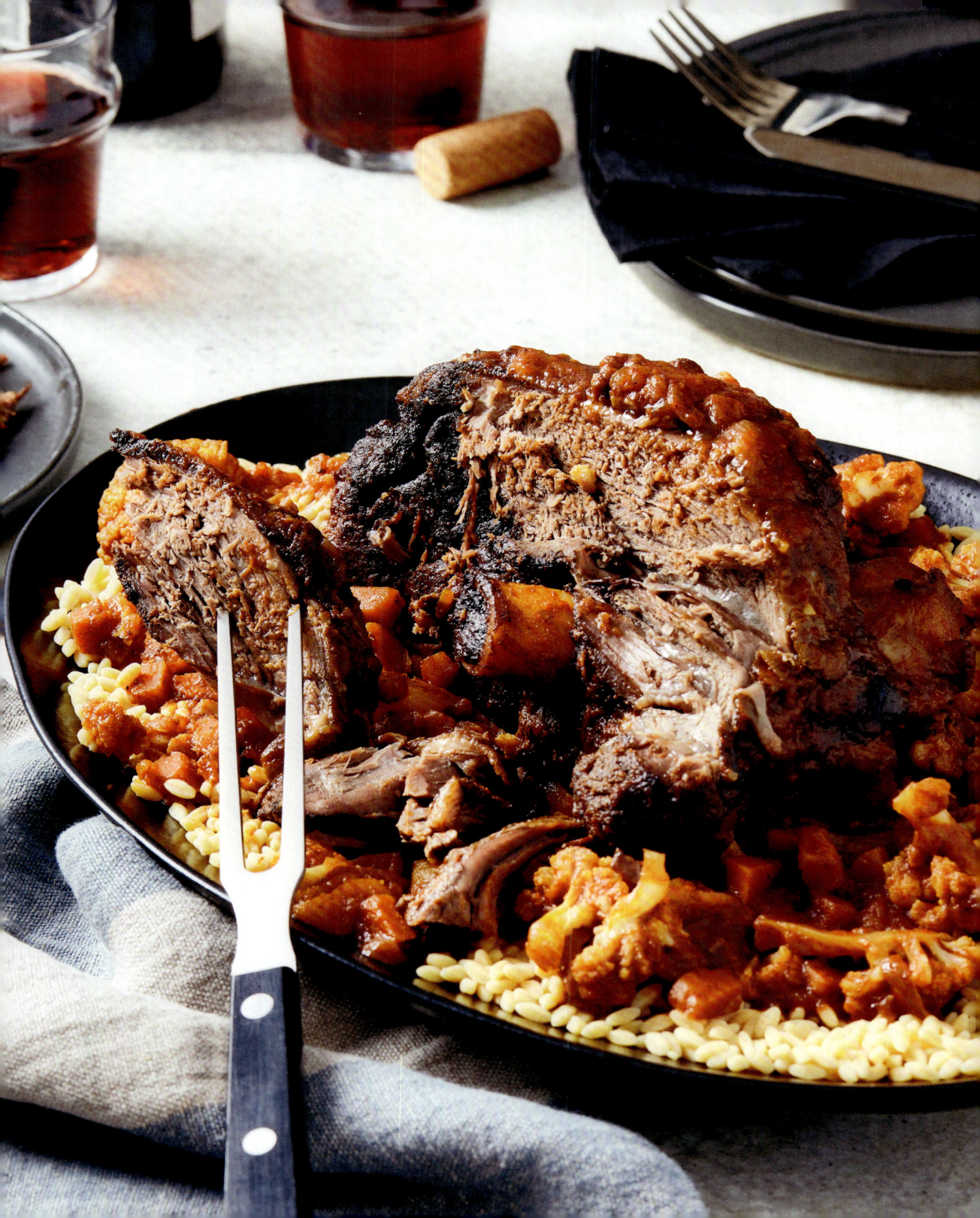

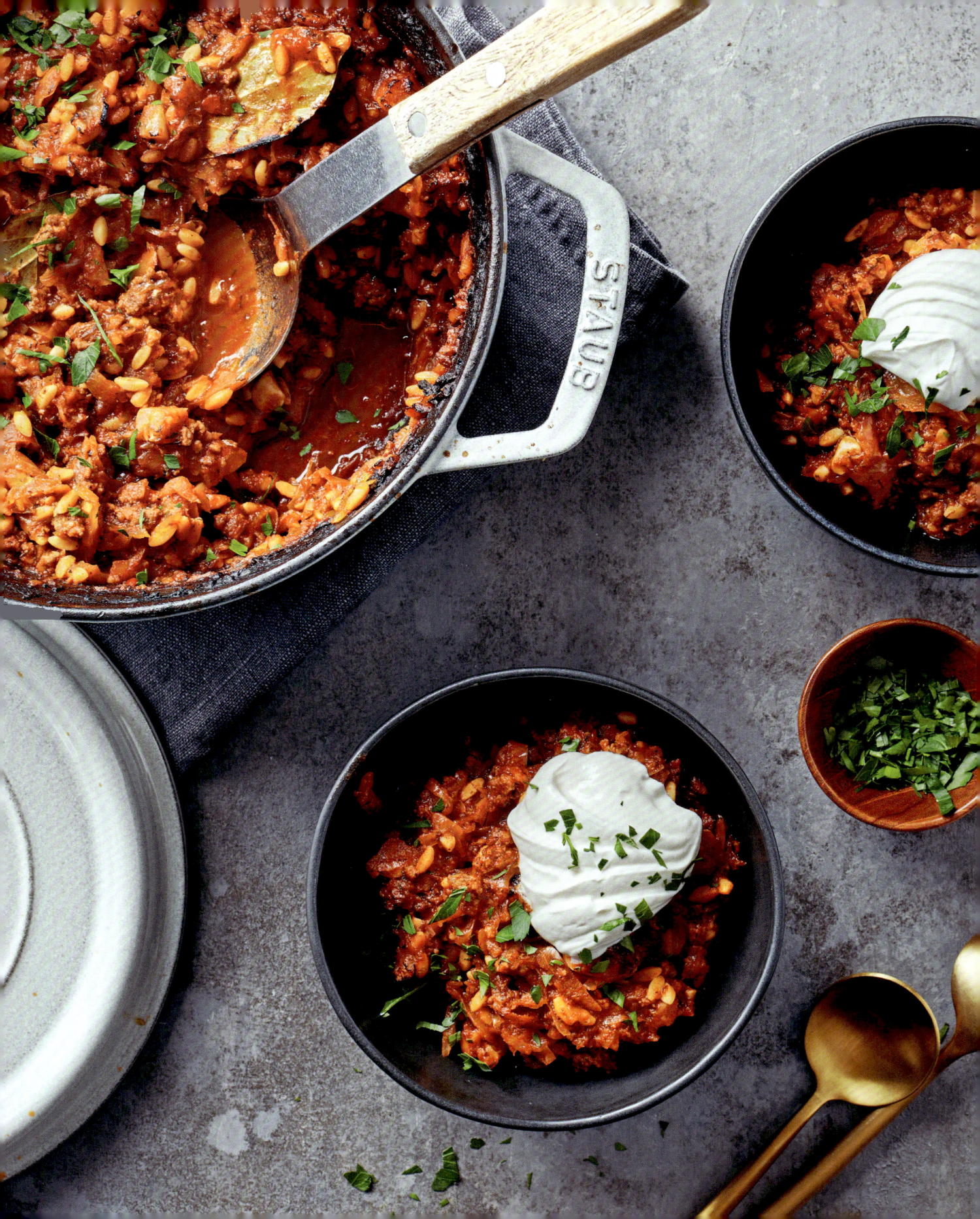

One-Pan Beef & Sauerkraut

This one-pan beef and sauerkraut dish reminds me of the Romanian dish *sarmale,* a staple usually cooked at Christmas. The unique flavor of the pickled cabbage, combined with the smokiness and rich texture of the beef and bacon, makes it one of my all-time favorites. This one needs a lot of time to get happy in the oven, but that'll allow you to chill out on the couch or take care of some things around the house while you wait. You've got to love a recipe that does most of the work for you!

1. Place a medium-size deep cast-iron pot or Dutch oven over medium heat. Add the olive oil. Once the oil is heated, add the onion and garlic and sauté for 3 to 4 minutes, until the onion turns golden brown. Add the thyme, dill, and red pepper flakes and cook for another minute.

2. Preheat the oven to 350°F.

3. Add the ground beef to the pot and use a spatula to break it up into smaller pieces as it cooks. Continue cooking until all the moisture evaporates and the meat starts to brown. Add salt and pepper to taste.

4. Add the rice. Add the bacon (if using—the bacon will give the dish a nice smoky flavor, but feel free to skip if you prefer). Mix the ingredients together and cook for another 2 to 3 minutes, until the rice is well coated and the bacon is soft.

5. Add the sauerkraut, the tomato puree, and 1 to 2 cups water. The sauerkraut should be just covered in the liquid. Cook for another 4 to 5 minutes, until it starts to simmer.

6. Add the bay leaves and cover the pot with a lid.

7. Move pot to the oven and bake for 1½ hours, until the sauerkraut is soft and tender. Check halfway along to ensure that there is enough liquid, and add more water if needed. The beef and sauerkraut should still be halfway immersed in liquid at this point.

8. After 1½ hours, switch the oven to broil on high and remove the lid. Broil for 5 minutes until a crust has formed on top.

9. Serve hot garnished with sour cream and fresh parsley, if desired.

PREP TIME: 20 MINUTES
COOK TIME: 2 HOURS
SERVINGS: 4 TO 6

2 tablespoons olive oil

1 medium onion, minced

4 garlic cloves, minced

2 teaspoons dried thyme

1 tablespoon dried dill

1 teaspoon crushed red pepper flakes

1 pound 80/20 ground beef

Salt and freshly ground black pepper

4 ounces Kaizen rice or regular rice

2 ounces smoked bacon, cut into ½-inch cubes (optional)

1 pound sauerkraut

2⅓ cups (16 ounces) canned tomato puree

3 or 4 bay leaves

OPTIONAL GARNISHES

Sour cream or plain Greek yogurt

Finely chopped fresh parsley

Greek Pasta Salad

WITH GRILLED SHRIMP

Adding shrimp to a Greek pasta salad is a delicious twist on a classic dish. The combination of wholesome ingredients like tangy feta cheese, sweet tomatoes, and crisp cucumbers with the juicy shrimp creates a burst of flavor and texture in every bite. Not only that, the shrimp give this dish a big protein boost, making it both filling and ultra-satisfying. I'm not shy with the ingredient list here—there are so many delicious elements that take this salad to the next level. Peperoncini, artichokes, kalamata olives, a homemade lemon Dijon dressing, and my Kaizen low-carb pasta all play a role in this summery main or side dish.

1. Bring a large pot of generously salted water to a boil. Add the pasta and cook according to the directions on the packaging. Drain and rinse with cold water.

2. In a large serving bowl, combine the pasta, cucumbers, cherry tomatoes, roasted red peppers, kalamata olives, artichokes, peperoncini, chives, dill, and feta.

3. For the dressing: In a small mason jar, combine the olive oil, lemon juice, mustard, Greek Spice Blend, and salt and pepper to taste. Secure the lid and shake well to mix.

4. Pour the dressing over the veggies and pasta and toss gently with a spatula or a large spoon. Set aside.

5. In a medium bowl, drizzle the shrimp with 1 tablespoon olive oil and season with the Greek Spice Blend and salt and pepper.

6. Heat the remaining olive oil in a pan over medium heat and cook the shrimp on each side for 1 to 1½ minutes, until they are pink and opaque throughout with a slight curl.

7. Remove from the heat and top the salad with the shrimp before serving.

PREP TIME: 15 MINUTES
COOK TIME: 15 MINUTES
SERVINGS: 4 OR 5

Salt

6 ounces Kaizen fusilli pasta or regular pasta

2 Persian or mini cucumbers, diced

1 cup cherry tomatoes, halved

½ cup roasted red peppers, chopped

⅓ cup kalamata olives, chopped

¼ cup marinated grilled artichokes

3 tablespoons sliced golden peperoncini

⅓ cup finely chopped fresh chives

⅓ cup finely chopped fresh dill

4 ounces feta cheese, crumbled

FOR THE DRESSING

6 tablespoons olive oil

2 tablespoons freshly squeezed lemon juice

1 teaspoon Dijon mustard

1 teaspoon Greek Spice Blend (page 221)

Salt and freshly ground black pepper

8 ounces raw shrimp, peeled and deveined

2 tablespoons olive oil

1½ tablespoons Greek Spice Blend

Freshly ground black pepper

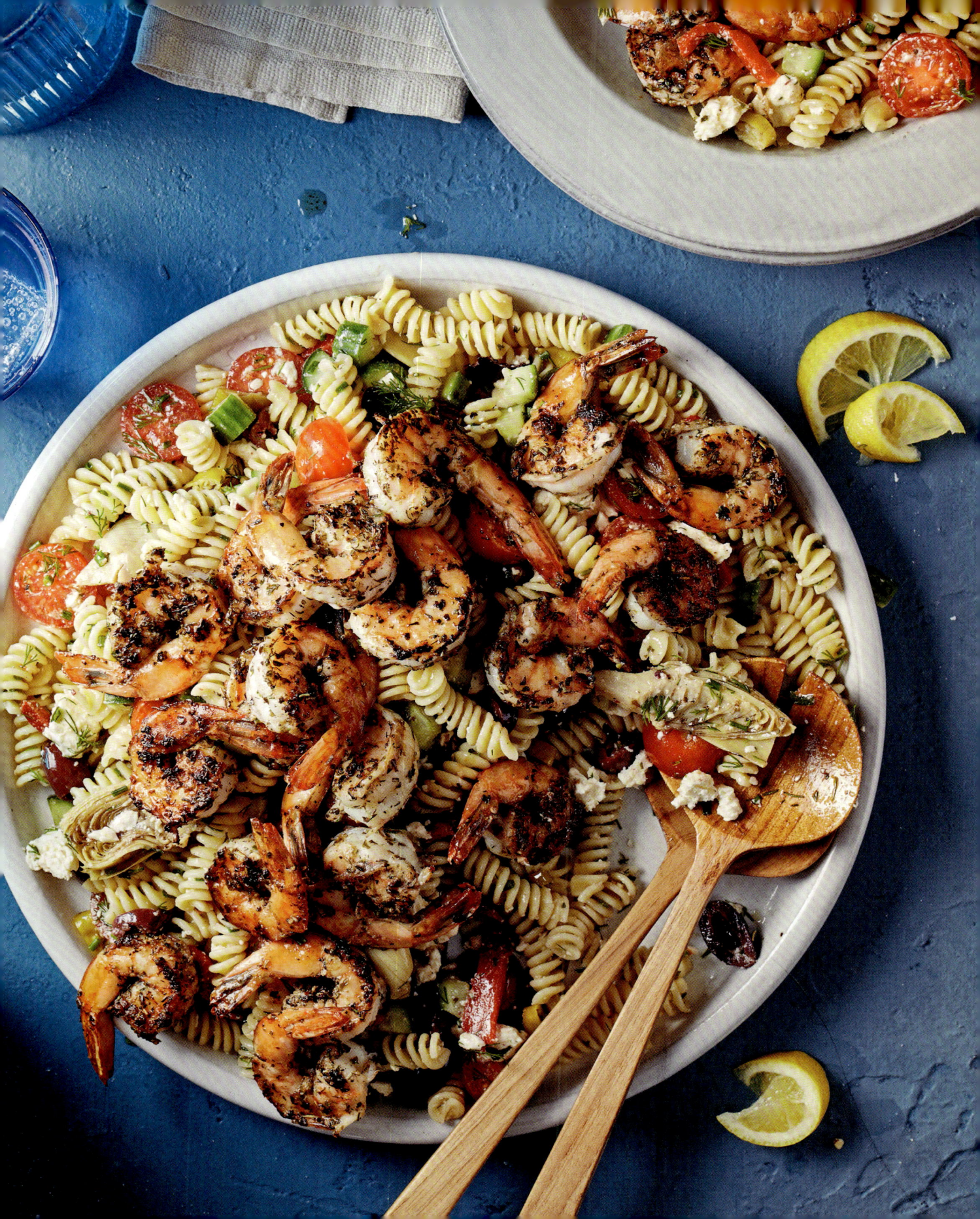

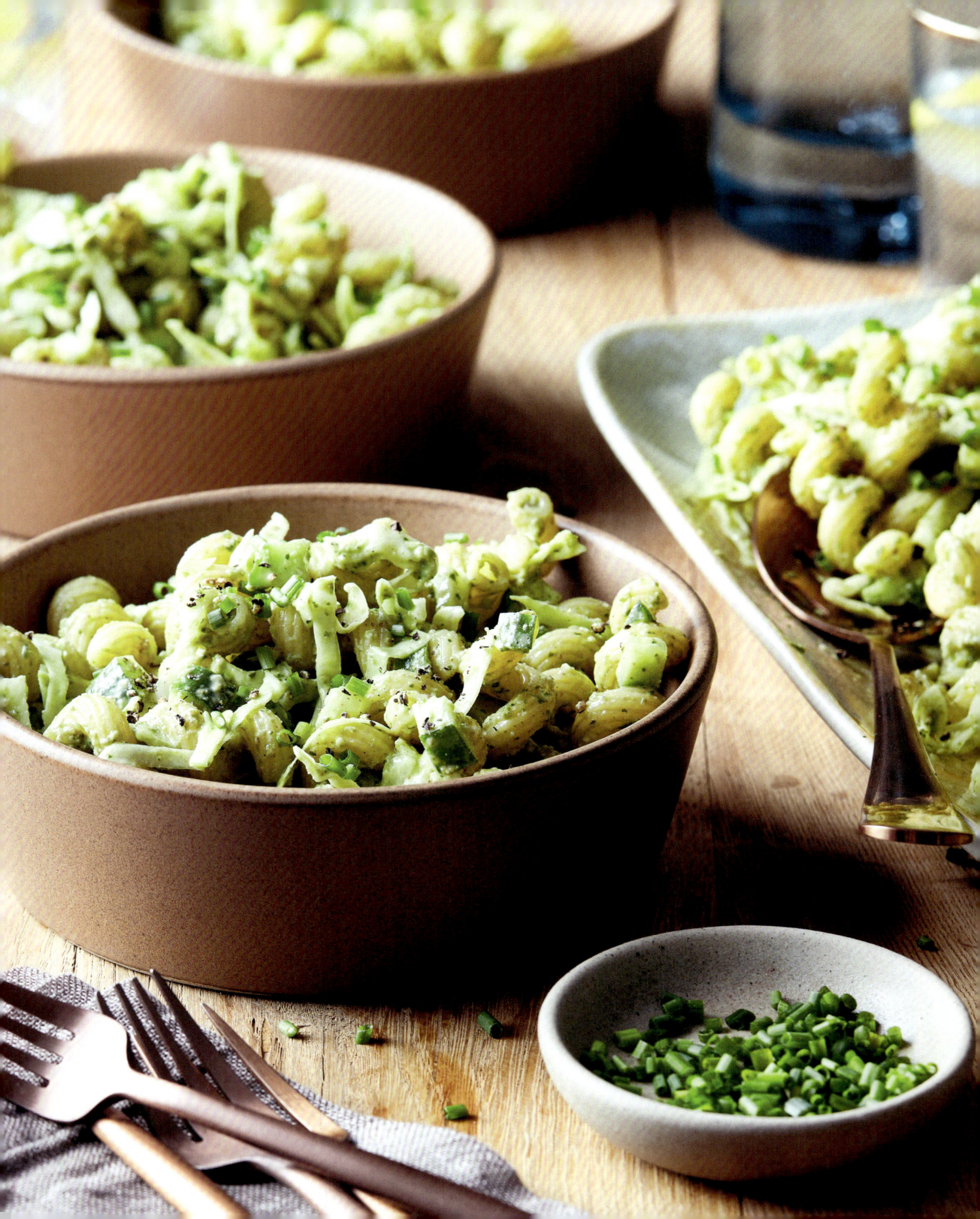

Green Goddess Pasta Salad

A big bowl of plant-based protein goodness, this green goddess pasta salad is what all your creamy pasta dreams are made of. If you are craving pasta but want to keep it low-carb, my Kaizen pasta is a great solution, as it is packed with protein and tastes like the real deal. But any other pasta substitute or even traditional pasta will work just great and is guaranteed to satisfy all cravings. For the dressing, all you have to do is toss the fresh ingredients into a food processor. It's one of those recipes that'll remind you that yes, you can have it all!

1. Place the cooked pasta in a large salad bowl. Add the cabbage, cucumbers, and chives. (Shredding and cutting them as I recommend helps coat everything with just the right amount of dressing, but you can vary the sizes if you prefer.)

2. **For the green goddess dressing:** In a food processor, combine the shallot, garlic, chives, basil, walnuts, olive oil, lemon juice, nutritional yeast, rice vinegar, and salt and pepper to taste. Blend well.

3. Pour the dressing over the salad and toss gently. Serve immediately.

PREP TIME: 30 MINUTES
SERVINGS: 4 TO 6

Salt

8 ounces Kaizen pasta or regular pasta, cooked, in shapes like cavatappi, fusilli, or penne

2½ cups finely shredded green cabbage

4 Persian or mini cucumbers, cut into ¼-inch cubes

Handful of finely chopped fresh chives

FOR THE GREEN GODDESS DRESSING

1 small shallot

2 garlic cloves

Handful of fresh chives

Handful of fresh basil

⅓ cup raw walnuts

⅓ cup olive oil

9 tablespoons freshly squeezed lemon juice

3 tablespoons nutritional yeast

3 tablespoons rice vinegar

Salt and freshly ground black pepper

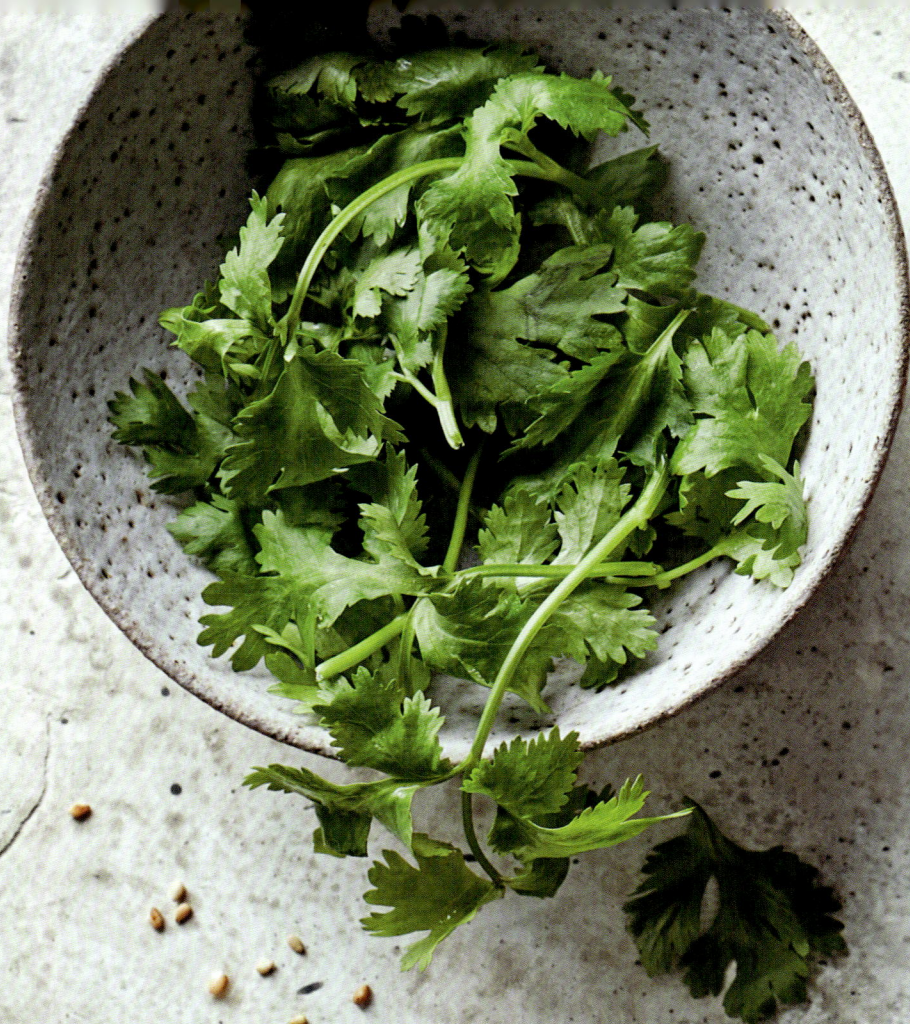

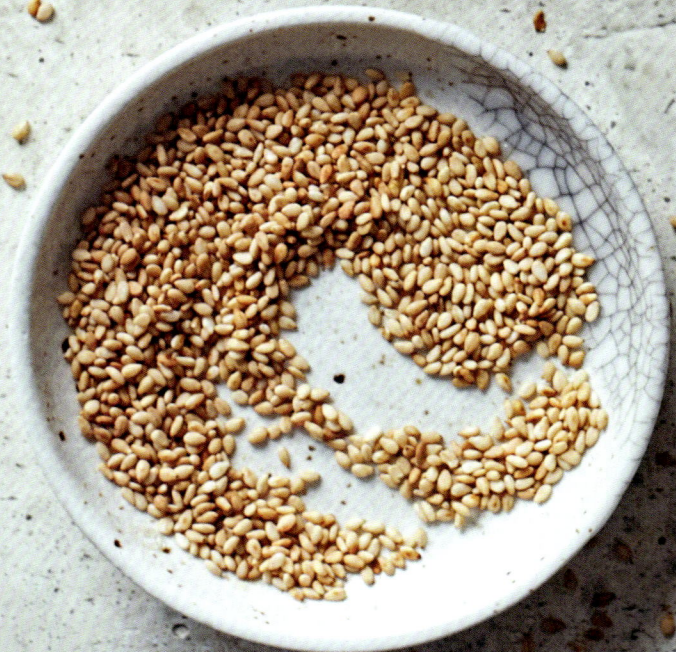

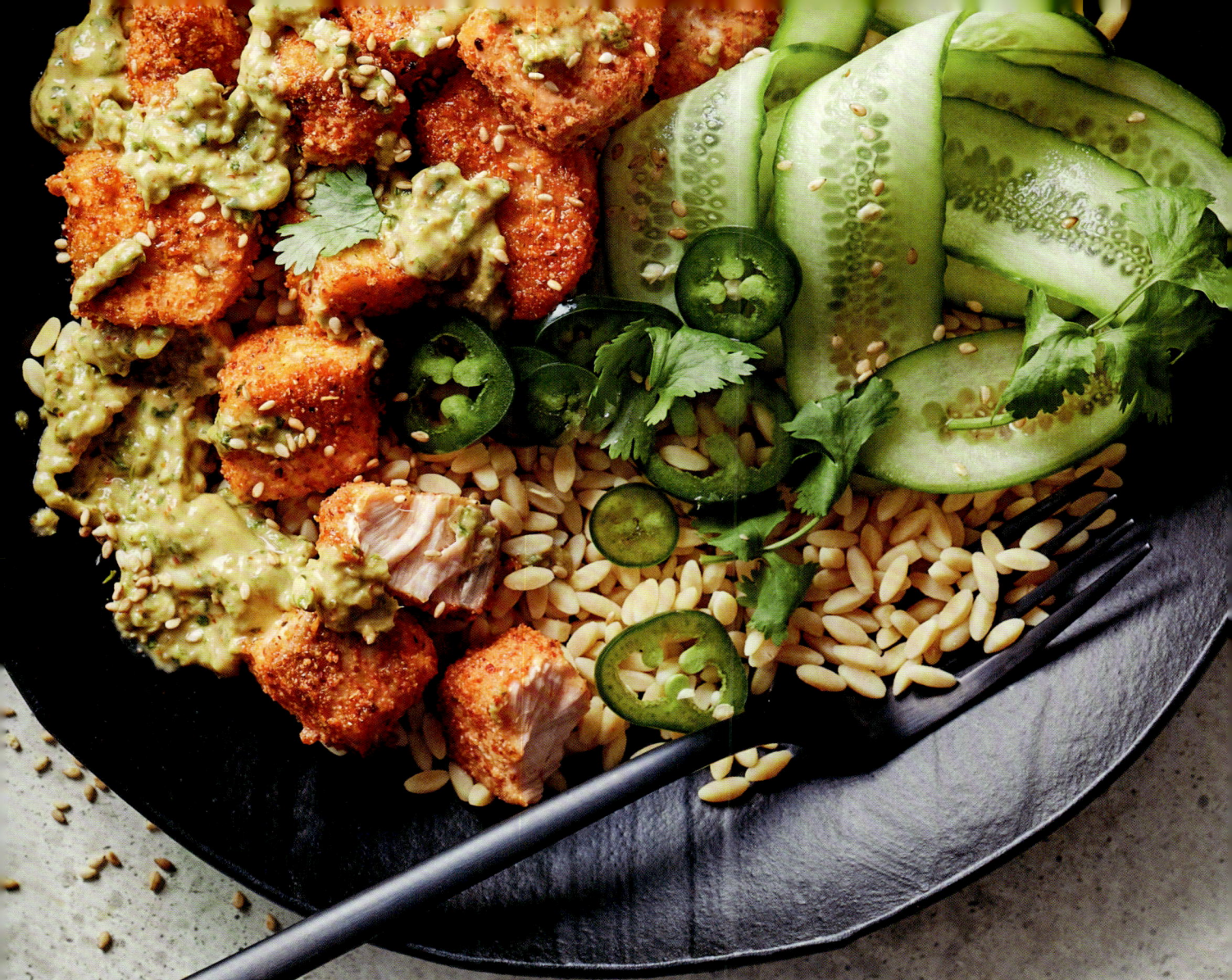

Power Bowls

Power bowls played a critical part in my hundred-pound-plus weight-loss journey. They are nutrient-dense meals that combine a variety of proteins, vegetables, healthy fats, and flavorful sauces into a single dish. These bowls are not only visually appealing but also incredibly nutritious and flavorful, making them great for those who want to fuel up with whole foods. They're also great for meal prep; make a big batch of your chosen protein and base on the weekend, chop up some veggies, and store them in separate containers.

You can use whichever base you prefer. Many power recipes use grains like quinoa or rice as their base, but the recipes I've included here were designed to be tasty with low-carb alternatives. Cauliflower rice is one of them, as the taste and texture are quite similar to couscous or quinoa. I also use fresh greens and my Kaizen low-carb rice, which is made with lupini beans.

For your protein, I've got flavors that range from Mediterranean to Asian. And then the toppings are where things get fun and creative! Feel free to use what you love and have on hand. Some of my go-tos are sliced avocado, nuts and seeds, fresh herbs, chopped or pickled vegetables, lemon juice, or feta cheese.

Middle Eastern Chicken & Rice Power Bowl

With bold spices and vibrantly fresh ingredients, this Middle Eastern–inspired power bowl ain't messing around when it comes to flavor and nutrition! Consider it your go-to meal for busy weeknights or lazy weekends when you want something hearty and healthy without spending long in the kitchen. Even better, make it ahead of time for a quick and easy lunch option throughout the week. The key here is the marinade, which is infused with Middle Eastern staples like cumin, paprika, yogurt, and lemon juice. Serve it over a salad with fresh veggies like red onion, tomatoes, and herbs, and top with a tangy, creamy white sauce for the perfect balance of flavor and texture.

1. Place the chicken thighs in a bowl and drizzle with 1½ tablespoons of the olive oil. Season with the smoked paprika, garlic powder, thyme, red pepper flakes, cumin, cinnamon, yogurt, lemon juice, and salt and pepper. Mix well.

2. This can be cooked right away, but ideally, let this marinate in the fridge for 4 to 6 hours before cooking it.

3. If marinating the chicken in the fridge, take it out 30 minutes before you want to cook it. While it's coming to room temperature, prepare your toppings.

4. **For the salad:** In a large bowl, combine the onion, cherry tomatoes, parsley, sumac, lemon juice, and salt and pepper. Mix well, then set aside.

PREP TIME: 30 MINUTES, PLUS 4 TO 6 HOURS MARINATING
COOK TIME: 15 MINUTES
SERVINGS: 4 TO 6

---

2 pounds boneless, skinless chicken thighs

2½ tablespoons olive oil

1 tablespoon smoked paprika

1 tablespoon garlic powder

1 tablespoon dried thyme

½ tablespoon crushed red pepper flakes

½ teaspoon ground cumin

¼ teaspoon ground cinnamon

2 tablespoons plain yogurt

5 tablespoons freshly squeezed lemon juice

Salt and freshly ground black pepper

FOR THE SALAD

1 red onion, thinly sliced

10 cherry tomatoes, cut in quarters

2 tablespoons finely chopped fresh parsley

2 tablespoons sumac

5 tablespoons freshly squeezed lemon juice

Salt and freshly ground black pepper

(recipe and ingredients continue)

5. **For the white sauce:** In a small bowl, combine the yogurt, mayo, pickle juice, dill, and salt and pepper to taste. Mix well, taste, and adjust. If you don't have pickle juice, you can replace it with half as much red wine vinegar.

6. Heat the remaining 1 tablespoon of olive oil in a cast-iron pan over medium heat.

7. When the oil is hot, add the chicken and sear it for about 4 minutes on each side first, then flip and cook for another 1 to 2 minutes on each side again, depending on the thickness of the thighs, until the outside is golden brown and the inside is fully cooked with no pink remaining.

8. Cook the rice per the instructions on the packaging.

9. When the rice is cooked, add a serving of it to a bowl, place 1 or 2 seared thighs on top, then pile it high with the salad, add some sliced mini cucumbers (if using), and drizzle it up with the white sauce.

FOR THE WHITE SAUCE

¼ cup plain yogurt

3 tablespoons mayonnaise

3 to 4 tablespoons pickle juice

2 tablespoons finely chopped fresh dill

Salt and freshly ground black pepper

8 ounces Kaizen rice or regular basmati rice

2 Persian or mini cucumbers, finely sliced (optional)

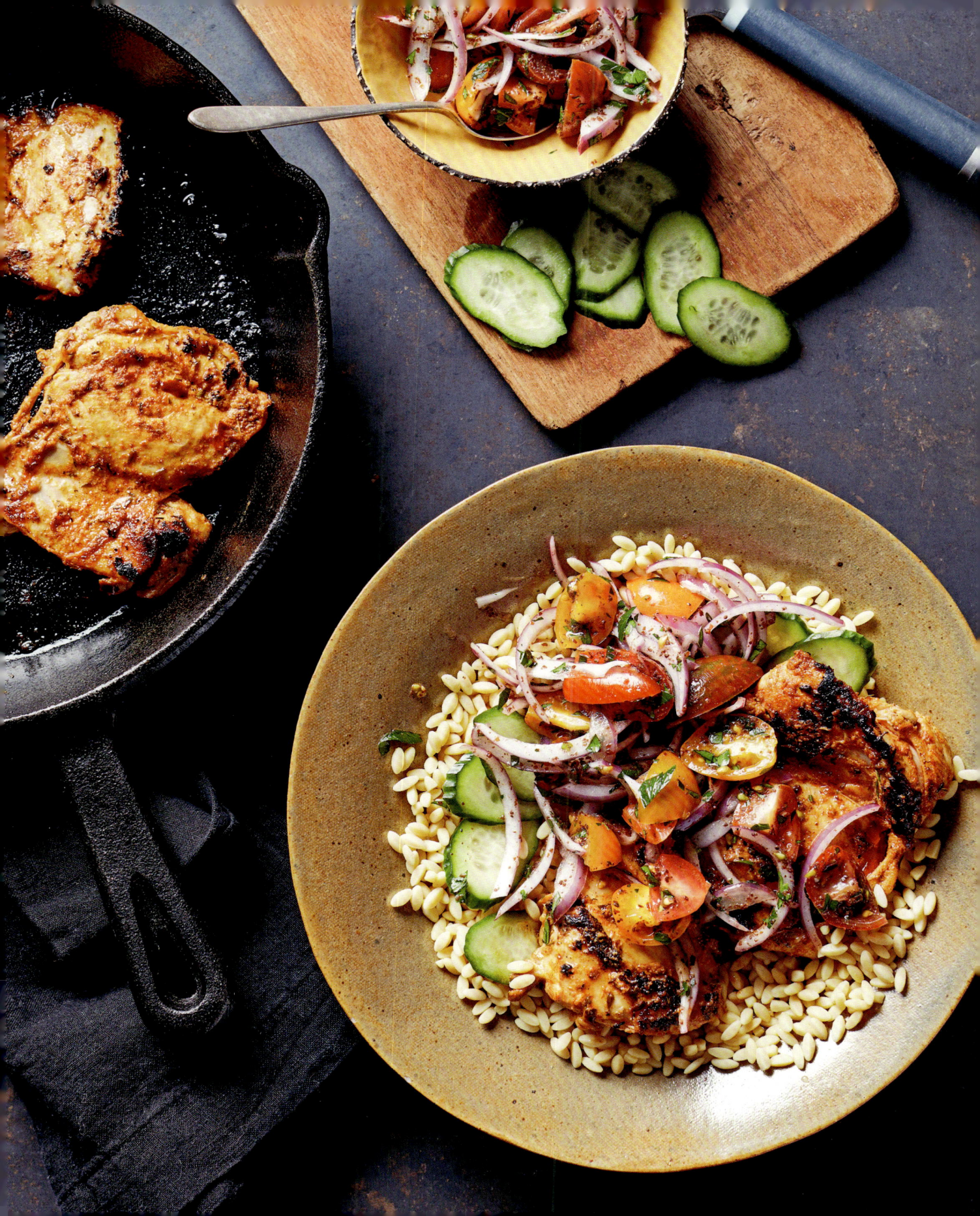

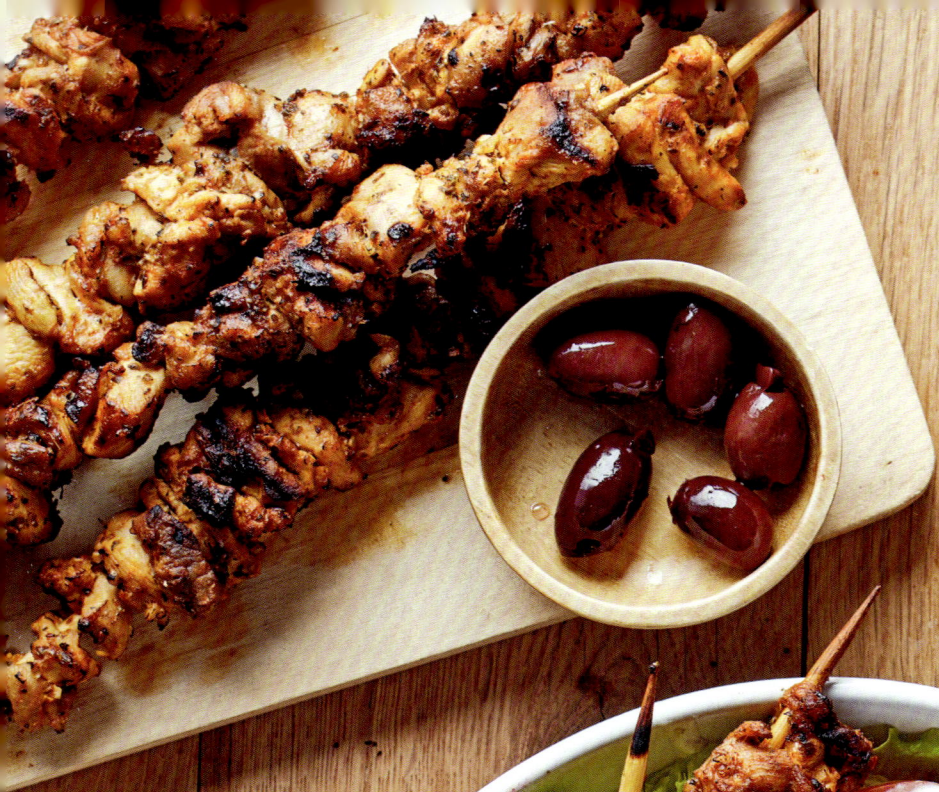

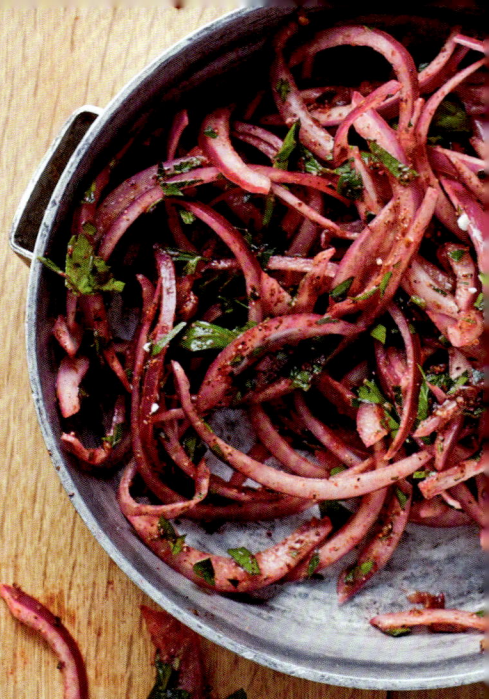

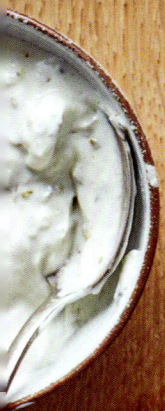

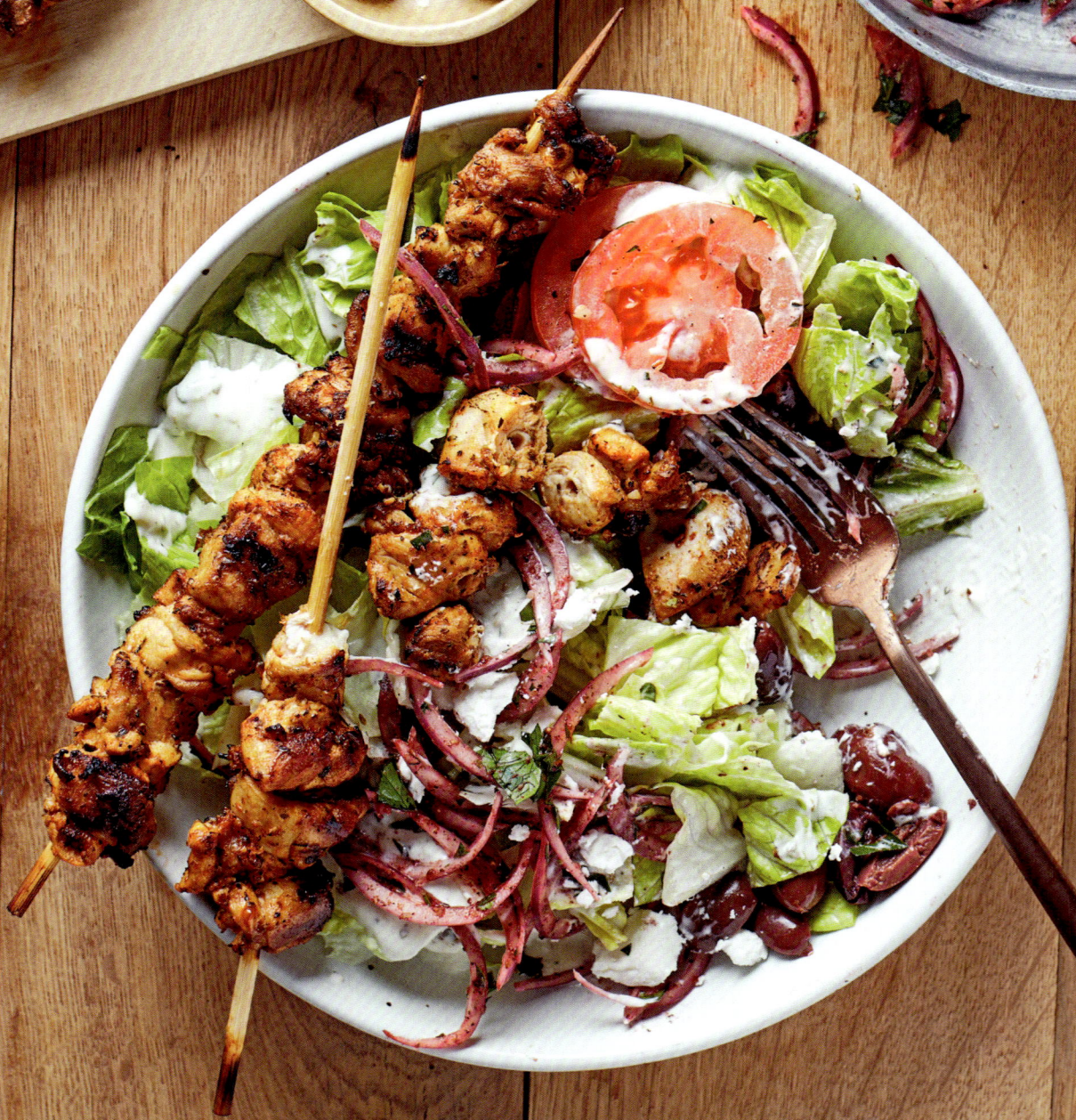

Mediterranean Chicken Power Bowl

This chicken power bowl was created out of a love of Mediterranean cuisine and a desire to eat healthy and filling food. The chicken is marinated in lemon juice and spices for a burst of tangy flavor, and cooked over the stovetop for an easy meal that tastes even better than takeout. No need for a carb-y base! This juicy chicken tastes superb over a bed of lettuce, tomato, and my easy homemade tzatziki, used as a sauce. Top it off with some red onion, sumac, lemon juice, and chopped parsley for an epic meal that will leave you feeling full and energized.

1. Cut the chicken thighs into 1-inch cubes and place in a bowl. Add the lemon juice, olive oil, garlic, smoked paprika, oregano, and cayenne. Season with salt and pepper. Massage the meat with the marinade and place it on skewers. Let it marinate for about an hour.

2. **For the pickled onion:** In a small bowl, combine the onion strips, sumac, lemon juice, parsley, and salt and pepper to taste. Give it a quick mix and set aside. (For meal prep, this is a topping you can make in larger batches and store in the fridge for a few days.)

3. Heat the olive oil on a griddle over medium heat. Once the griddle is hot, add the skewers and cook until the chicken is golden brown (5 to 7 minutes per side). Remove the chicken from the skewers before serving.

4. In a serving bowl, combine the chopped lettuce and sliced tomatoes, and drizzle the tzatziki over top.

5. Add the grilled chicken and top with the pickled onion, feta, olives, and more fresh parsley.

6. Serve as a standalone, with your favorite chips, or in a pita wrap.

PREP TIME: 45 MINUTES, PLUS 1 HOUR MARINATING
COOK TIME: 30 MINUTES
SERVINGS: 4

6 boneless, skinless chicken thighs, about 4 to 5 ounces each

5 tablespoons freshly squeezed lemon juice

1 tablespoon olive oil

4 garlic cloves, minced

1 teaspoon smoked paprika

1 tablespoon dried oregano

½ teaspoon cayenne pepper

Salt and freshly ground black pepper

FOR THE PICKLED ONION

1 red onion, cut into thin strips

1 tablespoon sumac

5 tablespoons freshly squeezed lemon juice

3 tablespoons chopped fresh parsley, plus extra for garnish

Salt and freshly ground black pepper

1 tablespoon olive oil

1 head of romaine lettuce, chopped

2 medium tomatoes, sliced

Tzatziki (page 71) (prep while the meat marinates)

4 ounces feta cheese, crumbled

2 tablespoons pitted kalamata olives, diced

Korean Beef Bowl

There's nothing quite like Korean cuisine, with its savory flavors and colorful dishes. If you're a fan of Korean-style beef like I am, then you definitely need to try this delicious Korean beef bowl recipe. The beef is cut super thin and marinated in a flavorful mixture of soy sauce, sesame oil, gochujang, garlic, and ginger, with monk fruit sweetener as the low-carb sugar substitute. Once you cook the meat and rice (I use my Kaizen low-carb rice for an added boost of protein), all that's left to do is assemble your power bowl with classics like kimchi, sliced avocado, cucumbers, red radishes, and sesame seeds. It's simple yet so satisfying!

1. **For the marinade:** In a medium bowl, combine the soy sauce, monk fruit sweetener, sesame oil, garlic, ginger, gochujang, and the white parts of the scallions and mix well.

2. Cut the beef into thin strips and add it to the bowl. Mix well and let the meat marinate for at least 1 hour.

3. **For the seasoned rice:** Prepare the rice per the instructions on the packaging. Combine the rice vinegar and monk fruit sweetener (if using) and drizzle over the rice. Gently fold the rice—lifting and folding it on top of itself, rather than stirring and smooshing the rice—until the vinegar is evenly mixed in.

4. When the meat is ready to cook, place the avocado oil in a skillet over medium-high heat. Once the oil is hot, add the meat (make sure all the marinade liquid is drained off). Sear for about a minute on each side. The meat should have a nice glazey caramelized look.

5. Grab a bowl and combine the rice, meat, kimchi, avocado, cucumbers, and radishes. Garnish with the sesame seeds and the green parts of the scallions.

PREP TIME: 30 MINUTES,
   PLUS 1 HOUR MARINATING
COOK TIME: 10 MINUTES
SERVINGS: 4 TO 6

___

FOR THE MARINADE

¼ cup soy sauce

2 tablespoons monk fruit sweetener, allulose, or regular sugar

1 tablespoon toasted sesame oil

4 garlic cloves, minced

2 teaspoons freshly grated ginger

1 tablespoon gochujang paste

2 scallions, thinly sliced, white and green parts separate

1 pound rib-eye steak

FOR THE SEASONED RICE

8 ounces Kaizen rice or regular short grain rice

¼ cup rice vinegar (optional)

1 tablespoon monk fruit sweetener (optional)

1 tablespoon avocado oil

5 ounces kimchi

1 medium avocado, sliced

2 mini cucumbers, thinly sliced

3 red radishes, thinly sliced

1 teaspoon toasted sesame seeds, for garnish

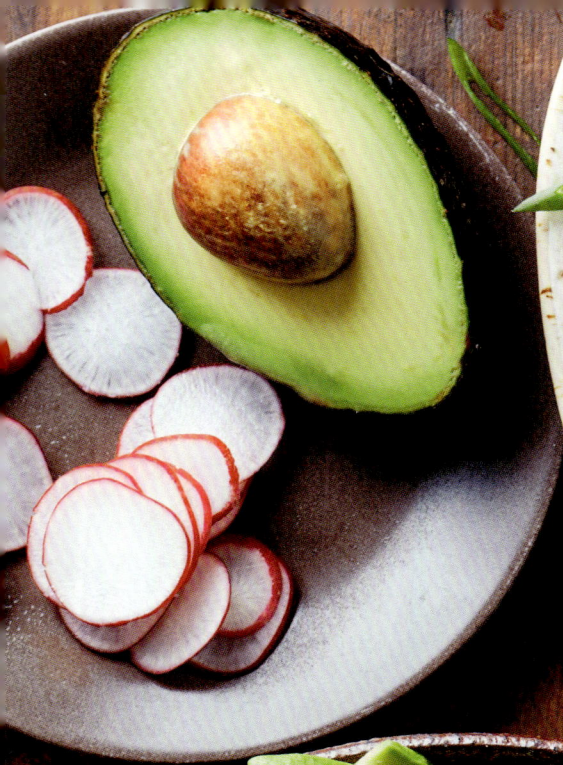

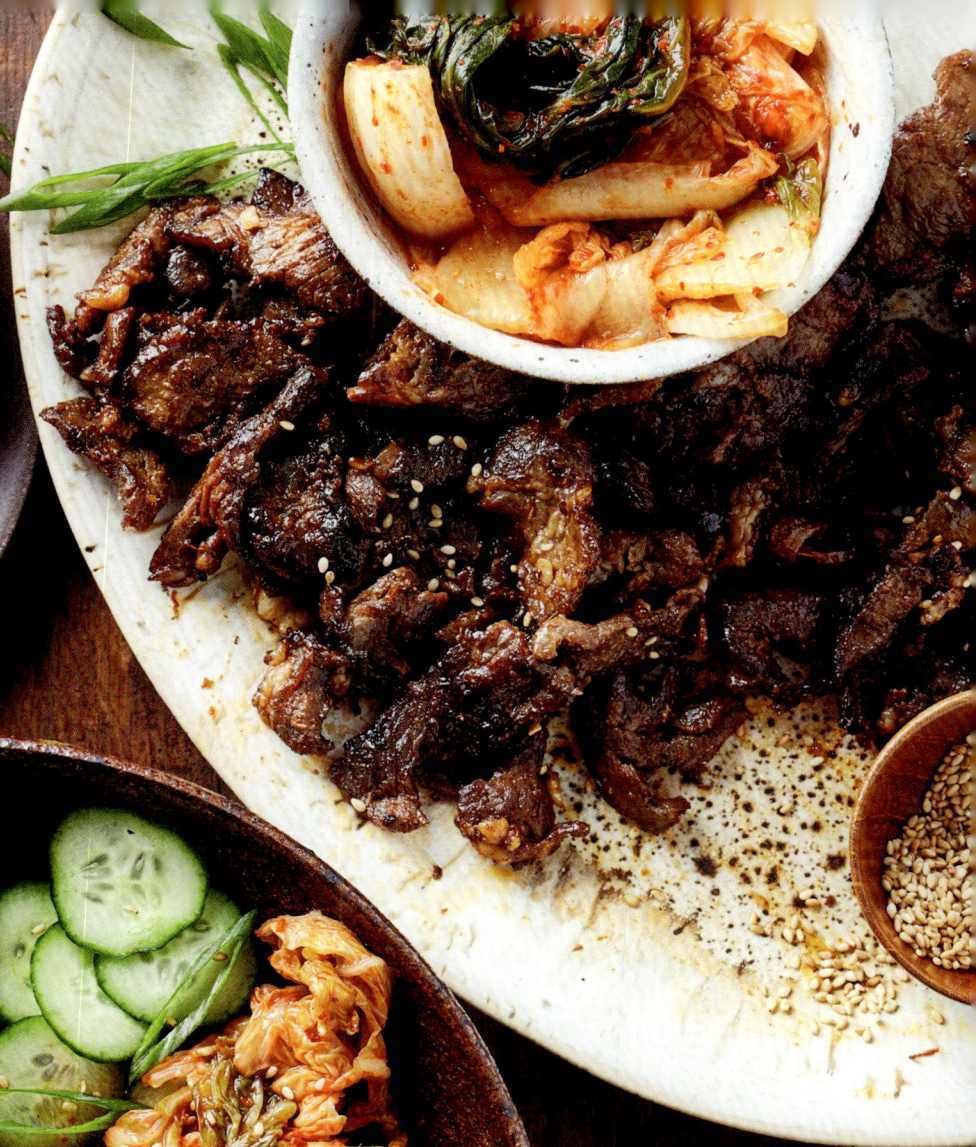

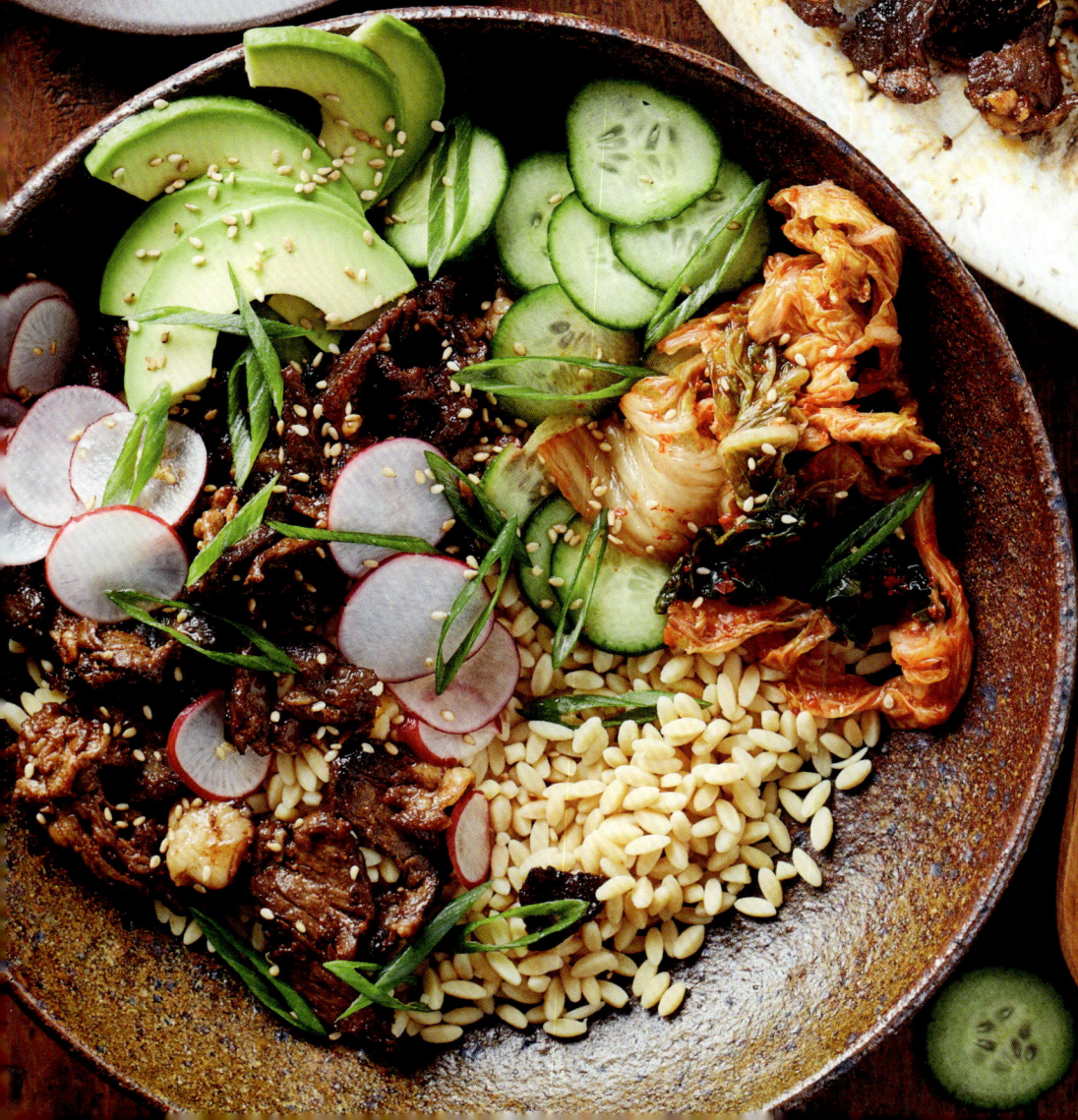

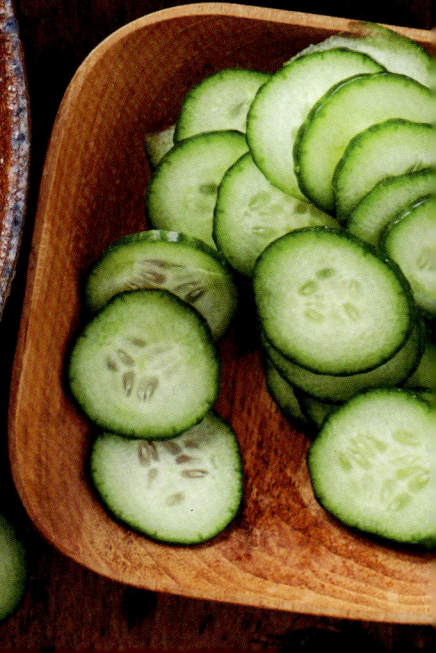

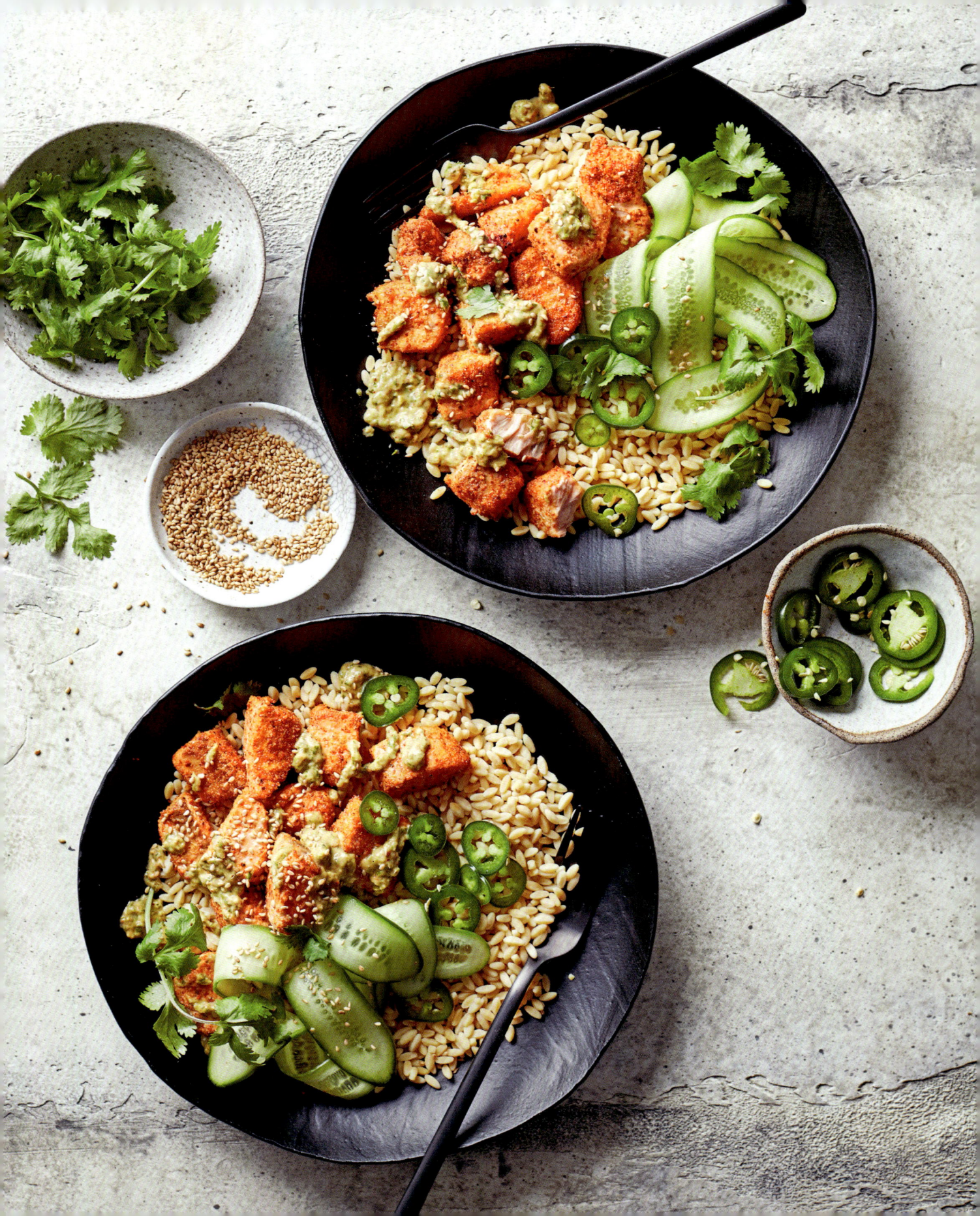

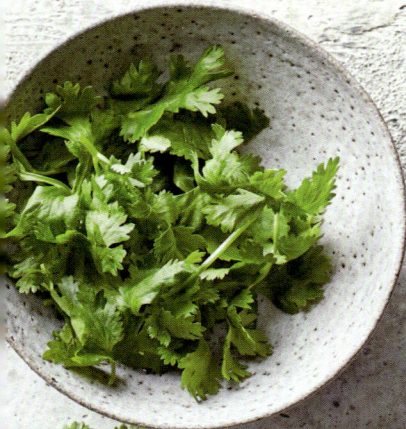

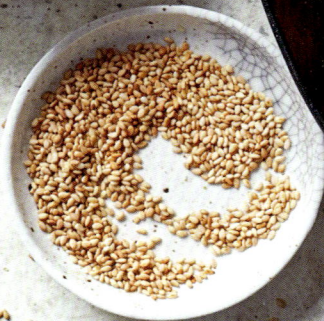

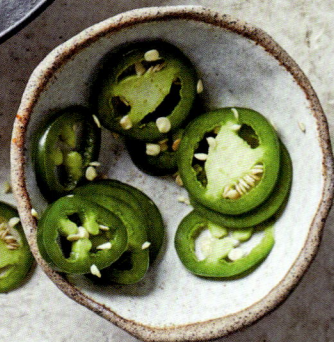

Salmon Power Bowl

This salmon power bowl is absolute perfection with every bite. The combination of flavors, textures, and colors is unreal! The dressing has a spicy kick from the jalapeño and ginger, balanced out by the sweetness of the coconut. Pour it over some air-fried salmon, and you've got a flavorful meal full of protein and healthy fats. It's easy to make and easy to adjust to your liking. Want it more citrusy? Add extra lime juice. Want more heat? Mix in extra jalapeño. Love the coconut element? Pour some more in! The flavor ratio is totally up to you.

1. Preheat the air fryer or oven to 400°F.

2. Cut the salmon into cubes, place in a mixing bowl, and drizzle with the avocado oil. Add the garlic powder, cayenne, and chili lime seasoning. Season with salt and pepper. Toss well so the salmon chunks are coated all over. Place on an air fryer tray or baking sheet.

3. If using the air fryer, cook for 10 to 12 minutes. If using the oven, bake for 8 to 10 minutes. Time varies by air fryer or oven and the size of your nuggets, so you may need to play around to find what works best for you. When gently pressed with a fork, the salmon should easily flake apart. Remove salmon nuggets from the air fryer or oven and let cool.

4. **For the dressing:** In a food processor, combine the ginger, jalapeño, avocado, shallot, chives, cilantro, lime juice, chili lime seasoning, and coconut cream. Blend well and add salt and pepper to taste.

5. Add your base of choice—I like to use raw cauliflower rice. I just add about half a head of cauliflower florets to a food processor and pulse it for a few minutes till I achieve a couscous-like size. I prefer it raw. Alternatively, you can use my Kaizen low-carb rice or any other rice of choice such as a short grain rice or a basmati rice. Just bring a large pot of salted water to a boil and cook the rice per the instructions on the packaging. Drain, rinse, and set as a base in your serving bowl.

6. Top your base with the salmon nuggets, the dressing, and any additional toppings you'd like, such as fresh sliced jalapeño, cucumbers, sesame seeds, fresh cilantro, and more chili lime seasoning.

PREP TIME: 25 MINUTES
COOK TIME: 15 MINUTES
SERVINGS: 4 TO 6

---

1 pound skinless wild salmon

1 tablespoon avocado oil

1½ tablespoons garlic powder

½ teaspoon cayenne pepper

1½ tablespoons chili lime seasoning, such as Tajín

Salt and freshly ground black pepper

FOR THE DRESSING

1-inch piece of fresh ginger

1 jalapeño pepper

½ avocado

⅓ medium shallot

Handful of fresh chives

Handful of fresh cilantro, plus extra for garnish

3 tablespoons freshly squeezed lime juice

1 tablespoon chili lime seasoning

⅓ cup coconut cream

Salt and freshly ground black pepper

BASE AND OPTIONAL TOPPINGS

2 cups raw cauliflower rice (about half a head of cauliflower) or 4 ounces Kaizen rice or regular short grain rice

Sliced jalapeño

Persian or mini cucumbers

Sesame seeds

Fresh cilantro

Chili lime seasoning

Baharat Steak Bowl

Baharat is a Middle Eastern spice blend that has become increasingly popular all over the world. It's mildly sweet and smoky and has a deep, rich flavor that goes so well with the juicy rib-eye steak in this recipe. Marinate the steak and cook it right away, or leave it for a few hours with the spices for bolder flavors. Grill it until perfectly charred on the outside and medium rare on the inside. The complex savory flavors of the meat taste amazing with the fresh, lemony, and herby veggie topping, and it's all placed over a bed of my Kaizen low-carb rice for a magnificent high-protein, low-carb meal.

1. Cut the meat against the grain in thin strips and place it in a medium bowl.

2. Slice the onion into thin strips and add to the meat.

3. **For the marinade:** In a small mixing bowl, combine the monk fruit sweetener, baharat, olive oil, lemon juice, garlic, baking soda, Aleppo pepper, and salt and pepper to taste and mix well.

4. Pour the marinade over the meat and onions and massage them until thoroughly coated. Set the meat aside to marinate while preparing the rest of the ingredients. For bolder flavors, let the meat marinate in the fridge for 2 hours or overnight.

5. In a medium bowl, combine the shallot, cucumbers, cherry tomatoes, mint, garlic, lemon juice, sumac, za'atar spice blend, olive oil, and salt and pepper to taste. Give it a mix.

6. Prepare the rice per the instructions on the package.

7. Cut the feta into ¼-inch cubes.

8. Place a medium grill skillet over medium-high heat. Once the skillet is hot, add the meat and sear it for a couple of minutes on each side. The meat should have a nice sear on the outside but still be moist and medium to medium rare on the inside.

9. Grab a serving bowl and add the rice or whatever base you're using with the seared meat and veggies. Top with the feta. Serve right away.

PREP TIME: 30 MINUTES, PLUS 2 HOURS TO OVERNIGHT MARINATING (OPTIONAL)
COOK TIME: 15 MINUTES
SERVINGS: 4 TO 6

---

1 pound rib-eye steak

½ medium onion

FOR THE MARINADE

1 teaspoon monk fruit sweetener or regular sugar

1 tablespoon baharat blend

2 tablespoons olive oil

2 tablespoons freshly squeezed lemon juice

3 garlic cloves, minced

1 teaspoon baking soda

½ teaspoon Aleppo pepper

Salt and freshly ground black pepper

1 medium shallot, minced

2 Persian or mini cucumbers, diced in ¼-inch cubes

10 cherry tomatoes, cut in quarters

1 tablespoon finely chopped fresh mint leaves

2 garlic cloves, minced

2 tablespoons freshly squeezed lemon juice

½ tablespoon sumac

½ tablespoon za'atar, homemade (page 222)

2 tablespoons olive oil

Salt and freshly ground black pepper

8 ounces Kaizen rice, couscous, regular basmati rice, or cauliflower rice

2 ounces feta cheese

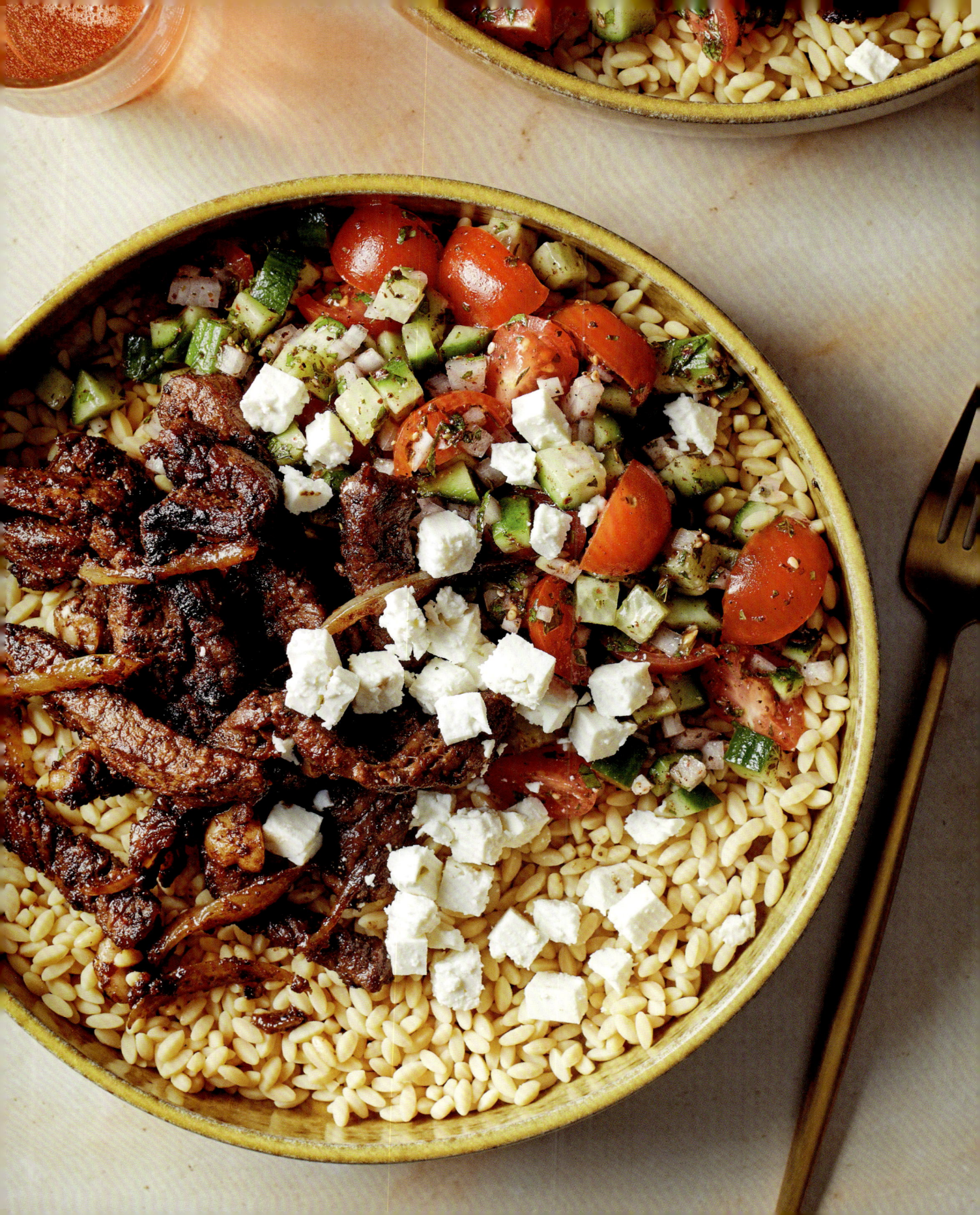

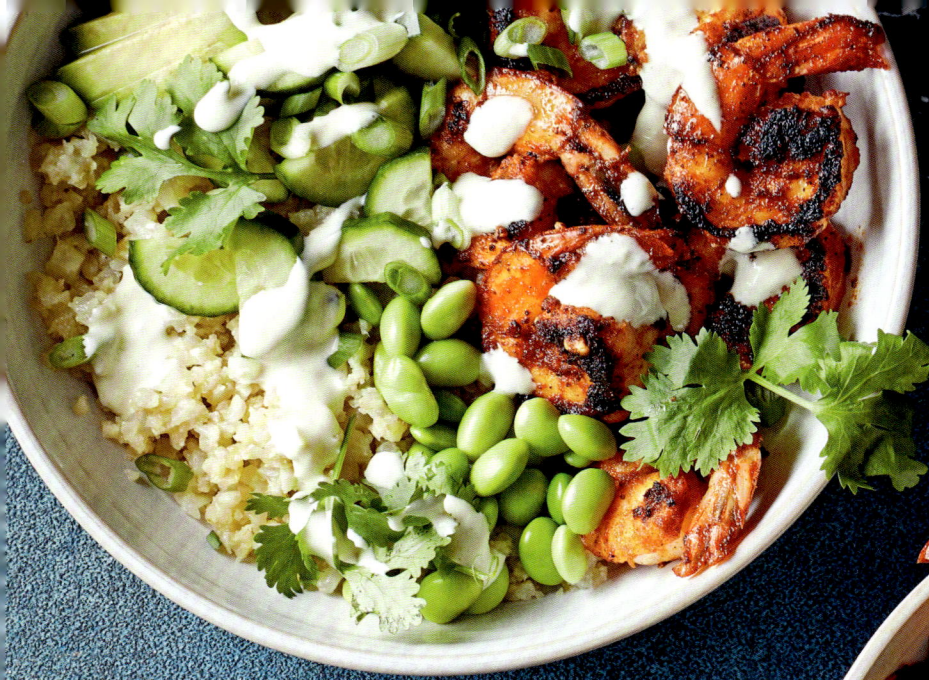

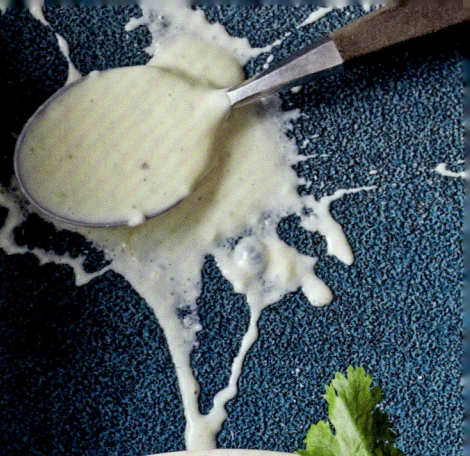

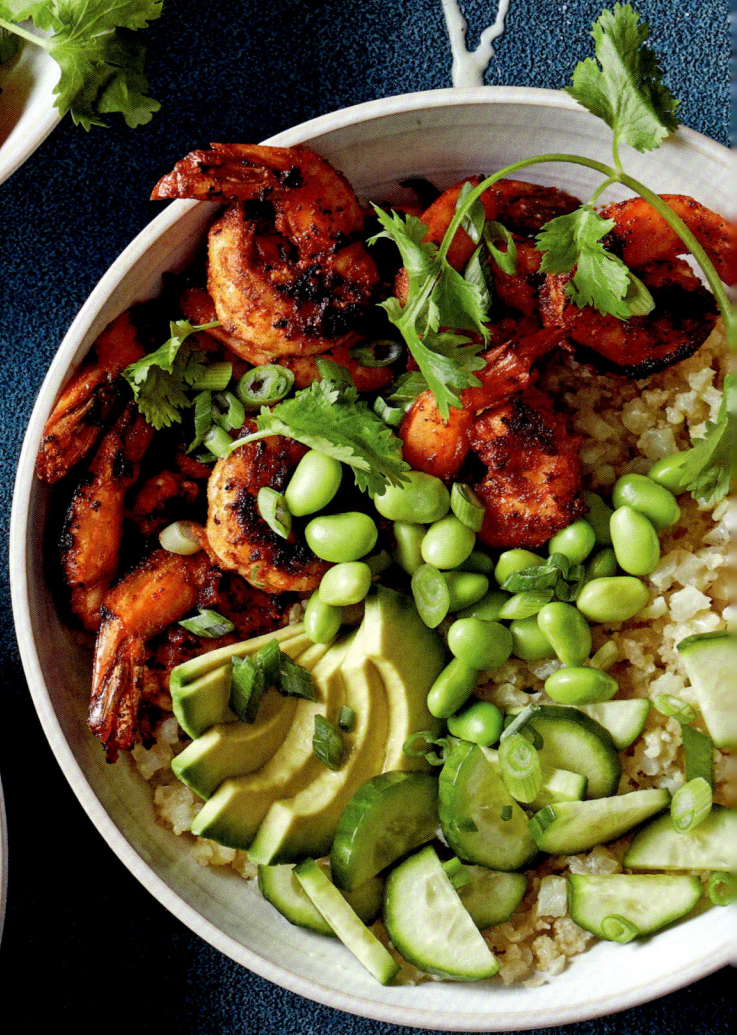

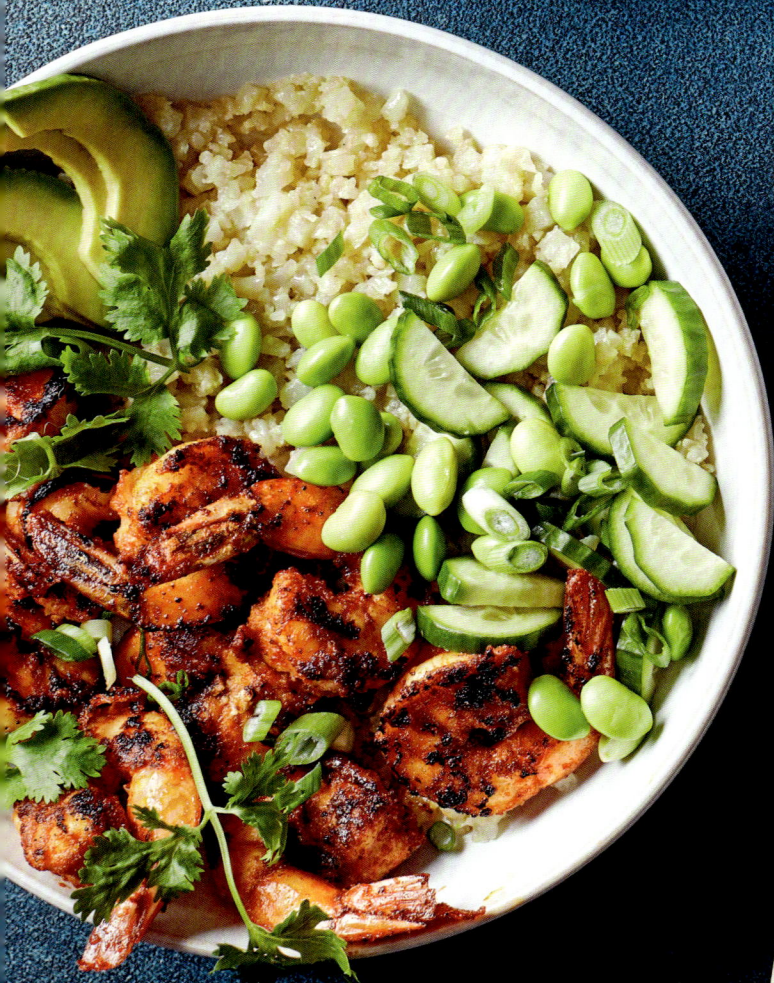

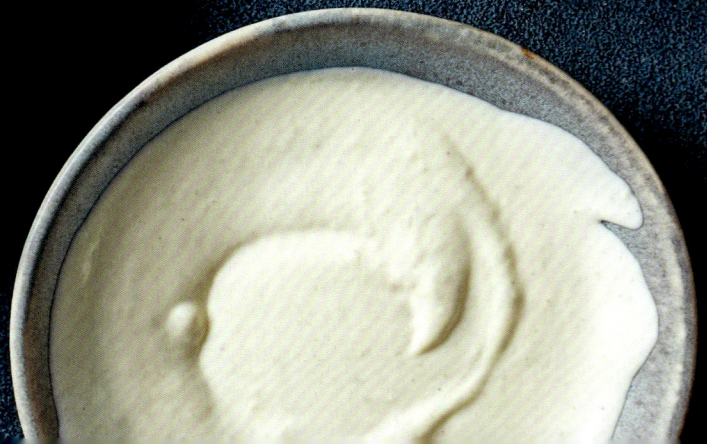

Shrimp Power Bowl

This shrimp power bowl is light, smoky, and so easy to make. The wasabi lime sauce and fresh toppings of Persian cucumber, cilantro, scallions, and avocado get whipped up in a matter of minutes, and the seasoned shrimp cooks quickly. It's great for those lazy cooking days when you're craving something healthy, filling, and flavorful. It's also great for meal prep.

1. Pat the shrimp dry with a paper towel and place them in a medium bowl. Add the avocado oil, cayenne, smoked paprika, garlic powder, and salt and pepper to taste. Toss well to coat the shrimp evenly. Set aside while you prep the sauce and toppings.

2. **For the wasabi lime sauce:** In a small bowl, combine the garlic, wasabi, mayo, rice vinegar, lime juice, and salt and pepper to taste. Mix well.

3. Dice the mini cucumbers into small cubes, chop the cilantro, slice the scallion and avocado, and set aside.

4. Set a pan over medium heat, drizzle with the oil, then add the shrimp and cook for about 1 minute on each side. (Tip: You don't want to overcook shrimp, as it becomes rubbery.) Remove the shrimp from the heat when they are pink and opaque throughout with a slight curl.

5. Add your base of choice—I like to use raw cauliflower rice. I just add about half a head of cauliflower florets to a food processor and pulse it for a few minutes till I achieve a couscous-like size. I prefer it raw. Alternatively, you can use my Kaizen low-carb rice or any other rice of choice, such as a short grain rice or a basmati rice. Just bring a large pot of salted water to a boil and cook the rice per the instructions on the packaging. Drain, rinse, and set as a base in your serving bowl.

6. Top with the shrimp, veggies, edamame, and wasabi lime sauce and serve right away.

PREP TIME: 20 MINUTES
COOK TIME: 10 MINUTES
SERVINGS: 4

1 pound raw shrimp, peeled and deveined

2 tablespoons avocado oil

2 teaspoons cayenne pepper

1 tablespoon smoked paprika

1 tablespoon garlic powder

Salt and freshly ground black pepper

FOR THE WASABI LIME SAUCE

2 garlic cloves, crushed

2 teaspoons wasabi paste

¼ cup mayonnaise

2 tablespoons rice vinegar

1 tablespoon freshly squeezed lime juice

Salt and freshly ground black pepper

2 Persian or mini cucumbers

Handful of fresh cilantro

1 scallion, white and green parts

1 medium avocado

1 tablespoon olive oil

2 cups raw cauliflower rice (about half a cauliflower head) or 4 ounces Kaizen rice or regular short grain rice

½ cup shelled edamame

Taco Power Bowl

This taco power bowl is packed with all your favorite Mexican-inspired flavors but with a healthy twist: my Kaizen low-carb rice as the base, generously seasoned lean ground beef, and fresh sautéed veggies topped with homemade guac and chipotle aioli. If you're a Chipotle regular, you're going to be obsessed with this dish.

PREP TIME: 40 MINUTES
COOK TIME: 30 MINUTES
SERVINGS: 4 TO 6

FOR THE GUAC

1 large avocado

2 tablespoons minced red onion

2 tablespoons finely chopped fresh cilantro

1 tablespoon minced jalapeño pepper

2 tablespoons freshly squeezed lime juice

1 garlic clove, minced

Salt and freshly ground black pepper

FOR THE SAUTÉED VEGGIES

1 tablespoon avocado oil

1 large red onion, thinly sliced

2 bell peppers, thinly sliced

½ tablespoon onion powder

½ tablespoon smoked paprika

Salt and freshly ground black pepper

FOR THE MEAT

1 tablespoon avocado oil

1 pound 80/20 ground beef

½ tablespoon chipotle powder

½ tablespoon smoked paprika

1 teaspoon ground cumin

½ teaspoon onion powder

½ teaspoon garlic powder

½ teaspoon dried oregano

Salt and freshly ground black pepper

BASE AND TOPPINGS

8 ounces Kaizen low-carb rice or regular basmati rice

1 head romaine lettuce, shredded

1 jalapeño pepper, sliced

Smoky Chipotle Aioli (page 208)

1. **For the guac:** In a small bowl, combine the avocado, red onion, cilantro, jalapeño, lime juice, garlic, and salt and pepper to taste. Mash the avocado, leaving some chunks to get that rough texture. (Or finely mash it, if you prefer, into a more paste-like consistency.) Set aside.

2. **For the sautéed veggies:** Heat the avocado oil in a pan over medium heat. Once the oil is hot, add the onion, bell pepper, onion powder, smoked paprika, and salt and pepper to taste. Cook until the onions and peppers turn golden brown around the edges. Remove from the pan and set aside.

3. **For the meat:** In the same pan over medium heat, add the avocado oil. Once the oil is hot, add the ground beef, chipotle powder, paprika, cumin, onion powder, garlic powder, oregano, and salt and pepper. Continue chopping the beef with a spatula to prevent it from clumping. Sauté until browned and crispy and set aside.

4. Cook the rice per the instructions on the packaging.

5. When the rice is cooked, place a serving of it in a bowl, add some taco meat and sautéed veggies, and pile it high with romaine, jalapeño, and a dollop of chunky guac. Drizzle some chipotle aioli on top and serve right away.

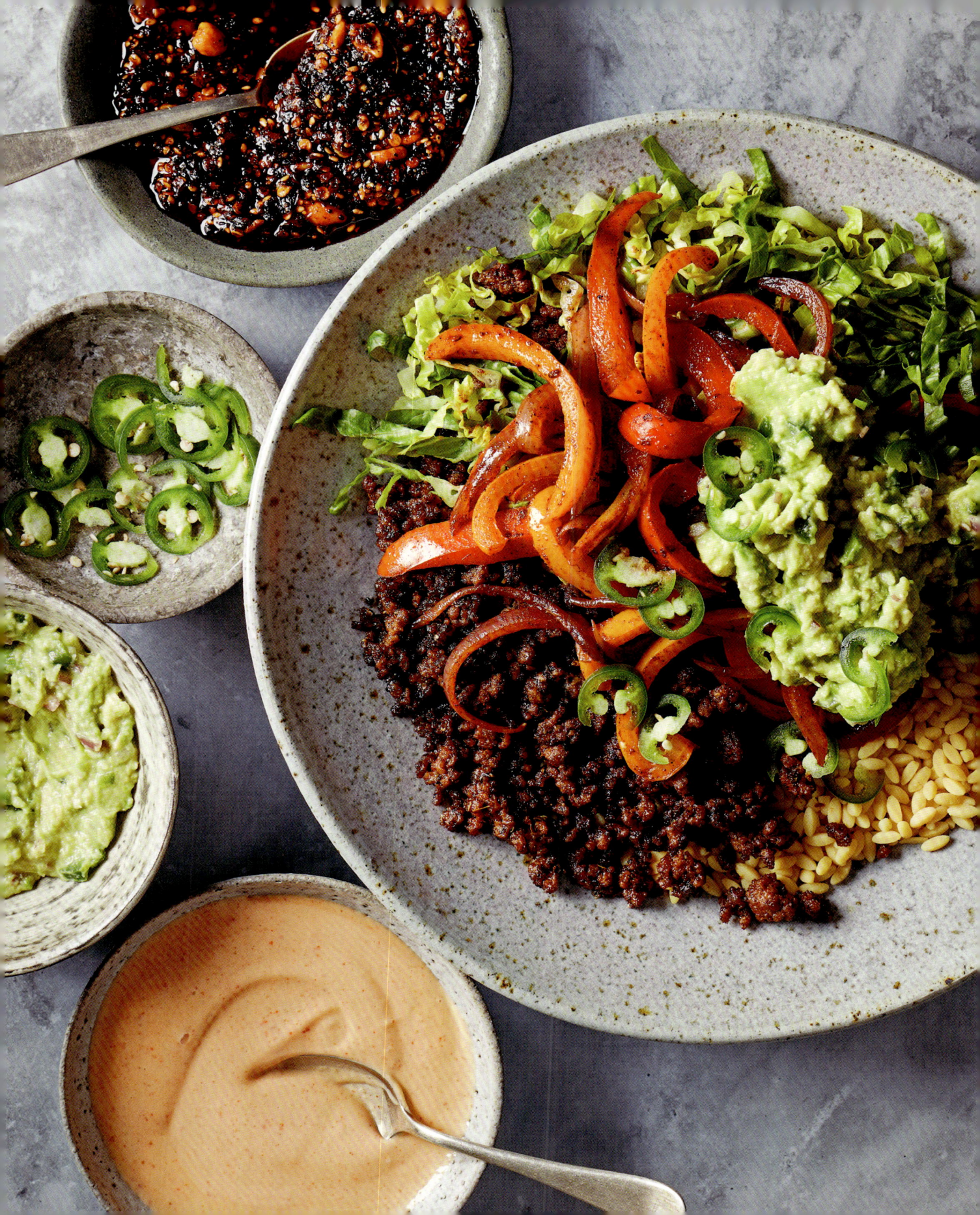

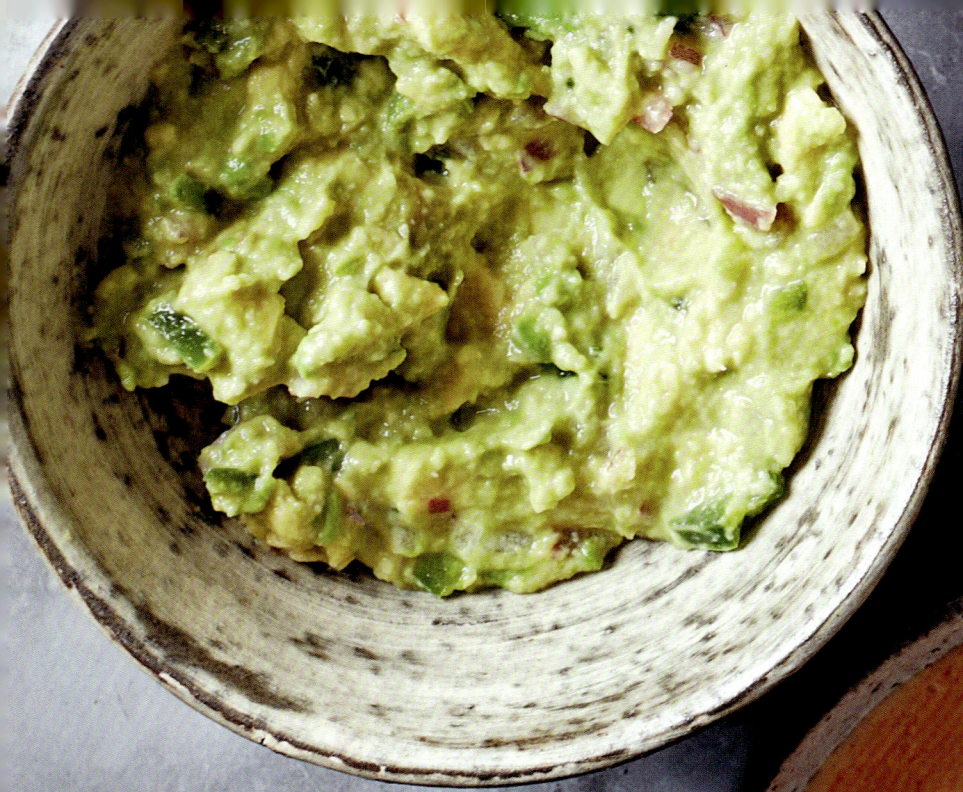

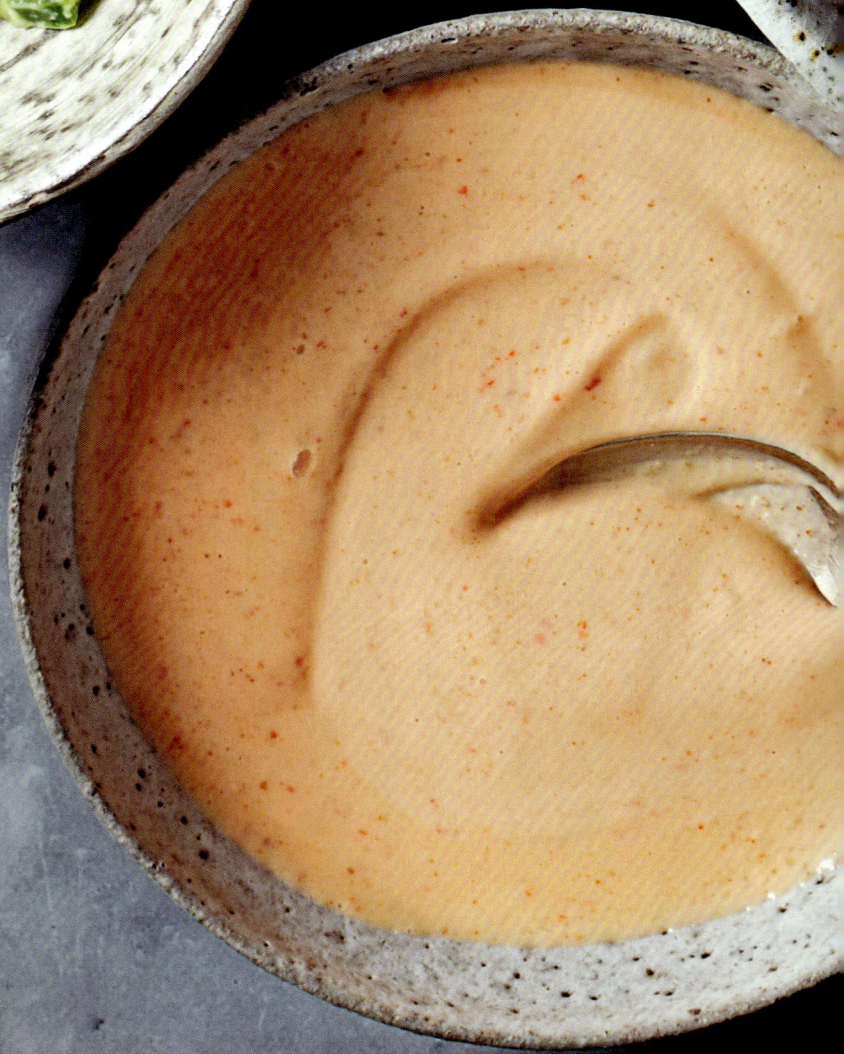

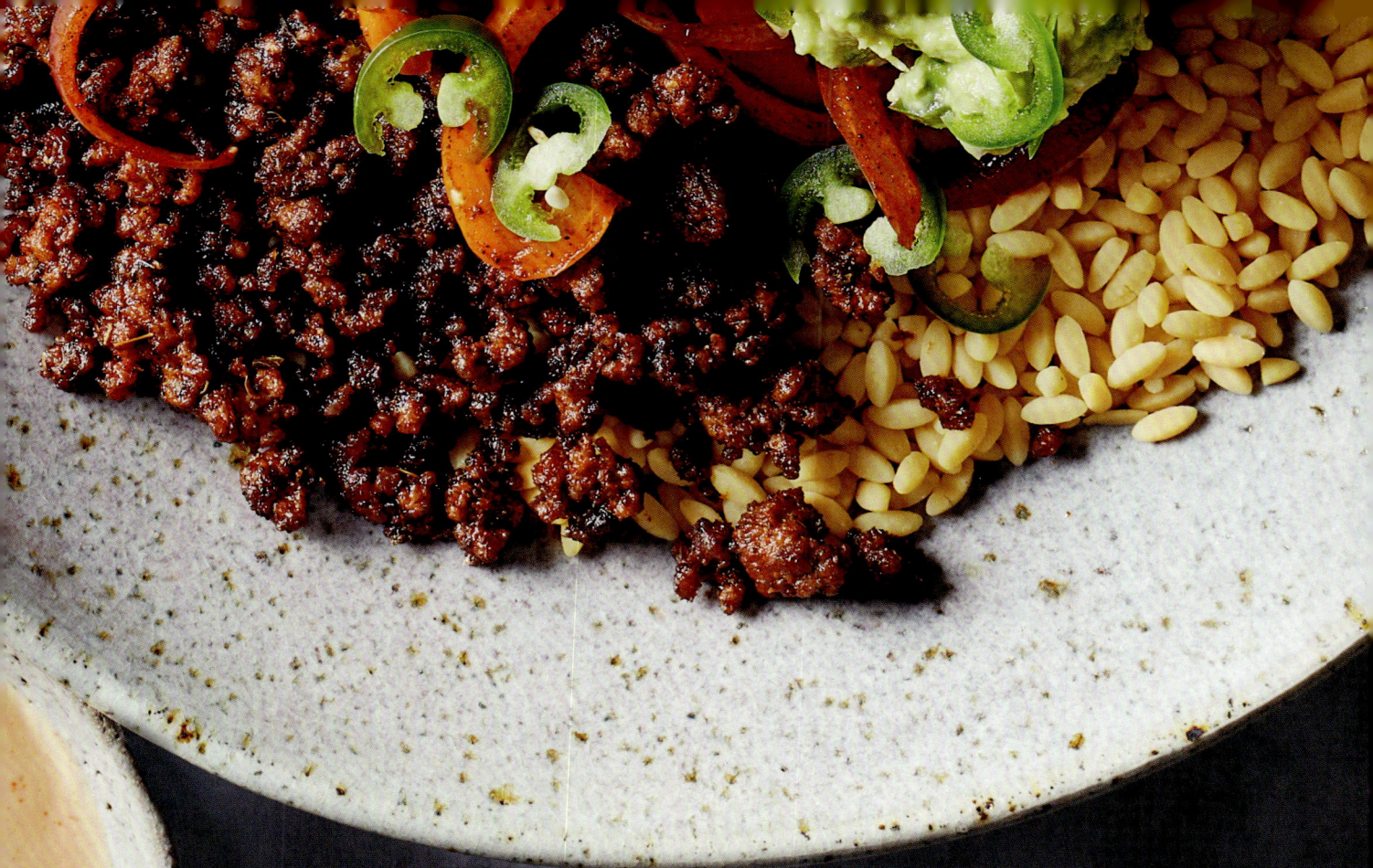

Sauces & Salsas

This chapter is an afterthought in many cookbooks, but not in this one. Sauces and salsas are central to my food philosophy. I keep many of these sauces and salsas in the fridge at all times because, with a scoop here and a drizzle there, they can take any meal to the next level. And I mean any meal—store-bought rotisserie chicken, frozen veggies zapped in the microwave, scrambled eggs with a side salad . . . the humblest dish is elevated into a flavor explosion by these sauces and salsas, and I encourage you to experiment to find your favorites to keep on hand for those busy days and nights.

While these recipes add deliciousness to practically anything they touch, they also hold their own as a dip for veggies or chips, a marinade for meats, or even as a salad dressing. So no, you don't have to worry about leftovers going to waste here! They're highly versatile and easy to repurpose for future meals.

These sauces and salsas are made with fresh ingredients, healthy fats, and spices that pack a punch. Some are creamy, some are tangy, some are refreshing, and some have a kick of heat. But all of them add their own special charm to whatever you're enjoying them with.

Spicy Yum Yum Sauce

Put it on your veggies, drizzle it over rice, dip your meat in it, slather it on bread . . . no matter what you do with Spicy Yum Yum Sauce, one thing is for sure: It brings the yum factor. I like to eat it with my Salmon Skewers (page 151) or drizzled on top of my Korean Beef Bowl (page 188) or in Spicy Tuna Salad (page 79). This recipe is a low-carb/keto-friendly variation of the popular Japanese steakhouse sauce. I use monk fruit sweetener or allulose instead of regular sugar to still give it that sweet touch without the carbs. And to give it some heat, I add cayenne pepper, because what's yum without a little spice? Mix it together in under 10 minutes and keep it handy in your fridge for when you need some extra yumminess in your life. This sauce pretty much goes with anything. Keeps well in the fridge for up to a week. PHOTO ON PAGE 202

PREP TIME: 10 MINUTES
MAKES: ABOUT 1½ CUPS

1 tablespoon unsalted butter

1 cup Kewpie mayonnaise or regular mayonnaise

½ tablespoon gochujang paste

1 teaspoon monk fruit sweetener or regular sugar

1 tablespoon sriracha

2 teaspoons garlic powder

1 tablespoon mirin

1 tablespoon rice vinegar

½ teaspoon cayenne pepper

Salt

1. In a small bowl, melt the butter in the microwave for 30 seconds. The butter should be liquid but not hot. If it is too hot, give it a couple of minutes to cool down.

2. In a medium bowl, combine the butter, mayo, gochujang, monk fruit sweetener, sriracha, garlic powder, mirin, rice vinegar, cayenne, and salt to taste. Mix well.

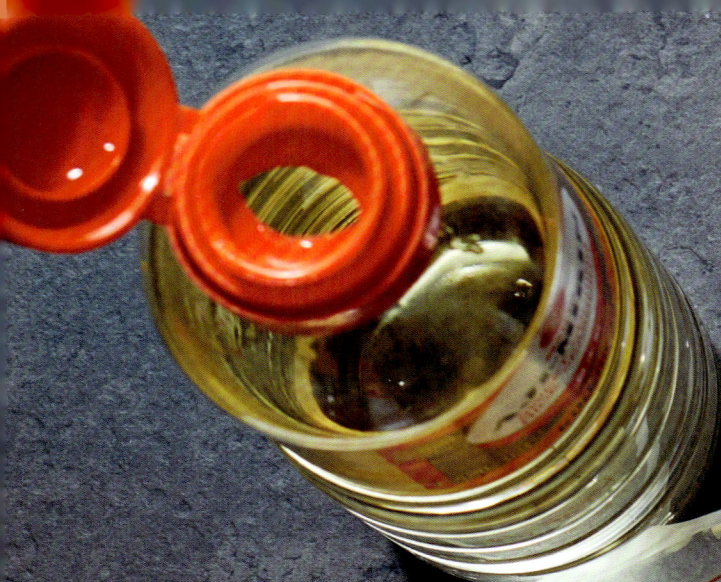

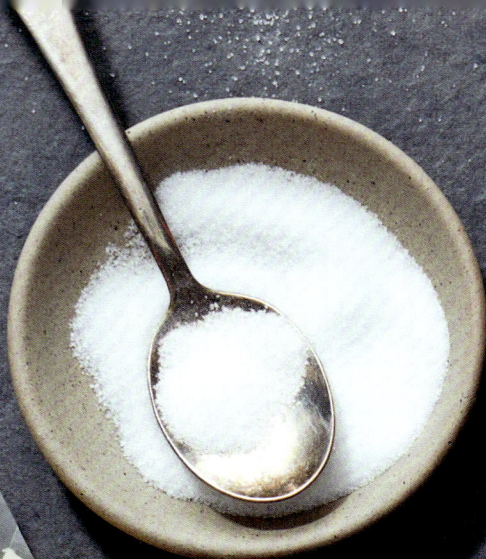

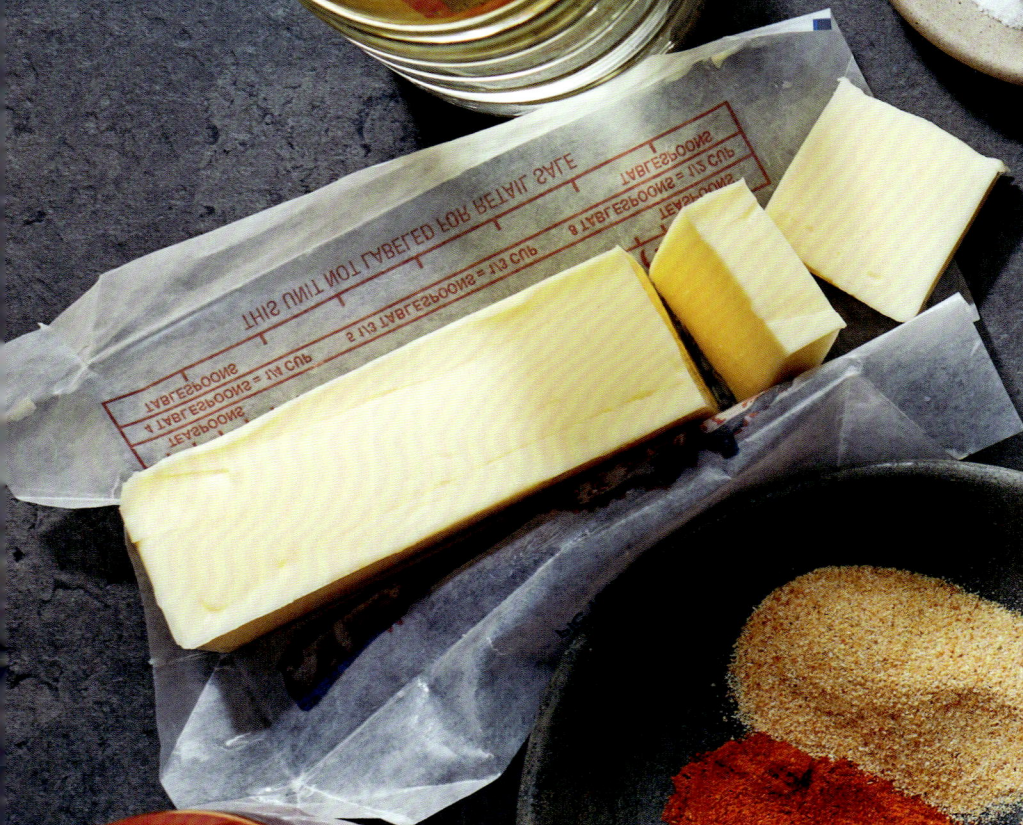

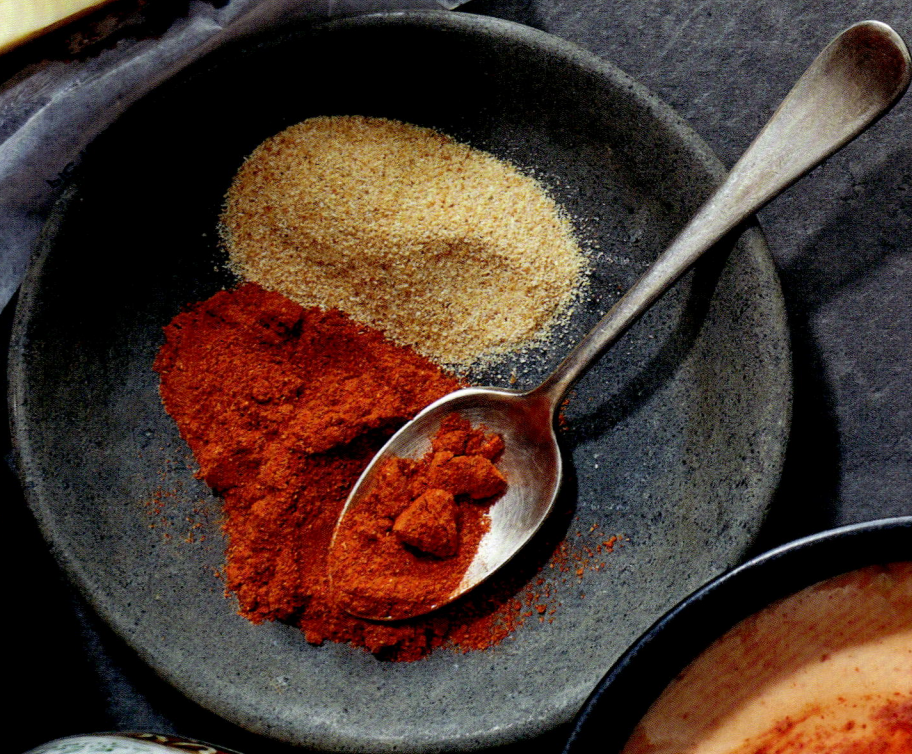

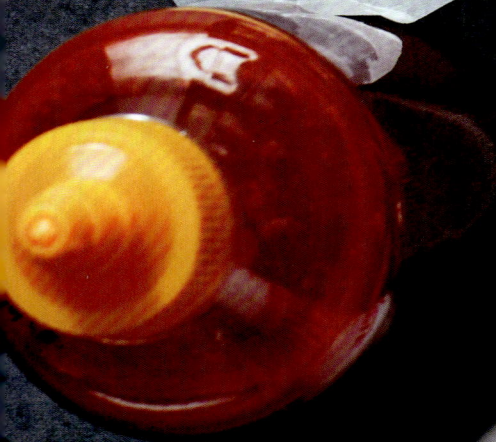

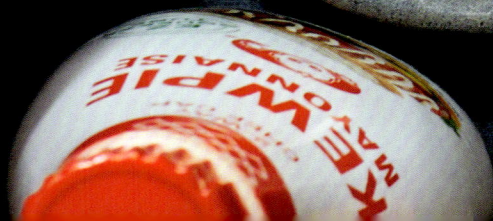

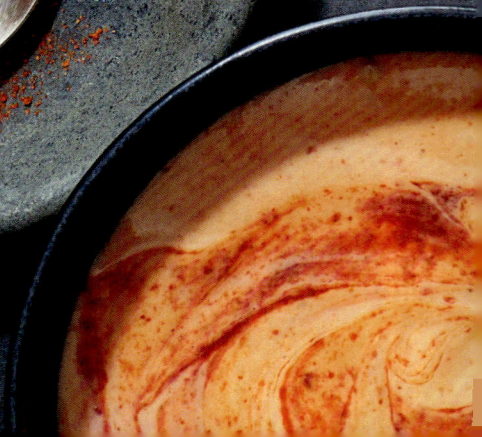

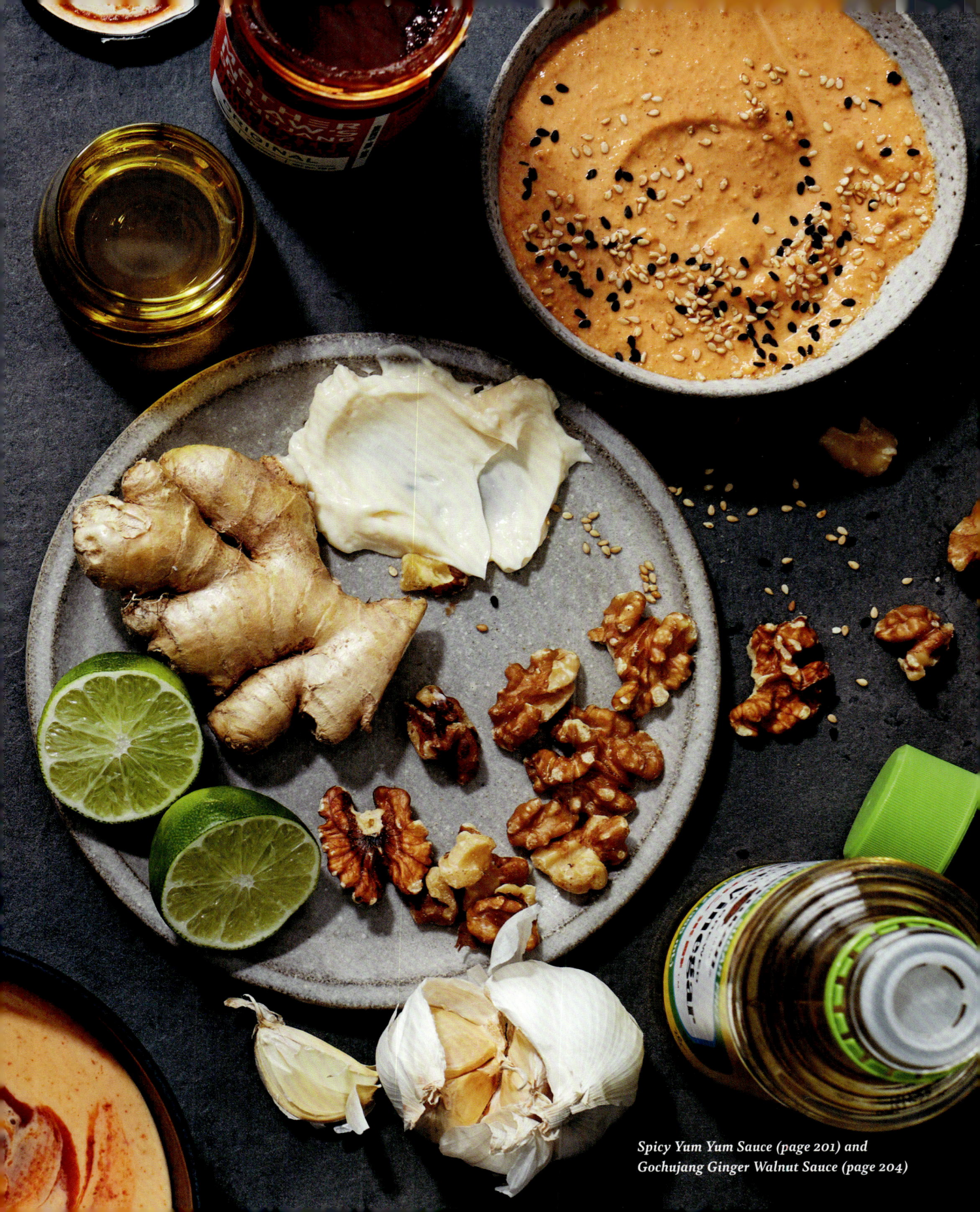

Spicy Yum Yum Sauce (page 201) and
Gochujang Ginger Walnut Sauce (page 204)

Gochujang Ginger Walnut Sauce

After a fun night of experimenting, this spicy gochujang ginger walnut sauce quickly became one of my favorite salad dressings. But the possibilities of this flavorful sauce go beyond salad—pour it over your favorite protein, drizzle it over roasted vegetables, or use it as a marinade to really take it to its full potential! It's made with soaked walnuts, fresh ginger, garlic, and some spicy gochujang, which is a Korean staple and one of my favorites. It adds a spicy, savory, and slightly sweet element that is truly one of a kind. This dressing goes well on any salad, but I like to serve it on a chopped salad with purple cabbage, cucumbers, red bell pepper, jalapeño, avocado, fresh chives, and parsley or cilantro, topped with toasted black or white sesame seeds and tossed well. Enjoy as is, or serve with your favorite protein (chicken or shrimp would be amazing).

PHOTO ON PAGE 203

PREP TIME: 30 MINUTES, PLUS AT LEAST 8 HOURS SOAKING
SERVINGS: 4 TO 6

¼ cup raw walnuts

1-to-2-inch piece of fresh ginger

2 garlic cloves

2 tablespoons avocado oil or olive oil

3 tablespoons rice vinegar

1½ tablespoons freshly squeezed lime juice

3 tablespoons mayonnaise or avocado mayonnaise

2 heaping teaspoons gochujang paste

Salt and freshly ground black pepper

Toasted white or black sesame seeds (optional)

1. Place the walnuts in water and let them soak in the fridge for at least 8 hours.

2. Once the walnuts are soaked, you can begin to prepare the dressing. In a food processor, combine the walnuts, ginger, garlic, oil, rice vinegar, lime juice, mayonnaise, gochujang, and salt and pepper to taste.

3. Give everything a pulse in the food processor, then taste the dressing to see if you want to add anything else. If you want the dressing to be more gingery, add more ginger. If you want the dressing less gingery, add more oil or mayo. If you want the dressing to be more acidic, add more lime.

4. Place in a serving bowl and top with toasted sesame seeds.

Pepitas Salsa Macha

If you're like me and put chili oil on practically everything, you're going to be obsessed with this pepitas salsa macha. This particular recipe is my own take on the classic Mexican condiment. It's made with four kinds of dried chile as well as garlic, to give it lots of flavor and heat. Then I add sesame seeds, toasted peanuts, and pepitas to give it that satisfying crunch. Put it on everything from eggs to pizza, and get ready to fall in love!

PREP TIME: 10 MINUTES
COOK TIME: 30 MINUTES
SERVINGS: 35 TO 40

---

2 ounces dried chile de árbol

½ ounce dried chile morita

1 ounce dried chile guajillo

½ ounce dried chile ancho

1½ cups olive oil

6 garlic cloves

6 teaspoons toasted sesame seeds

1½ ounces toasted peanuts

1 ounce toasted pepitas (pumpkin seeds)

Salt

1. Remove the stems from the chiles. Either toast each type of chile separately or cut the larger chiles (morita, guajillo, and ancho) into smaller pieces to match the chile de árbol.

2. In a medium-size shallow pan, heat ¾ cup of the olive oil over medium-low heat. Once the oil is hot, add the garlic cloves and sauté them for a few minutes, until the garlic is golden brown. Remove from the pan and set aside.

3. Using the same pan, sauté the chiles (either in batches or, if you've cut up the larger ones, together) for 60 to 90 seconds, until fragrant. The chiles are already dry and they can burn fast, so keep an eye on them and continue to stir them with a slotted spoon to prevent burning.

4. Remove the pan from the heat and add the chiles, together with the oil in the pan, the garlic, and half the seeds (sesame, peanuts, and pepitas) to a food processor or blender. Gradually add the remaining ¾ cup olive oil with the machine running. The goal is to obtain a runny consistency, so adjust the oil quantity as needed. Add salt to taste.

5. Once the chiles are well mixed, pour the liquid into a jar, add the remaining sesame seeds, peanuts, and pepitas and give it another mix with a spoon. This can be stored in the pantry for up to a week but best stored in the fridge for up to 3 weeks.

Homemade Lime Aioli

Bright, tangy, and flavorful, my homemade lime aioli is an irresistible sauce that adds a burst of flavor to any dish. This yummy condiment can be used in so many ways—as a dip for fries or veggies, as a sandwich spread, on tacos, in power bowls, or even as a dressing for salads. The best part about it? It's incredibly easy to make at home with just a few ingredients. Just mix everything with an immersion blender, and you'll have a jar of deliciousness ready to go in minutes.

PREP TIME: 15 MINUTES
SERVINGS: 8 TO 10

2 egg yolks, at room temperature

1 tablespoon Dijon mustard

2 tablespoons freshly squeezed lime juice

½ teaspoon lime zest

3 garlic cloves, minced

1 tablespoon finely chopped fresh cilantro

½ teaspoon salt

¼ teaspoon freshly ground black pepper

⅔ cup avocado oil

1. In the mixing jar of an immersion blender, combine the egg yolks, mustard, lime juice, lime zest, garlic, cilantro, salt, and pepper. (You can also use a pint jar that fits the blade end of the blender snugly; at least three-quarters of the jar bottom should be covered by the end of the blender.)

2. Pour in the oil and then allow it to separate and rise to the top, which will take about 30 seconds.

3. Place the immersion blender into the mixing container, so that the bottom of the blender touches the bottom of the container. Hold vertically and blend until the bottom of the mixture has substantially emulsified, about 1 minute.

4. Slowly raise the blender to allow a little more oil at a time to be drawn into the emulsion. Continue until all the oil is incorporated, 3 to 4 minutes.

5. Give the aioli a final stir with the immersion blender, and it is ready to serve.

6. Store in the fridge for up to 4 days.

OPPOSITE FROM TOP TO BOTTOM: *Pepitas Salsa Macha (page 205), Smoky Chipotle Aioli (page 208), and Homemade Lime Aioli.*

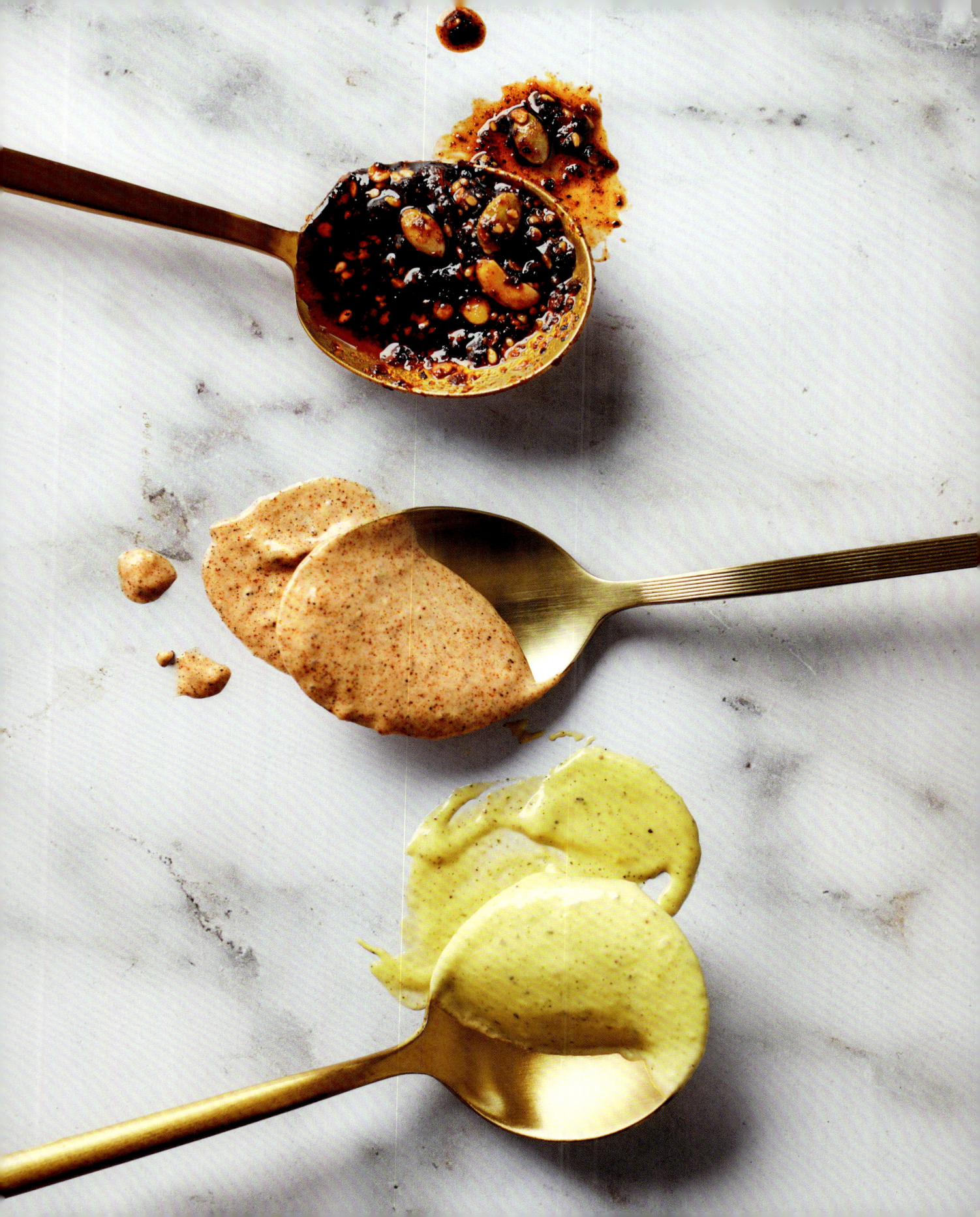

Smoky Chipotle Aioli

I don't know about you, but I always get excited when the restaurant menu mentions anything involving aioli. The creamy, garlicky goodness that accompanies dishes like fries, burgers, or sandwiches is always a welcome addition. Naturally, I had to make my own version so I could have it on hand whenever the craving strikes. This smoky chipotle aioli is quick and easy to make and tastes phenomenal with your favorite veggies or grilled meats. You could even serve it over nachos or tacos to elevate your Taco Tuesday game. It's definitely something you're going to want handy for all your meals!

PREP TIME: 5 MINUTES
SERVINGS: 3 OR 4

¼ cup mayonnaise

1 tablespoon freshly squeezed lime juice

½ teaspoon chipotle powder

1 teaspoon minced garlic

¼ teaspoon onion powder

¼ teaspoon dried oregano

¼ teaspoon ground cumin

½ teaspoon sweet paprika

Salt and freshly ground black pepper

1. In a small bowl, combine the mayonnaise, lime juice, chipotle powder, garlic, onion powder, oregano, cumin, and paprika. Mix well, and add salt and pepper to taste.

2. Serve right away or store in the fridge for 3 to 4 days.

Garlicky Sesame Harissa Sauce

Elevate the taste of your meal with this garlicky sesame harissa sauce. The tahini mixed with the harissa creates a unique flavor profile that is deliciously smoky and earthy. I add in some lemon juice for the perfect dose of acidity, and garlic for a savory kick. I strongly recommend using a high-quality olive oil and a velvety, high-quality tahini to ensure that you get a sauce that is equally rich in flavor and texture. Fantastic on just about anything, this harissa sauce is sure to become a staple in your kitchen! Try it as a dip for vegetables, as a topping for roasted meats, or even mixed in with your favorite pasta dish. It'll rock your world.

PREP TIME: 5 MINUTES
SERVINGS: 6

½ cup tahini

2 tablespoons olive oil

¼ cup freshly squeezed lemon juice

1 large garlic clove, minced

½ cup harissa paste

Large pinch of salt

In a mason jar, combine the tahini, olive oil, lemon juice, garlic, harissa, and salt with ¼ cup water. Shake well. Taste, and adjust as desired with more salt or lemon juice. Store in the fridge for up to 3 days.

Herbs & Caraway Seed Sauce

(ZHOUG)

Bright, fresh, and spicy, this zhoug sauce will transform any dish from ordinary to extraordinary. This traditional Yemeni herb and caraway sauce is known for its vibrant green color and bold flavors. Some of the most notable are caraway seeds, which add a unique earthy taste, and a combination of jalapeños and Aleppo pepper, which gives the sauce a spicy kick. Its versatility makes it an essential condiment in many Middle Eastern and Israeli cuisines. Use it for dipping, for marinating, or as a sauce for meats and vegetables. Just toast the spices before blending with the herbs and aromatics for an irresistible savory sauce that will elevate any dish.

PREP TIME: 10 MINUTES
COOK TIME: 5 MINUTES
SERVINGS: 8 TO 10

1 teaspoon caraway seeds

1 teaspoon black peppercorns

¾ teaspoon ground cumin

½ teaspoon ground cardamom

1 teaspoon Aleppo pepper

3 whole jalapeño peppers
(seeds removed for less heat)

4 garlic cloves

2 ounces fresh cilantro

½ ounce fresh mint leaves

½ cup olive oil

2 tablespoons lemon juice

Salt

1. Heat a small dry pan over medium heat. Once the pan is hot, add the caraway seeds and peppercorns and toast them for 1 minute, tossing frequently. The spices are done toasting when they become aromatic and slightly darker in color. Add the cumin, cardamom, and Aleppo pepper and continue toasting for another minute, until fragrant. Remove from the heat and let cool for a few minutes.

2. In a food processor, combine the toasted spices with the jalapeños, garlic, cilantro, mint, olive oil, and lemon juice. Process for a couple of minutes to get everything blended into a runny sauce. Add salt to taste and adjust any other spices to your preferences. For extra heat, add more Aleppo pepper.

3. Serve right away or store in the fridge for up to 3 days.

OPPOSITE FROM TOP TO BOTTOM: *Herbs & Caraway Seed Sauce (Zhoug), Moroccan Herbs Sauce (Chermoula) (page 212), and Garlicky Sesame Harissa Sauce (page 209).*

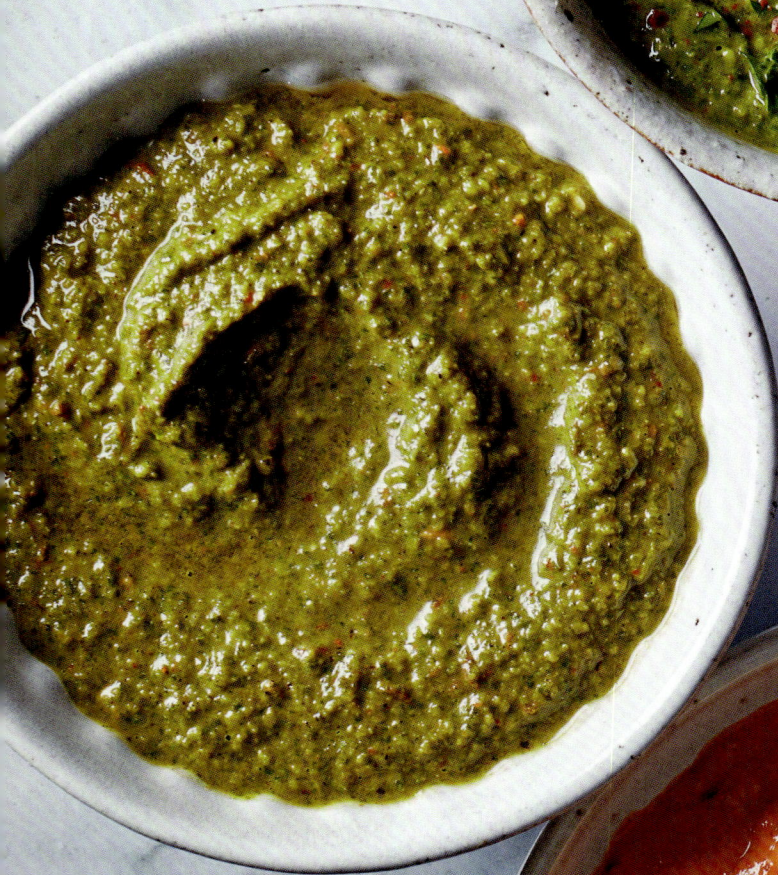

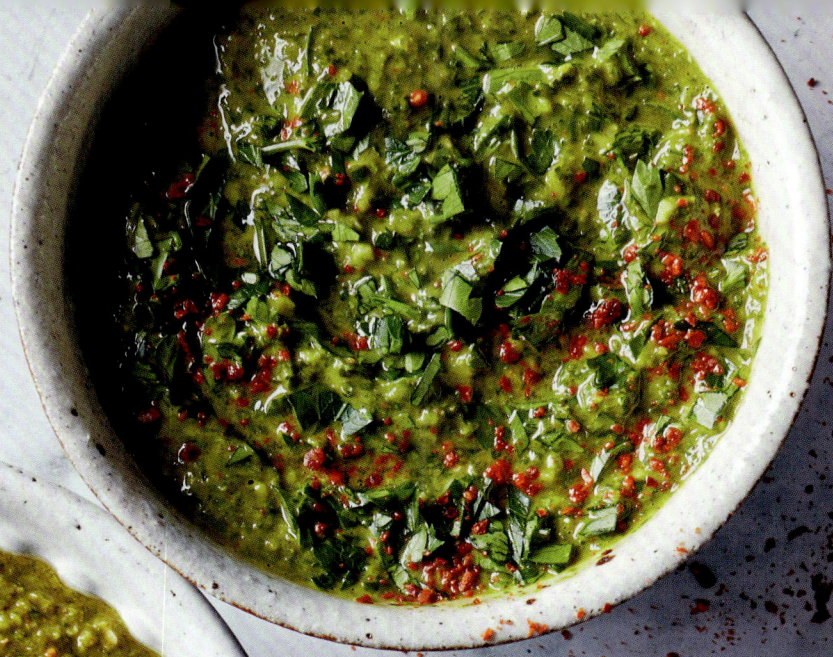

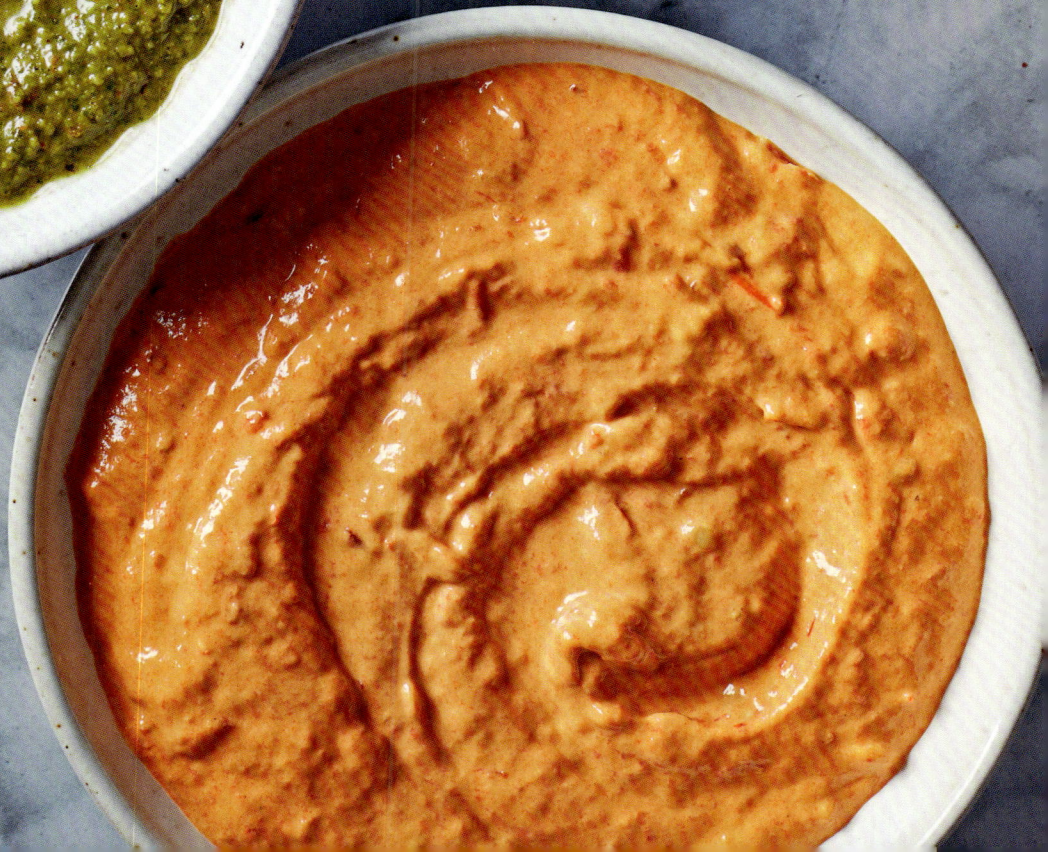

Moroccan Herbs Sauce (CHERMOULA)

Chermoula is a versatile sauce found in almost every Moroccan household. This flavorful and aromatic mixture of herbs and spices is used as both a marinade and a condiment to season salads, stews, tagines, grilled foods—you name it. Just like a true Moroccan, you can brush chermoula over meat, chicken, fish, and vegetables or add it as a flavor enhancer to fillings for stuffed fish, bread, and poultry. You can even use it to add an extra kick to ground and roasted meat of all sorts—the flavor potential of this tasty sauce is endless!

PREP TIME: 15 MINUTES
SERVINGS: 6 TO 8

1½ bunches fresh parsley

1½ bunches fresh cilantro

6 garlic cloves

¼ teaspoon ground cumin

¼ teaspoon ground cinnamon

½ teaspoon Aleppo pepper

1½ teaspoons lemon zest

5 tablespoons freshly squeezed lemon juice

1 cup olive oil

Salt and freshly ground black pepper

1. In a food processor, combine the parsley, cilantro, garlic, cumin, cinnamon, Aleppo pepper, lemon zest, lemon juice, and ½ cup of the olive oil and blend for a couple of minutes.

2. Gradually add the remaining oil until the chermoula sauce is thin enough to drip from a spoon.

3. Add salt and pepper to taste and adjust the seasoning if needed.

4. Use right away or store in the fridge for 2 to 3 days.

Chili Lime Everything Sauce

I call this an everything sauce because it truly does taste phenomenal on everything. This chili lime sauce is a unique blend of spicy, tangy, and sweet flavors that will revive your taste buds and elevate any dish it touches. Zesty limes, spicy cayenne pepper, and aromatic garlic mingle with rich and creamy mayo and sour cream for a perfect balance of flavors. It's incredibly versatile and can be used as a dip, dressing, or marinade, or even just drizzled on top of your favorite foods. An easy way to take grilled or roasted veggies, burgers, or tacos to a whole new level. I particularly like drizzling it over barbacoa or fish tacos or using it to dip roasted butternut squash. Just pop all the ingredients into a food processor, blend, and adjust to your personal taste.

1. In a food processor, combine the lime juice, lime zest, garlic, scallions, mayonnaise, sour cream, olive oil, cayenne, paprika, onion powder. Process well and add salt and pepper to taste. Adjust as desired with more lime juice or mayonnaise.

2. Keeps well in the refrigerator for 2 to 3 days.

PREP TIME: 5 MINUTES
SERVINGS: 6 TO 8

3 tablespoons freshly squeezed lime juice

1 teaspoon lime zest

1 garlic clove

2 scallions (green parts only)

3 tablespoons mayonnaise

3 tablespoons sour cream

1 tablespoon olive oil

¼ to ½ teaspoon cayenne pepper

½ teaspoon sweet paprika

½ tablespoon onion powder

Salt and freshly ground black pepper

Green Herbs Salsa

There are lots of fresh herbs in this dish, and they taste wonderful with the jalapeño, shallot, garlic, and lemon juice. It's also a ridiculously easy recipe, as everything is tossed into a food processor and blended until you get your ideal salsa consistency. Pair it with practically any grilled protein or roasted veggies—especially my Baked Whole Cauliflower (page 30)—to elevate your meal with a bright, herbaceous flavor that'll leave your taste buds singing. This will keep for 3 to 4 days in an airtight container in the fridge.

In a food processor, combine the olive oil, parsley, cilantro, tarragon, basil, mint, jalapeño, shallot, garlic, and lemon juice. Blend until a coarse texture is obtained, and add salt and pepper to taste.

PREP TIME: 10 MINUTES
SERVINGS: 4 TO 6

3 tablespoons olive oil

⅓ bunch fresh parsley

⅓ bunch fresh cilantro

½ bunch fresh tarragon leaves

⅓ bunch fresh basil

⅓ bunch fresh mint leaves

½ jalapeño pepper, seeds removed

1 shallot, chopped

3 garlic cloves

5 tablespoons freshly squeezed lemon juice

Salt and freshly ground black pepper

Tahini Sauce

(TARATOR)

This is my take on *tarator,* a Lebanese variation of tahini sauce that is commonly used in Middle Eastern and Mediterranean cuisine. It's super creamy and bright while being completely dairy-free! Making it is a breeze, as you just mix everything together in a bowl until smooth. I love having this condiment on hand for dipping vegetables into, spreading on sandwiches, or drizzling over grilled meats. This goes particularly well with my Minced Lamb Lettuce Cups (page 42) or drizzled over the Baharat Steak Bowl (page 192). I sprinkle on my za'atar spice blend at the end for a little extra flavor, but that's totally optional.

PREP TIME: 5 MINUTES
SERVINGS: 6 TO 8

½ cup tahini

2 garlic cloves, minced

5 tablespoons freshly squeezed lemon juice

Salt

½ teaspoon finely chopped fresh parsley

½ teaspoon za'atar, homemade (page 222) or store-bought (optional)

1. In a small bowl, combine the tahini, garlic, and lemon juice. Give it a mix using a fork or a small whisk. The sauce will harden right away, so gradually add up to 3 tablespoons of water to dilute it to a runny consistency. Add the salt to taste and parsley. Mix it again to blend all the ingredients.

2. Sprinkle with za'atar (if using) and serve right away or store in the fridge for up to 4 days in an airtight container.

Everyday Cilantro Sauce

This cilantro sauce makes elevating any dish effortless. Whether I pour it over fish tacos or use it as a base for a smoked salmon sandwich, drizzle it over my fried eggs in the morning or dip veggies into it as an afternoon snack, this flavorful sauce will deliver absolute deliciousness in every bite. Fresh cilantro combines with garlic, jalapeño, lime, sour cream, and chili lime seasoning for a burst of flavor. This recipe is made entirely in a food processor, so there is no need to worry about chopping up veggies or dirtying multiple dishes. Use it on any protein, on eggs, as a spread on a sandwich, or as a dip with veggies—you're going to fall in love. It's easy, delicious, and your new secret weapon in the kitchen!

PREP TIME: 15 MINUTES
SERVINGS: 3 TO 5

2 ounces fresh cilantro

2 garlic cloves

1 jalapeño pepper

2 tablespoons freshly squeezed lime juice

2 tablespoons sour cream

1 to 2 tablespoons olive oil

1 tablespoon chili lime seasoning, such as Tajín

Salt

1. In a small food processor or blender, combine the cilantro, garlic, jalapeño, lime juice, sour cream, 1 tablespoon of the olive oil, chili lime seasoning, and salt to taste. (I remove about half the jalapeño seeds to control the spiciness. You can remove all or, if you are feeling particularly bold, leave them all in.)

2. Close the lid and process until the mixture becomes a creamy sauce. Give it a good taste, and adjust as you like with more creaminess, citrusy vibes, salt, or spice! Adding enough salt is key.

3. Store in the fridge for 2 to 3 days.

Spicy Peanut Sauce

This spicy peanut sauce is perfect for adding a kick of flavor to any meal. Whether you are in a time crunch and looking for a sauce to dip your store-bought rotisserie chicken or tofu into, or you need to spice up a stir-fry veggie dish, this is the sauce for you. It will take any basic meal to the next level! It has just the right amount of heat, sweetness, and nuttiness that'll make you want to pour it over everything. The key ingredient in this sauce is peanut butter. It provides a rich and creamy base for the sauce. All you have to do is combine the ingredients in one pan over the stove, and in just a few minutes, you'll have a delicious sauce ready to be enjoyed.

PREP TIME: 15 MINUTES
COOK TIME: 10 MINUTES
SERVINGS: 6 TO 8

―――――

1 tablespoon sesame oil

3 garlic cloves, minced

1 small shallot, minced

1 tablespoon crushed red pepper flakes

1 tablespoon monk fruit sweetener or regular sugar

2 tablespoons soy sauce

½ cup peanut butter

¾ cup coconut cream

1 tablespoon freshly squeezed lime juice

1 tablespoon crushed roasted peanuts, for garnish (optional)

1. Heat the sesame oil in a pan over medium heat. When the oil is hot, add the garlic, shallots, and red pepper flakes and sauté for 1 to 2 minutes, until golden brown.

2. In a food processor, combine the garlic and shallots with the monk fruit sweetener, soy sauce, peanut butter, coconut cream, and lime juice. Blend for a couple of minutes, until a smooth consistency is achieved.

3. Place in a bowl and garnish with the crushed roasted peanuts (if using) for some extra crunch.

4. Keeps well in the fridge for up to a week.

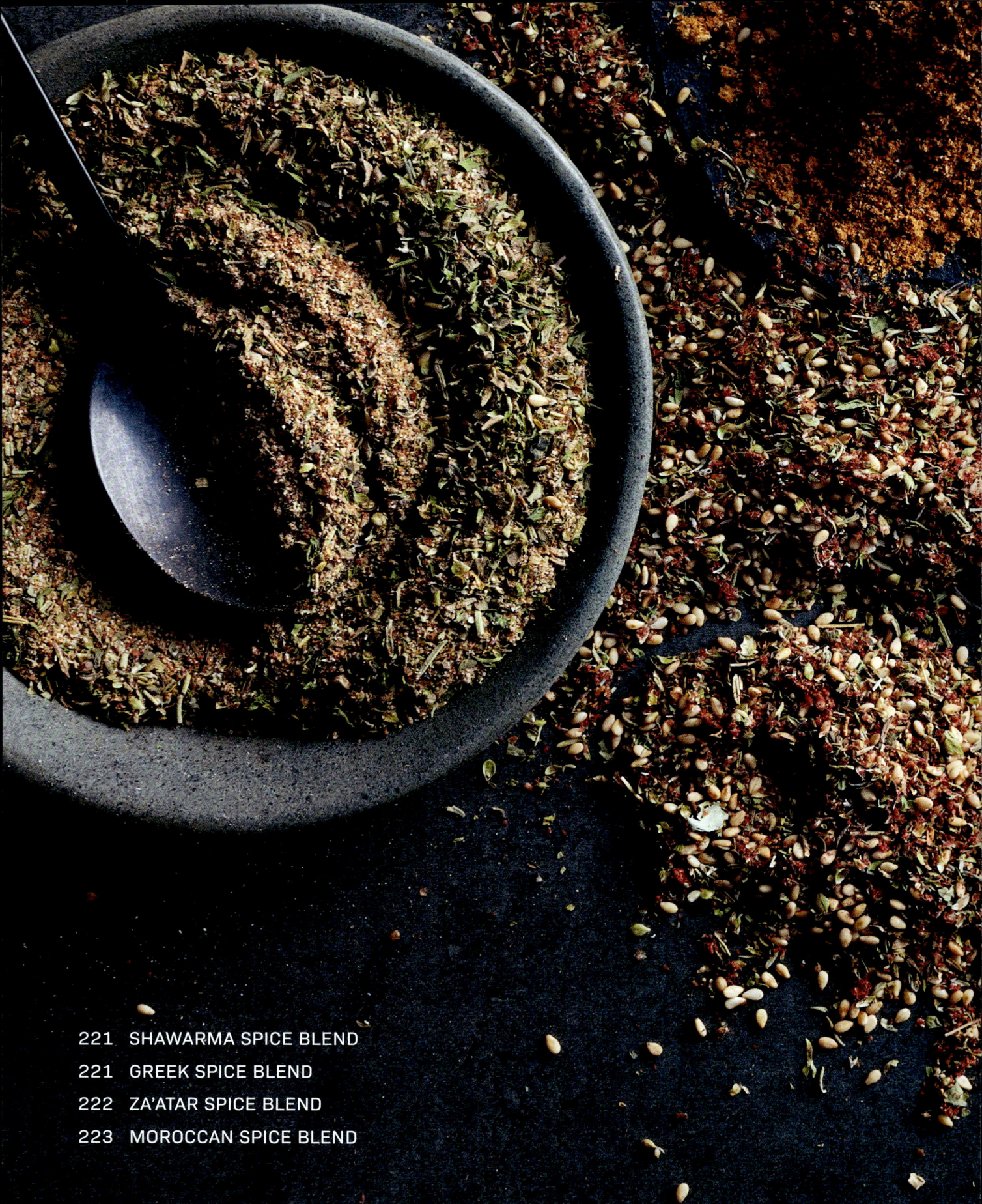

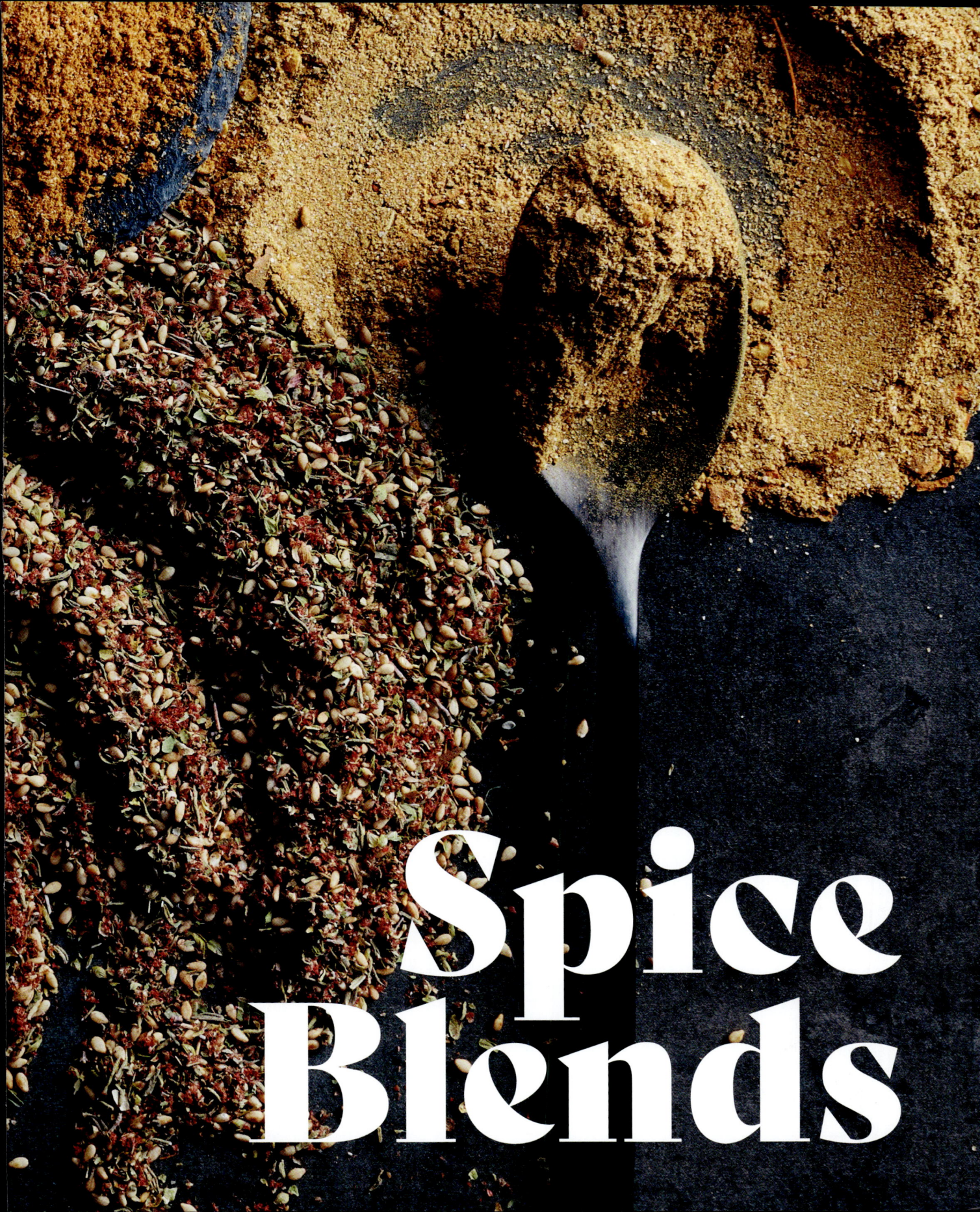

Spice
Blends

Deck out your spice cabinet with these easy-to-
make spice blends. They're such an effortless way to level up
your cooking game, as they not only provide amazing flavor but
also eliminate the need to measure out individual spices every
time you cook.

Many store-bought spice blends contain added sugar,
preservatives, and other ingredients you may not want in
your diet. They're also quite expensive! But with these
homemade versions, you can control what goes into them
and save money in the long run. As a bonus, you'll feel like a
true chef when you whip out your own custom spice blend.

Making spice blends yourself also allows you to adjust the
flavors and heat levels to your liking. Not a fan of cayenne
pepper? Simply leave it out or reduce the amount. Want more
oregano in your Greek seasoning? Go for it!

These spice blends taste fantastic with meats, vegetables,
soups, and stews, or even as a rub for grilling. They're versatile
and easy to store, and make adding flavor to your meals simple
and efficient.

Shawarma Spice Blend

Make your shawarma dish that much easier with this shawarma spice blend. With its bold flavors and aromatic spices, this blend adds a delicious kick to your favorite protein, whether it be chicken, beef, or lamb. But this spice blend isn't only limited to shawarma—it can also be used in a variety of dishes, like soups, stews, and even roasted vegetables, making it a must-have in your kitchen.

1. In a small bowl, combine the cinnamon, cardamom, cloves, coriander, turmeric, ginger, paprika, cumin, cayenne, sumac, and garlic powder and mix well.

2. Add them to an airtight jar, and done! Store in a dark dry place for up to 3 months.

PREP TIME: 10 MINUTES
MAKES: ½ CUP
SERVINGS: 15 TO 20

1 teaspoon ground cinnamon

½ teaspoon ground cardamom

½ teaspoon ground cloves

2 teaspoons ground coriander

1 tablespoon ground turmeric

1 teaspoon ground ginger

4 teaspoons sweet paprika

6 teaspoons ground cumin

1 teaspoon cayenne pepper

1½ teaspoons sumac

2 teaspoons garlic powder

Greek Spice Blend

If you love Greek food, you're going to want to have this Greek spice blend in your pantry at all times. I did all the taste testing for you, so you can trust that it's the perfect combination of herbs and spices for your next Greek-inspired dish. It'll be a major game-changer in your cooking, making Greek dishes taste even more authentic and flavorful. Use it on anything from grilled meats to fish and vegetables. To start, try the Mediterranean Chicken with Olive Feta Salsa (page 111) or Greek Pasta Salad with Grilled Shrimp (page 176).

1. In a small bowl, combine the basil, garlic powder, oregano, pepper, cinnamon, dill, marjoram, parsley, rosemary, nutmeg, thyme, sumac, and mint and mix well.

2. Add them to an airtight jar, and done! This is an easy blend that can be used on any protein, whether cooked on a grill or in a stew, as well as on your favorite veggies or in a soup. Store in a dark dry place for up to 3 months.

PREP TIME: 10 MINUTES
SERVINGS: 15 TO 20

1 tablespoon dried basil

2 tablespoons garlic powder

1 tablespoon dried oregano

1 teaspoon freshly ground black pepper

1 teaspoon ground cinnamon

1 teaspoon dried dill

1 teaspoon dried marjoram

1 tablespoon dried parsley

1 teaspoon dried rosemary

½ teaspoon nutmeg

1 teaspoon dried thyme

1 teaspoon sumac

½ teaspoon dried mint

Za'atar Spice Blend

One of my most used and loved spice blends is za'atar. This aromatic blend of herbs and spices has been a staple in Middle Eastern cuisine for centuries, and it's easy to see why. It's versatile and fragrant and adds a ton of flavor to any dish. Not only that, but it has a lot of health benefits too! The sumac, oregano, and sesame seeds make it a rich natural source of vitamins and antioxidants. I like to use za'atar in a variety of dishes, from roasted vegetables to meats, and even sprinkled on top of dips and spreads for an extra kick. Add it to high quality olive oil or labneh to enjoy with a low-carb pita or your favorite bread. Use it to season salads or marinate any protein, however you plan to cook it. Try it in my Za'atar Chicken (page 148), Honey Grilled Halloumi with Pistachios & Za'atar (page 54), Baharat Steak Bowl (page 192), or Sautéed Mushrooms over Tahini Labneh (page 45). It's a pantry essential that every Mediterranean-food lover should have on hand.

PREP TIME: 5 MINUTES
SERVINGS: 15

1 tablespoon dried marjoram

2 tablespoons dried thyme

2 tablespoons dried oregano

½ teaspoon dried mint

2 tablespoons sumac

3 tablespoons toasted sesame seeds

1. In a small bowl, combine the marjoram, thyme, oregano, mint, sumac, and sesame seeds and mix well.

2. Add them to an airtight jar, and done! Store in a dark dry place for up to 3 months.

Moroccan Spice Blend

Elevate your cooking by adding a touch of Moroccan flavor with this versatile spice blend. Made with a combination of aromatics and spices, this blend adds depth and complexity to any dish. With roots in North African cuisine, Moroccan spice blends are known for their warm and rich flavors. The unique combination of spices creates a balance of sweet, spicy, and savory notes that are sure to take your taste buds on a journey. I love how this spice blend tastes on everything from meats and vegetables to dips and dressings. I recommend you try my Moroccan Braised Lamb Leg (page 172) to start, but this also makes a great addition to lamb burgers, roasted chicken, lentil stews, dry rubs, or roasts.

1. In a small bowl, combine the ginger, cardamom, red pepper flakes, turmeric, cumin, coriander, cinnamon, onion powder, and garlic power and mix well.

2. Add them to an airtight jar, and done! Store in a dark dry place for up to 3 months.

PREP TIME: 10 MINUTES
SERVINGS: 35

2 teaspoons ground ginger

1 teaspoon ground cardamom

4 teaspoons crushed red pepper flakes

2 teaspoons ground turmeric

4 teaspoons ground cumin

4 teaspoons ground coriander

2 teaspoons ground cinnamon

1 tablespoon onion powder

1 tablespoon garlic powder

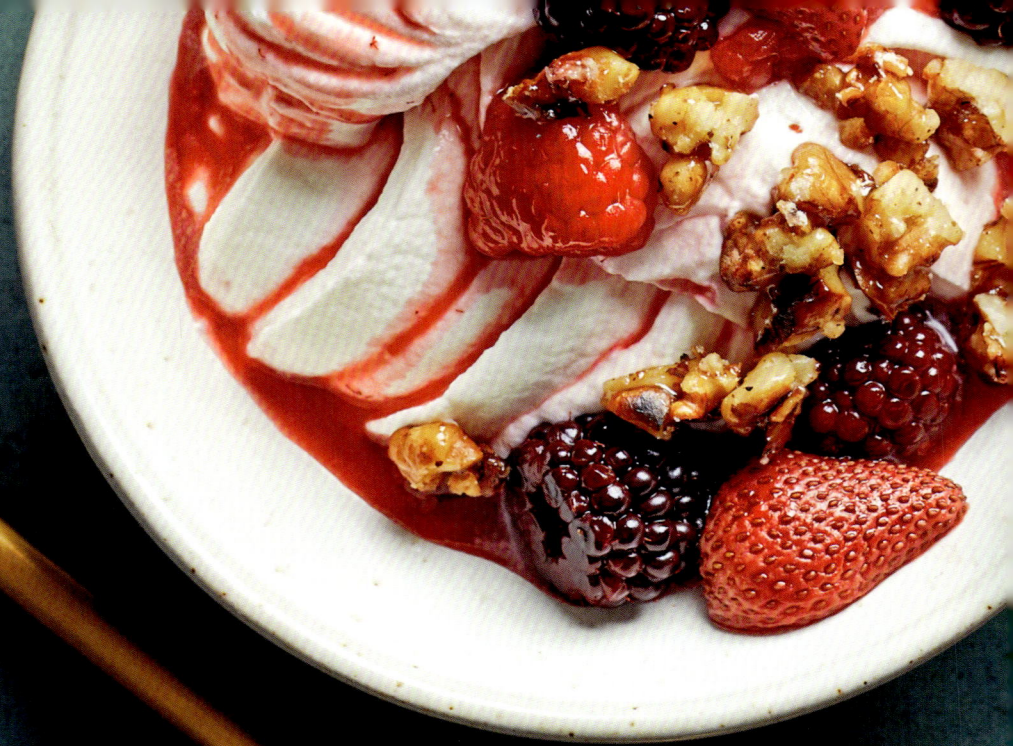

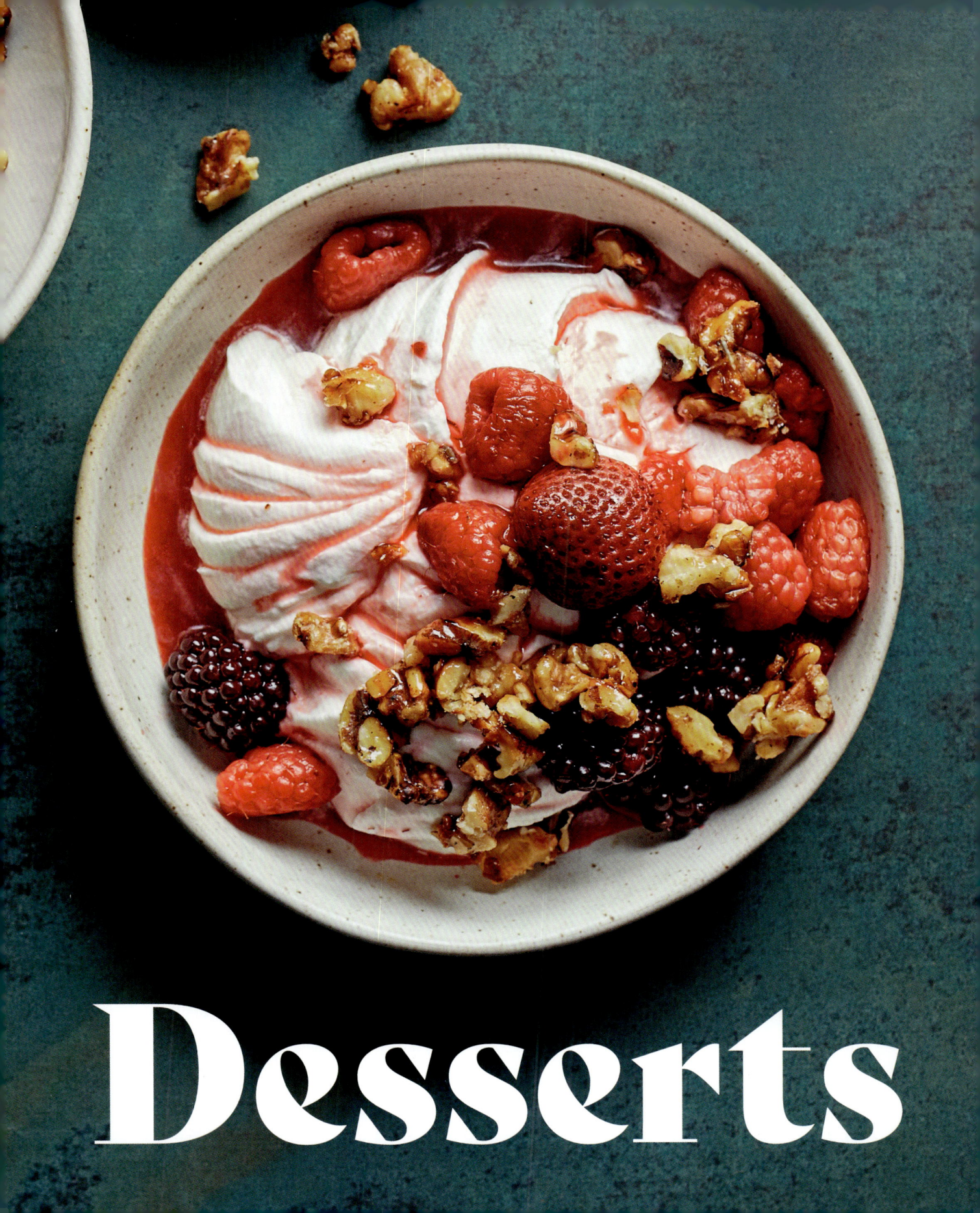

Desserts

We all know making desserts, especially low-carb ones, can be intimidating. But they don't have to be! With a little creativity and some simple swaps, you can still enjoy sweet treats without compromising your health goals.

Sugar? Nah, we don't need that here. Instead, these desserts use natural sweeteners like monk fruit and allulose. These are both must-have sweeteners for any low-carb kitchen, as well as alternative flour options like almond flour, coconut flour, and flaxseed meal. With these ingredients, you've got practically everything you need to make delicious low-carb desserts that are just as—if not *more*—decadent and satisfying as their carb-filled counterparts.

The desserts in this chapter range from quick indulgences like mug cakes, yogurt bowls, and cookies to more elaborate treats like cheesecake and tiramisu. But the one thing they all have in common is that they use basic ingredients and are simple in preparation. And let me tell you, these recipes are so good, I'm sure no one will even notice they're low-carb!

Tiramisu

Just because you're eating low-carb doesn't mean you can't indulge in the classics! This tiramisu tastes so much like the sugary, carb-filled sensation that it'll fool even the most sophisticated palate. Almond flour swoops in for the flour and, as usual, allulose gets the job done in place of sugar. Egg yolks and mascarpone cheese make up the layers of creamy goodness, while coffee and cocoa powder are sprinkled on top for that signature tiramisu flavor. This dessert takes a bit more effort than some of my other dessert recipes, but you'll be amazed at how close the end result is to the original.

1. Preheat the oven to 350°F.

2. **For the cake:** In a mixing bowl, combine the butter, allulose, almond flour, eggs, sour cream, vanilla, and baking powder. Using a hand mixer, blend the ingredients for about 3 minutes or until the mixture is smooth and well incorporated.

3. Line a 9-inch springform baking pan with parchment paper. Add the batter to the pan. The mixture should be smooth and level across the surface before placing in the oven. Bake in the preheated oven for about 30 minutes, or until the cake is golden brown and a toothpick inserted into the center comes out clean.

4. Remove from the oven and place on a rack to cool to room temperature.

5. **For the filling:** Separate the egg yolks and egg whites into two mixing bowls.

6. Clean and dry the beaters for the hand mixer. Add the allulose to the yolks and, using the hand mixer, mix into a light yellow paste, 3 to 4 minutes. Add the mascarpone and mix for another 2 to 3 minutes or until the mixture is smooth and creamy with no lumps. Set aside.

7. Clean and dry the beaters for the hand mixer. With the hand mixer on medium speed, beat the egg whites until soft peaks form, then beat on high until stiff, glossy peaks form.

8. Using a rubber spatula, scoop about one-third of the whipped egg whites at a time and add to the mascarpone mix. Fold gently using a flipping motion. This will ensure an airy, fluffy consistency. The important part here is not to stir. Set aside.

9. Combine the coffee, allulose, and rum in a medium measuring cup.

PREP TIME: 40 MINUTES, PLUS 2 HOURS CHILLING
COOK TIME: 30 MINUTES
SERVINGS: 8 TO 10

FOR THE CAKE

¼ cup unsalted butter, melted

⅓ cup allulose

2 cups almond flour

4 eggs

⅓ cup sour cream

2 teaspoons vanilla extract

2 teaspoons baking powder

FOR THE FILLING

3 eggs

½ cup allulose

2 cups mascarpone cheese

1 cup strong coffee or cold brew

3 tablespoons allulose

2 teaspoons rum, rum extract, or vanilla extract

2 tablespoons cocoa powder

(recipe continues)

10. Once the cake has cooled down, cut it in half horizontally to get 2 thinner round layers.

11. Line the same 9-inch springform with plastic wrap. Lower in the first cake layer. Gradually pour part of the coffee syrup over the first layer until it is fully saturated with liquid. Spread half of the mascarpone filling on top. Add the second cake layer and repeat the process.

12. Using a small strainer, dust the top layer of mascarpone with cocoa powder.

13. Place in the fridge for at least 2 hours before serving. This will allow all the flavors to infuse the cake.

14. Serve chilled.

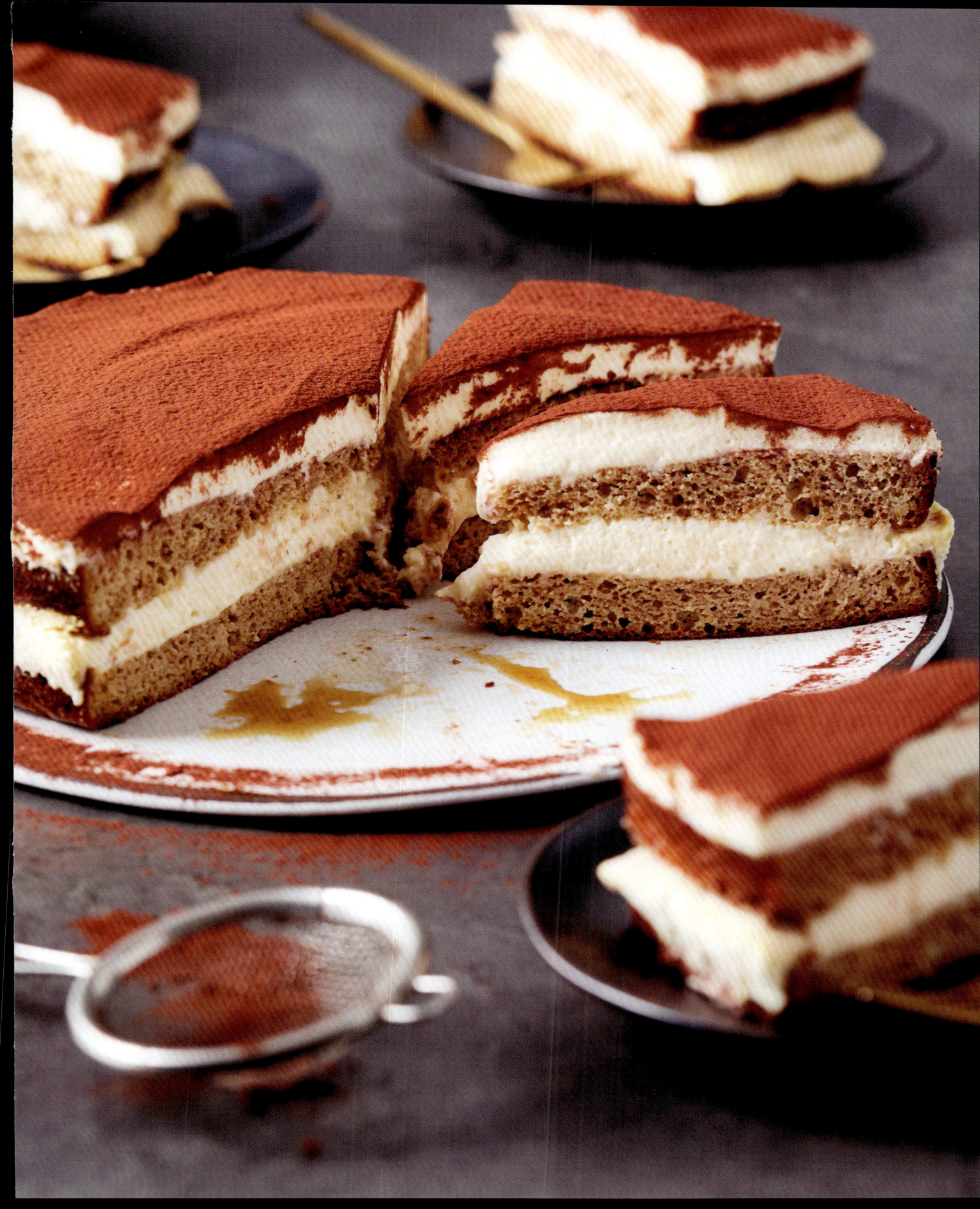

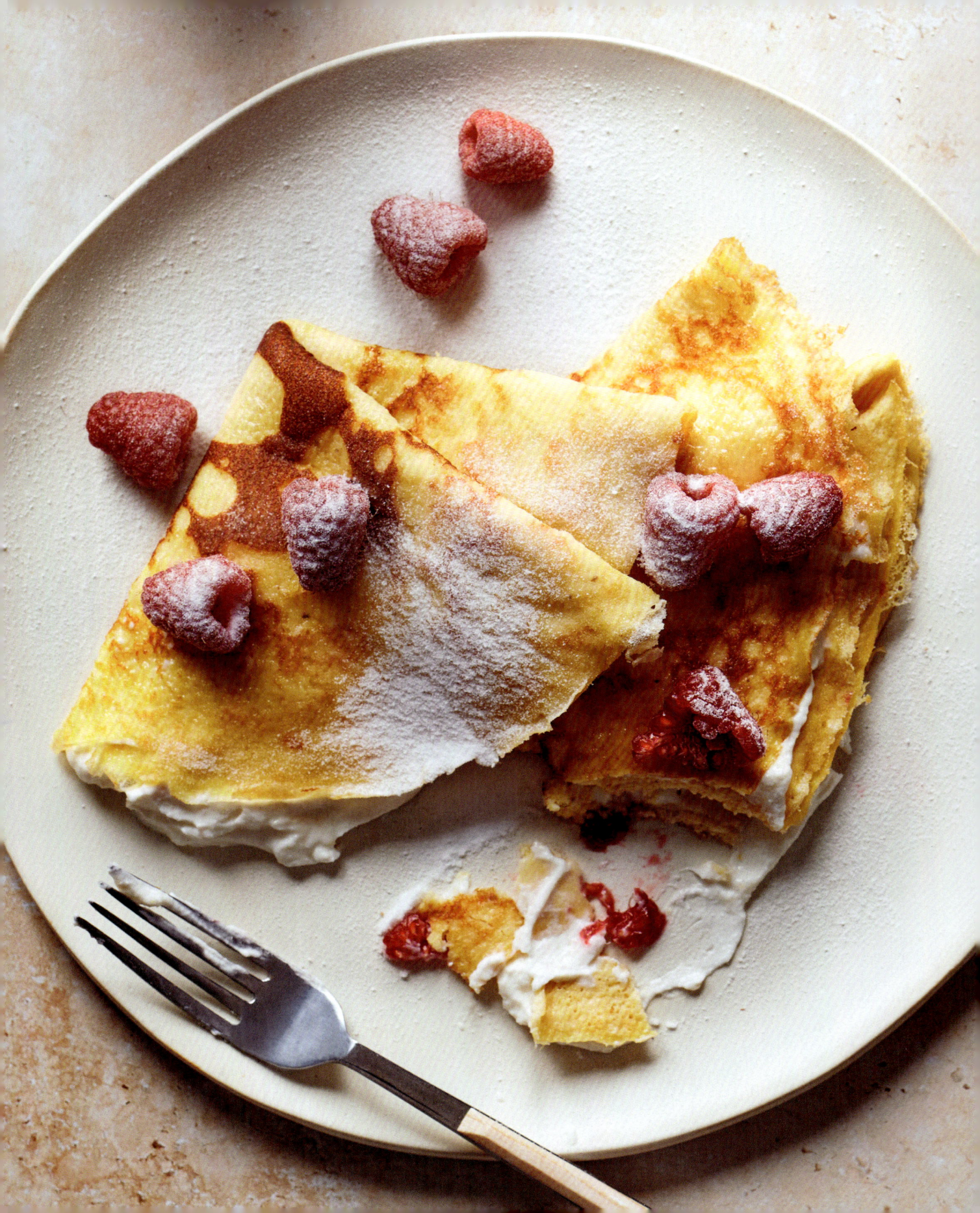

Lemon Ricotta Crepes

You haven't had crepes like these lemon ricotta–filled crepes. Ricotta cheese introduces a lovely creamy texture and mild flavor that pairs well with the tanginess of the lemon and the Greek yogurt. I like topping these crepes with fresh raspberries for some added sweetness and color, but feel free to use any fruit you like. The filling comes out super creamy, and the crepes add a slightly crispy outer layer, making it the perfect balance of textures and flavors. If you've never made crepes before, you're in good hands.

PREP TIME: 15 MINUTES
COOK TIME: 30 MINUTES
SERVINGS: 4 TO 6

2 large eggs

¼ cup almond flour

½ cup milk or almond milk

1 teaspoon vanilla extract

1 tablespoon allulose

¼ teaspoon baking powder

⅛ teaspoon salt

Nonstick cooking spray

FOR THE FILLING

½ cup ricotta cheese

¼ cup plain Greek yogurt

½ teaspoon lemon zest

1 teaspoon freshly squeezed lemon juice

2 tablespoons allulose, plus extra for garnish

¼ cup fresh raspberries, for garnish (optional)

1. In a food processor, combine the eggs, almond flour, milk, vanilla, allulose, baking powder, and salt. Process until smooth and free of lumps (1 to 2 minutes). Let sit for 5 minutes to allow the ingredients to properly hydrate. This will help thicken up the batter.

2. Heat a nonstick skillet over medium-low heat. Lightly coat with nonstick cooking spray. Test if the pan is hot by dropping water onto the surface. If it sizzles, you're ready to go.

3. Pour about ¼ cup of the batter into the center of the skillet. Tilt the pan with a circular motion so that the batter coats the surface evenly. Cook the crepe for 1 to 2 minutes, until the bottom is light brown. Loosen with a spatula, flip, and cook the other side.

4. Continue with the remaining batter, spraying the pan as needed. This should yield about 6 crepes. Set the finished crepes aside.

5. **For the filling:** In a bowl, combine the ricotta, yogurt, lemon zest, lemon juice, and allulose and mix with a fork.

6. Fill the crepes with the mixture and fold them in quarters, or roll them if you prefer.

7. Garnish with the raspberries (if using) and use a small strainer to dust some more allulose on top. Serve right away.

Chocolate Hazelnut Bonbons

Full of delicious, chocolatey goodness, these bite-sized chocolate hazelnut bonbons are a must-try for any chocolate lover. They've got the perfect combination of rich, creamy chocolate and crunchy hazelnuts to satisfy your sweet tooth and then some. Low-carb chocolate chips and allulose are essential here. While a bit labor-intensive, these bonbons are still relatively easy to make and totally worth the time investment. They last a while in the fridge, so make a big batch, and you can have them handy whenever you need a quick, on-the-go treat.

1. Place ¾ cup of the hazelnuts in a food processor and blend until it turns into a paste.

2. Add the allulose, vanilla, and cocoa powder and blend for another 2 minutes. Add the coconut oil and blend again for another minute. Set aside.

3. Bring a small pot of water to a boil. Place the chocolate chips in a heat-safe bowl and set over the boiling water. Be sure the bowl is not touching the water. Heat the chocolate chips until barely melted, to a paste-like consistency.

4. Add the chocolate to the food processor and blend all ingredients together for another minute. The mixture should be ready to shape, but if it is too soft, place it in the refrigerator for 10 to 15 minutes.

5. Using your hands, grab some of the mixture and roll it into a 1½-inch disk. Wrap the disk around a hazelnut, rolling it between your palms to create a perfectly round ball. You should get about 12 balls.

6. Place the balls on a baking sheet in the freezer for about an hour to harden.

7. In a clean food processor bowl or using a mortar and pestle, coarsely crush the remaining ¼ cup of hazelnuts. Set aside.

PREP TIME: 30 MINUTES, PLUS 2 HOURS CHILLING TIME
COOK TIME: 20 MINUTES
MAKES: ABOUT 12 BONBONS

1 cup toasted whole hazelnuts

½ cup allulose

2 teaspoons vanilla extract

1 tablespoon cocoa powder

2 tablespoons unrefined cold-pressed coconut oil

2 ounces low-carb dark chocolate chips

FOR THE COATING

3 ounces dark low-carb chocolate chips

2 tablespoons heavy cream

8. **For the coating:** In a heat-safe bowl over boiling water, melt the chocolate chips with the heavy cream. Be sure the bowl is not touching the water. Once fully melted, the mixture should have a thick sauce-like consistency.

9. Remove the balls from the freezer. Using a fork, roll each ball in the melted chocolate mixture and place it onto a cooling rack.

10. Sprinkle the crushed hazelnuts on top while the chocolate is still soft.

11. Place the balls in the fridge for another 30 minutes to allow the chocolate to harden.

12. Serve chilled or store in the fridge for up to a week.

Crème Caramel

This crème caramel may be fancy by name, but it's surprisingly easy to make. You don't have to be a pastry chef to make this recipe—with just a handful of ingredients, you'll have an elegant and delicious dessert that will impress any crowd. Allulose is used instead of regular sugar in this recipe to help create that perfect caramelization without the added carbs. It's creamy and decadent, with just the right amount of sweetness to satisfy your cravings.

PREP TIME: 20 MINUTES, PLUS 2 TO 3 HOURS CHILLING
COOK TIME: 1 HOUR
SERVINGS: 4

FOR THE CARAMEL

¾ cup granulated allulose

FOR THE FILLING

4 large eggs

½ cup granulated allulose

1¾ cups whole milk

2 teaspoons vanilla extract

1. **For the caramel:** Combine 3 tablespoons water and the allulose in a small pan. Give it a mix and set the pan over medium heat. Cook for 5 to 8 minutes, until the mixture turns golden brown. Remove from the heat right away and pour it into four 3-inch oven-safe ramekins. Coat the bottom and sides of each ramekin with the sauce either by slowly turning and swirling the sauce in each ramekin or with a spatula. You need to move fast, as the caramel hardens rather quickly. Set aside and allow it to cool to room temperature.

2. Preheat the oven to 320°F.

3. **For the filling:** In a large mixing bowl or bowl of a stand mixer, combine the eggs and allulose. Using a hand mixer or the stand mixer, mix on high speed for 3 to 5 minutes, until the sugar is fully dissolved.

4. Add the milk and vanilla and mix on low for another 30 seconds.

5. Divide the filling evenly between the caramel-coated ramekins.

6. Place the ramekins in a deep oven-safe dish. Pour water into the dish until the ramekins are half submerged. (Make sure not to pour water into the actual ramekins.)

7. Place the dish with the ramekins in it into the oven and bake for 50 to 60 minutes, until the tops are set.

8. Let cool to room temperature, then place in the fridge for at least 2 to 3 hours. Serve chilled.

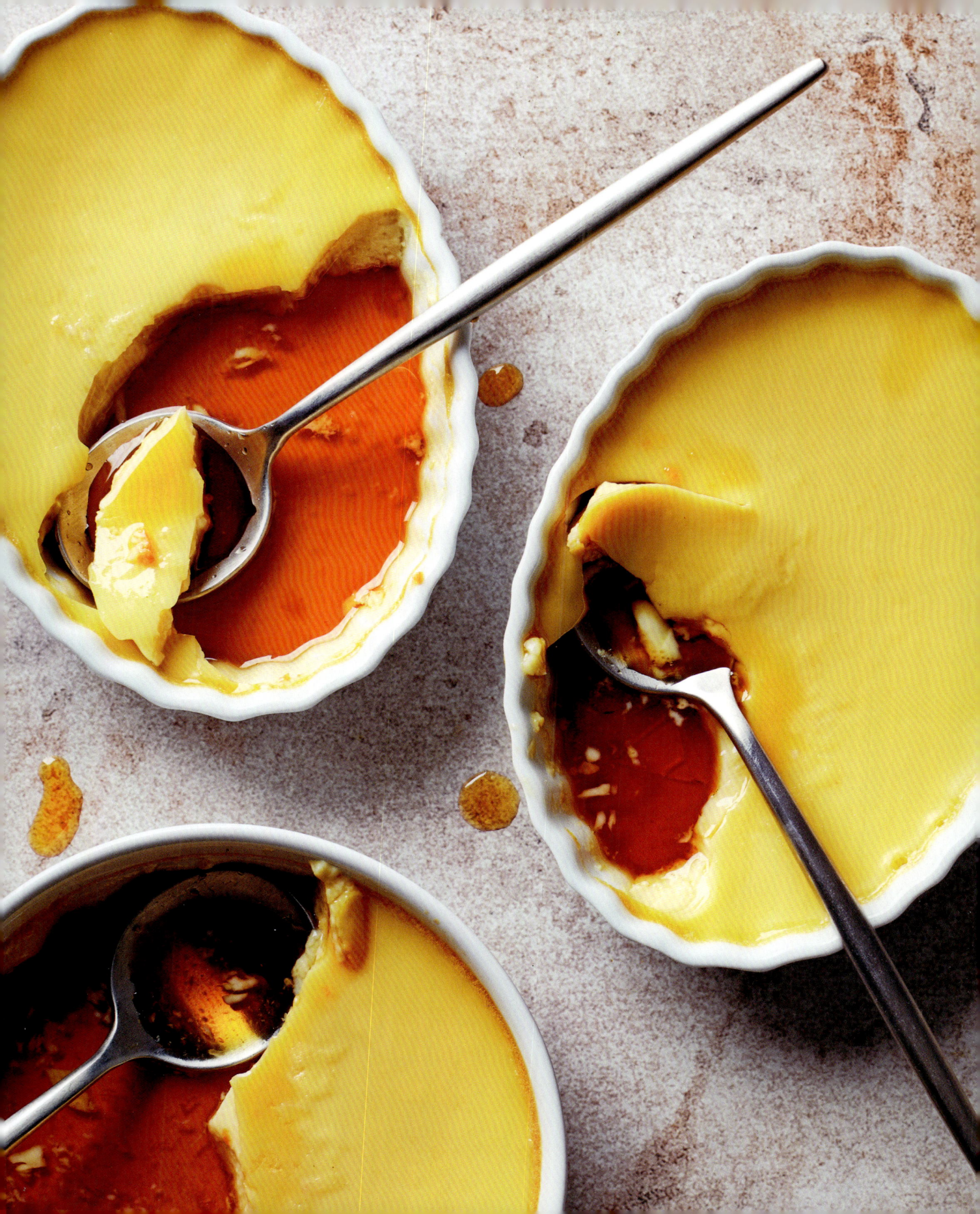

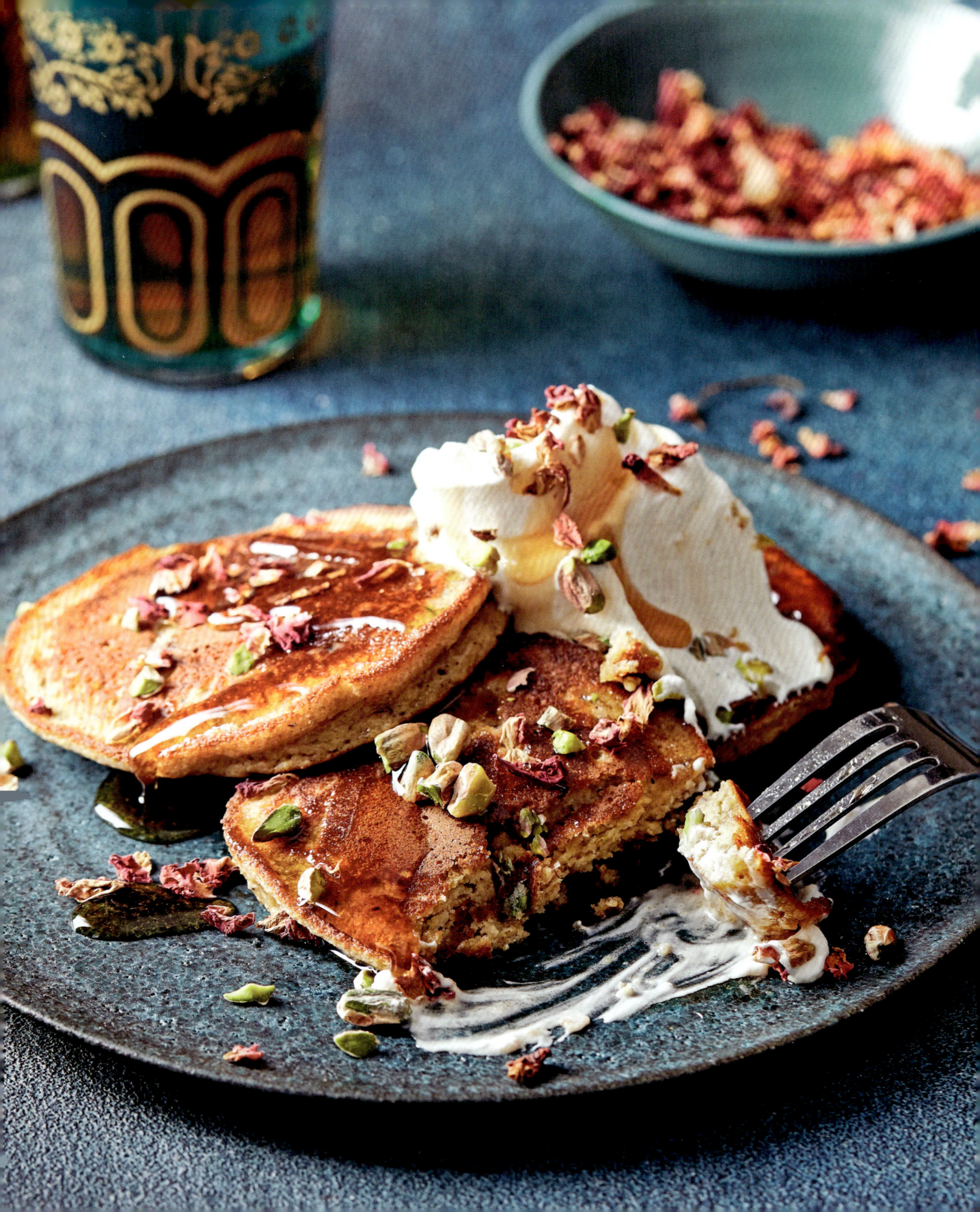

Baklava Pancakes

Love baklava? Love pancakes? Well, you're in for a treat! These baklava pancakes are a completely foolproof, low-carb breakfast (or dessert!) that taste just as impressive as they look. The batter is made with ingredients like almond milk, almond flour, and allulose to keep things low-carb, while warm spices and blended pistachios bring the wow factor of a classic baklava. I went a bit extra and topped my pancakes with some easy homemade whipped cream, a sprinkle of pistachios, and crushed rose petals—the extra flavor and presentation is so worth it.

PREP TIME: 15 MINUTES
COOK TIME: 30 MINUTES
SERVINGS: 2 TO 4

2 large eggs

⅓ cup almond milk

1 teaspoon vanilla extract

1 tablespoon coconut oil, melted

1¼ cups almond flour

2 tablespoons allulose

1 teaspoon baking powder

¼ teaspoon salt

½ teaspoon ground cinnamon

⅛ teaspoon ground cardamom

⅛ teaspoon ground nutmeg

¼ cup toasted pistachios

1 tablespoon avocado oil

FOR THE WHIPPED CREAM TOPPING

½ cup heavy cream

⅛ teaspoon ground cardamom

2 teaspoons allulose

GARNISHES

2 tablespoons toasted pistachios, crushed

1 teaspoon dried rose petals, crushed (optional)

¼ cup low-carb maple syrup (optional)

1. In a medium bowl or a food processor, combine the eggs, almond milk, vanilla, and coconut oil and mix.

2. Add the almond flour, allulose, baking powder, salt, cinnamon, cardamom, nutmeg, and pistachios and mix or blend for another minute. (Almond flour can be grainy, and I find that using a food processor to blend the batter for this recipe helps create a smoother consistency. But you can also mix it in a bowl using a regular whisk.)

3. Let the batter sit for 5 minutes to allow the ingredients to properly hydrate. This will help thicken it.

4. **For the whipped cream topping:** In a mixing bowl, combine the heavy cream, cardamom, and allulose. Using a hand mixer, whip the cream until stiff peaks form. Refrigerate until ready to serve.

5. Once you're ready to make the pancakes, heat a nonstick pan over medium-low heat. Drizzle in some of the avocado oil to lightly coat the pan.

6. Use a ladle to pour in enough batter to make your preferred size of pancake.

7. Cook for 2 to 3 minutes on the first side, until bubbly. Flip and cook for another 1 to 2 minutes on the other side. Continue with the rest of the batter, adding more oil to the pan between pancakes as needed.

8. Enjoy warm with the whipped cream and pistachios, rose petals, low-carb maple syrup, and any other toppings you like.

Wild Blueberry Bliss Labneh Cheesecake

This wild blueberry cheesecake has "bliss" in the name for a reason. The blueberry sauce is out of this world, and with the ultra-creamy, lemony vanilla cheesecake filling, it's a match made in heaven. For the crust, I use almond flour and finely ground flaxseed meal to keep things healthy and low-carb. Top it with some lemon zest for a pop of color and extra lemony flavor, and you have yourself a simple and nutritious dessert that tastes like a healthier dessert you actually crave!

1. Preheat the oven to 350°F and line a 9 x 9–inch baking dish with parchment paper.

2. **For the crust:** Add the almond flour to a large skillet over medium-low heat. Use a spatula to toss the flour continuously, moving the bottom layer to the top so it doesn't burn, until most of the flour is very lightly browned, 5 to 7 minutes. Transfer immediately to a mixing bowl.

3. Whisk in the flaxseed meal, allulose, cardamom, and salt. Add the melted butter and stir to combine.

4. Press the crust into the lined baking dish. Bake for 6 to 8 minutes, until the edge of the crust is golden. Set aside to cool.

5. **For the filling:** In a small bowl, hydrate the gelatin by adding the unflavored powder to 1 cup of water, whisking as its being added to prevent clumps. Let it sit for 10 minutes. In a small pot, bring ½ cup of water to a boil. Once it starts boiling, remove from the heat and add the hydrated gelatin and whisk well. Let it cool for 5 minutes, until it's cool enough to touch.

6. In the bowl of a stand mixer fitted with the whisk attachment or in a bowl using a hand mixer, beat the heavy cream and ½ cup of the allulose until stiff peaks form, 3 to 5 minutes.

PREP TIME: 15 MINUTES
COOK TIME: 15 MINUTES, PLUS 4 TO 8 HOURS CHILLING
SERVINGS: 12 TO 16

FOR THE CRUST

1½ cups almond flour

1 tablespoon finely ground flaxseed meal

½ cup allulose

¼ teaspoon ground cardamom

⅛ teaspoon salt

4 tablespoons unsalted butter, melted

FOR THE FILLING

2 tablespoons unflavored gelatin powder

1 cup heavy whipping cream

¾ cup allulose

2 cups labneh

1 tablespoon freshly squeezed lemon juice

1 teaspoon lemon zest

½ teaspoon vanilla extract

(recipe and ingredients continue)

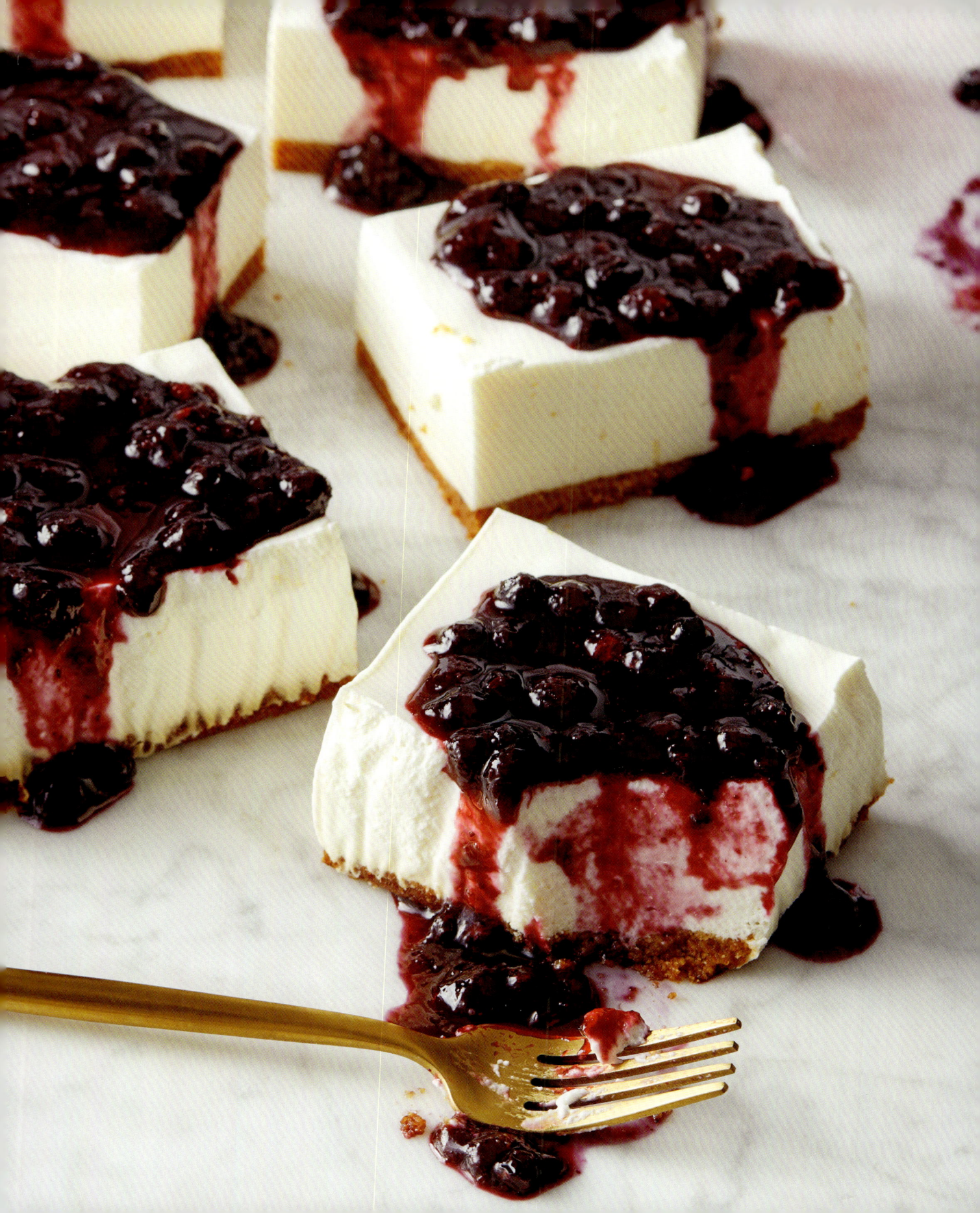

7. In a separate bowl, combine the remaining ¼ cup of allulose, labneh, lemon juice, lemon zest, and vanilla and mix well. Add the gelatin and mix. (The liquid should be warm, not yet hardened).

8. Add the labneh mixture to the whipped cream and mix on low speed just until combined, about 30 seconds.

9. Pour the filling into the cooled crust and smooth the top. Refrigerate for 4 to 8 hours or overnight.

10. For the blueberry sauce: Just before serving, in a pan over medium heat, combine the blueberries, allulose, and lemon juice and bring to a boil. Reduce the heat to medium-low and cook for another 10 to 15 minutes to reduce it to a sauce-like consistency.

11. Slice the cheesecake into bars, pour the blueberry sauce on top, and sprinkle with lemon zest.

FOR THE BLUEBERRY SAUCE

3 cups fresh or frozen wild blueberries

1 cup allulose

3 tablespoons freshly squeezed lemon juice

2 teaspoons lemon zest, for garnish

Dark Chocolate Chip Tahini Cookies

Ready in under 20 minutes, these low-carb dark chocolate chip tahini cookies are an effortless way to satisfy your cookie cravings. These rich, chewy, and chocolatey cookies are made with tahini, which gives them a nutty and slightly sweet flavor and delightfully soft texture that'll last even after a couple of days. If you like a crispier cookie, use erythritol instead of monk fruit sweetener. It'll give the cookies a firmer texture that crisps as it cools and a deeper, more caramelized flavor reminiscent of your favorite store-bought cookies. Dunk 'em in coffee or milk, or enjoy them on their own!

1. Preheat the oven to 350°F and line a large baking sheet with parchment paper.

2. In a large bowl, whisk together the egg, monk fruit sweetener, tahini, butter, and vanilla until smooth.

3. In a separate bowl, combine the almond flour, coconut flour, baking powder, and salt. Mix well.

4. Add the dry mix to the wet and mix with a silicone spatula until a sticky dough forms. Fold in two-thirds of the chocolate chips (save some to put on top of the cookies) and refrigerate for 10 minutes.

5. Scoop about 1 tablespoon of the chilled dough and form it into a thick, round disk, similar to what you want your finished cookie to look like, and place it on the baking sheet. Add a couple of extra chocolate chips on top. Repeat with the remaining dough.

6. Bake for 8 to 10 minutes, until the edges just begin to brown, aiming for a slightly underbaked center.

7. Remove the cookies the oven, sprinkle with flaky salt, and let cool for 10 minutes. They will firm up as they cool.

8. Once the cookies are no longer warm, store them in an airtight container to prevent them drying out.

PREP TIME: 20 MINUTES
COOK TIME: 10 MINUTES
MAKES: ABOUT 12 COOKIES

---

1 large egg

½ cup monk fruit sweetener

¼ cup tahini

2 tablespoons unsalted butter, melted and cooled

½ teaspoon vanilla extract

1 cup almond flour

2 tablespoons coconut flour

¼ teaspoon baking powder

¼ teaspoon salt

½ cup low-carb dark chocolate chips

Pinch of flaky salt, to finish

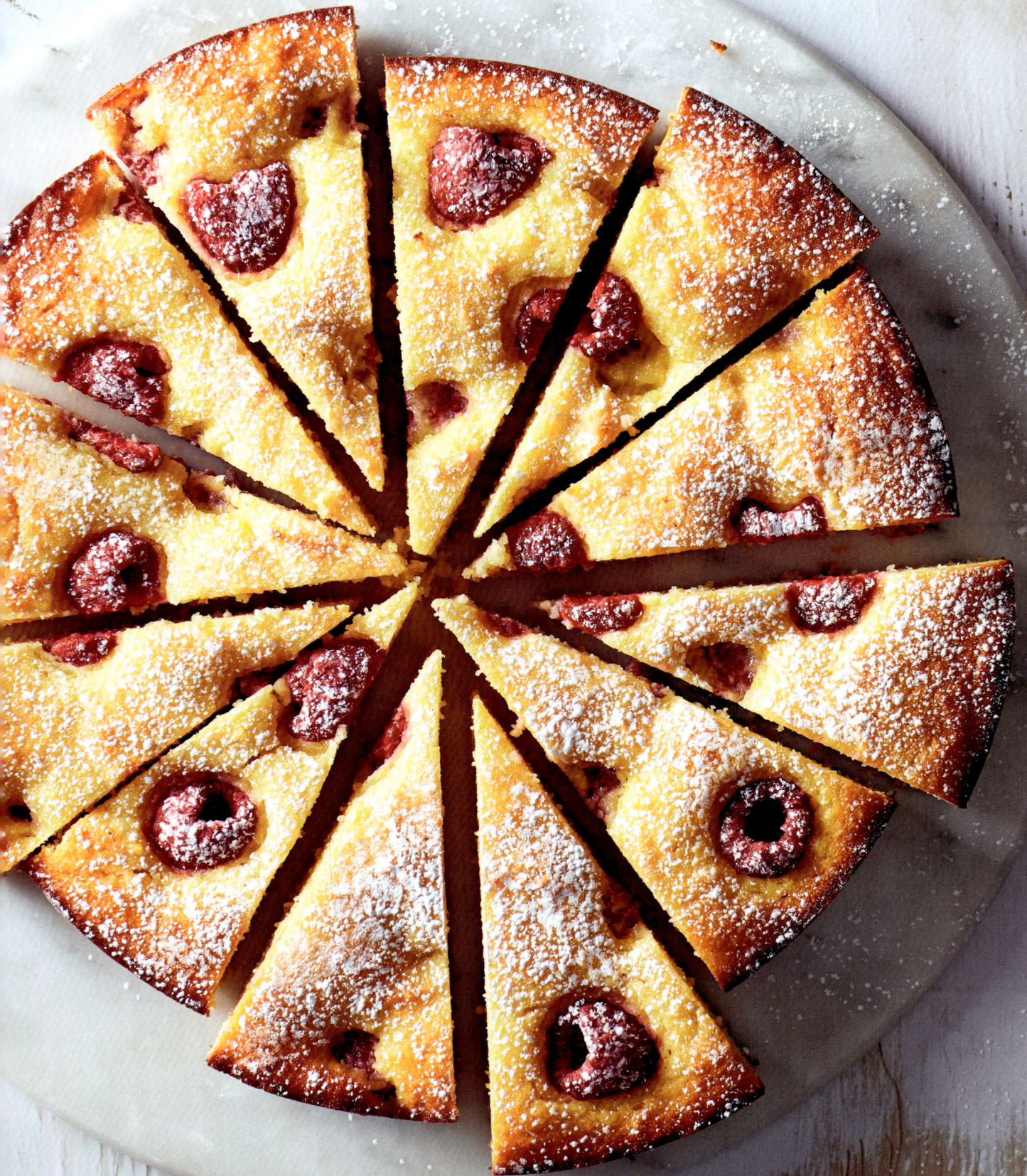

Low-Carb Raspberry Lemon Ricotta Cake

When the sweet cravings strike, a slice of this moist and flavorful heaven is all you need to feel satisfied and pampered. The prep work is super basic, and it's made with low-carb ingredients like allulose, almond flour, and coconut flour so that it tastes like the real deal. However, ricotta cheese is the secret ingredient that keeps this cake extra moist, fluffy, and delicious. It tastes superb with the fresh raspberries, lemon juice, and zest, adding a burst of flavor with every bite.

PREP TIME: 15 MINUTES
COOK TIME: 30 MINUTES
SERVINGS: 12

3 large eggs

½ cup ricotta cheese

⅔ cup monk fruit sweetener

1 teaspoon vanilla extract

2 tablespoons freshly squeezed lemon juice

1 teaspoon lemon zest

1 cup almond flour

3 tablespoons coconut flour

1 teaspoon baking powder

½ teaspoon arrowroot powder

⅛ teaspoon salt

1 cup fresh raspberries

Powdered monk fruit sweetener, for dusting (optional)

1. Preheat the oven to 350°F and line a 9-inch round cake pan with parchment paper.

2. In a large bowl, use a hand mixer to beat the eggs, ricotta, and monk fruit sweetener until combined. Add the vanilla, lemon juice, and lemon zest and mix well.

3. In a separate bowl, whisk together the almond flour, coconut flour, baking powder, arrowroot powder, and salt.

4. Add the dry mixture to the wet and mix well by hand. Fold in half of the raspberries, then pour the batter into the prepared pan, smoothing the top with a spatula.

5. Top with the remaining raspberries, pressing them firmly into the top of the cake batter.

6. Bake for 20 to 30 minutes, until the center is set and the edges are golden.

7. Let rest for 10 minutes. Generously dust the cake with powdered monk fruit sweetener (if using) before serving.

Whipped Greek Yogurt

WITH ROASTED BERRIES & CANDIED WALNUTS

One of my favorite ways to enjoy Greek yogurt is by making a whipped version that is light and airy. Add roasted berries and candied walnuts, and you've got yourself a flavor party! Why roast the berries? Roasting berries brings out their natural sweetness and intensifies their flavor. Toasting the walnuts also brings out their nutty flavor, and the candied coating adds a nice crunch and hint of sweetness. It's simple techniques like these that'll easily elevate your yogurt game and keep you full and satisfied for hours. Enjoy this whipped yogurt as a breakfast, snack, or dessert!

1. Preheat the oven to 375°F.

1. **For the roasted berries:** Trim any stems and wash the berries. Pat dry. Leave small berries whole, but halve any larger berries to ensure even roasting. Add the berries to a large mixing bowl and sprinkle with the monk fruit sweetener, lemon juice, and salt. Toss to coat.

2. Arrange the berries on a small rimmed baking sheet lined with parchment paper and roast for 20 minutes, tossing halfway through, until the natural juices begin to thicken and the berries are soft.

3. While the berries roast, prepare the rest of the toppings.

4. **For the candied walnuts:** In a small dry pan over medium heat, toast the walnuts for 2 minutes, stirring constantly until they turn golden brown on the edges. Add the monk fruit sweetener and continue stirring until the sweetener melts and coats the nuts, 3 to 4 minutes. Transfer the nuts to a plate to cool.

5. **For the whipped Greek yogurt:** In a mixing bowl or the bowl of a stand mixer, combine the heavy cream, monk fruit sweetener, and vanilla. Using a hand mixer or the stand mixer's whisk attachment, whip on medium-high speed until stiff peaks form, about 3 minutes. Be careful not to overbeat. Add the Greek yogurt and whip on medium just until incorporated, about 30 seconds.

6. To serve, add ¾ cup of whipped Greek yogurt to a small bowl and top with 2 to 3 tablespoons of the roasted berries and a sprinkle of the candied walnuts.

PREP TIME: 10 MINUTES
COOK TIME: 35 MINUTES
SERVINGS: 3 OR 4

FOR THE ROASTED BERRIES

1 pound mixed fresh berries

2 tablespoons monk fruit sweetener or regular sugar

2 tablespoons freshly squeezed lemon juice

⅛ teaspoon salt

FOR THE CANDIED WALNUTS

½ cup raw walnuts, chopped

1 tablespoon monk fruit sweetener

FOR THE WHIPPED GREEK YOGURT

½ cup heavy cream

½ cup monk fruit sweetener

½ teaspoon vanilla extract

1 cup plain Greek yogurt

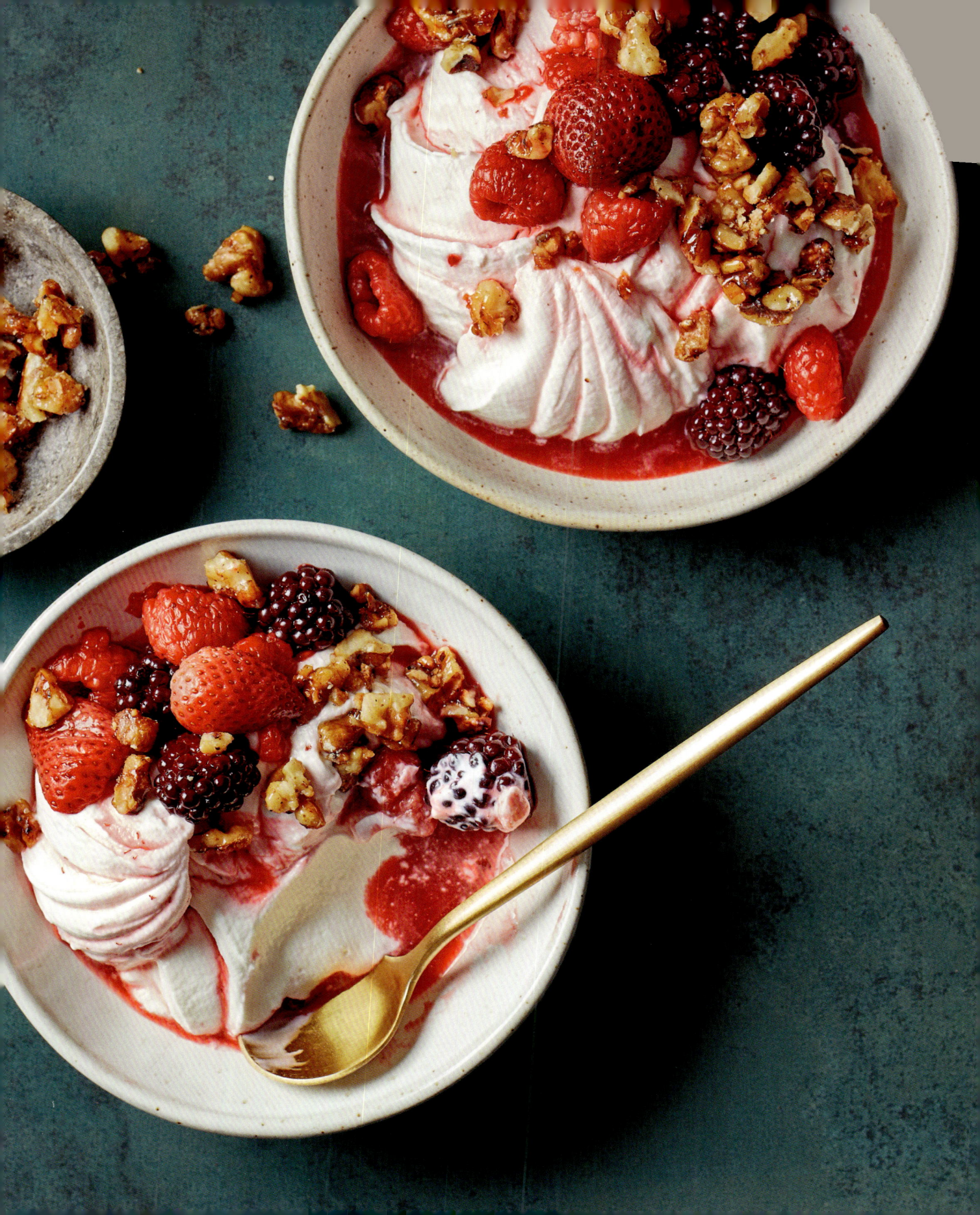

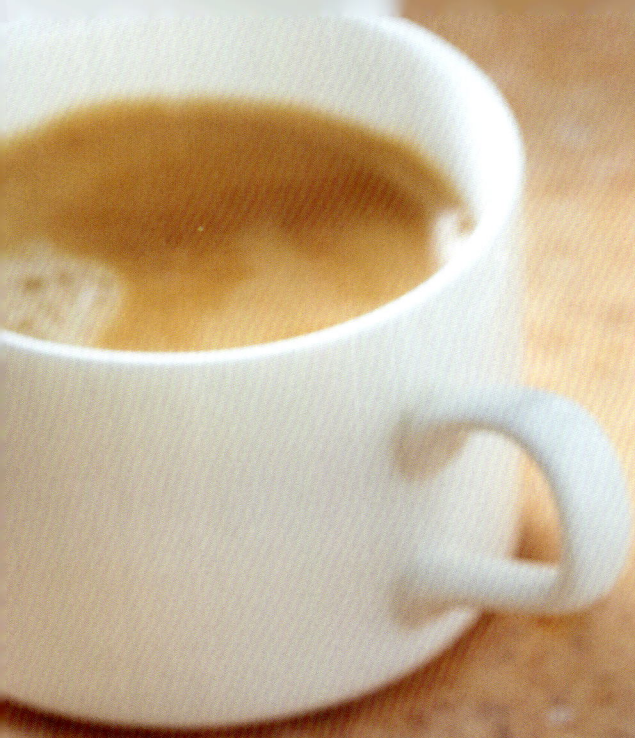

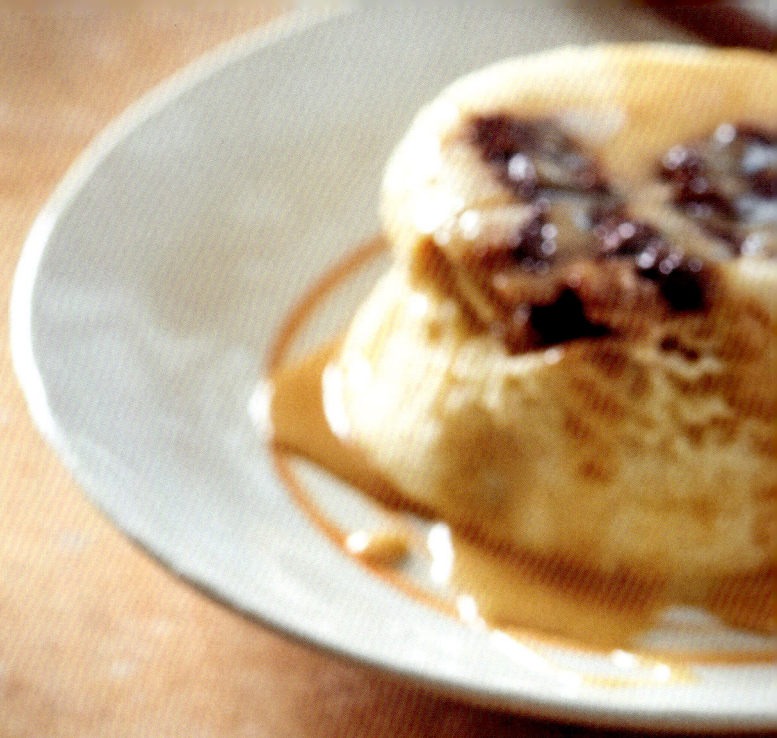

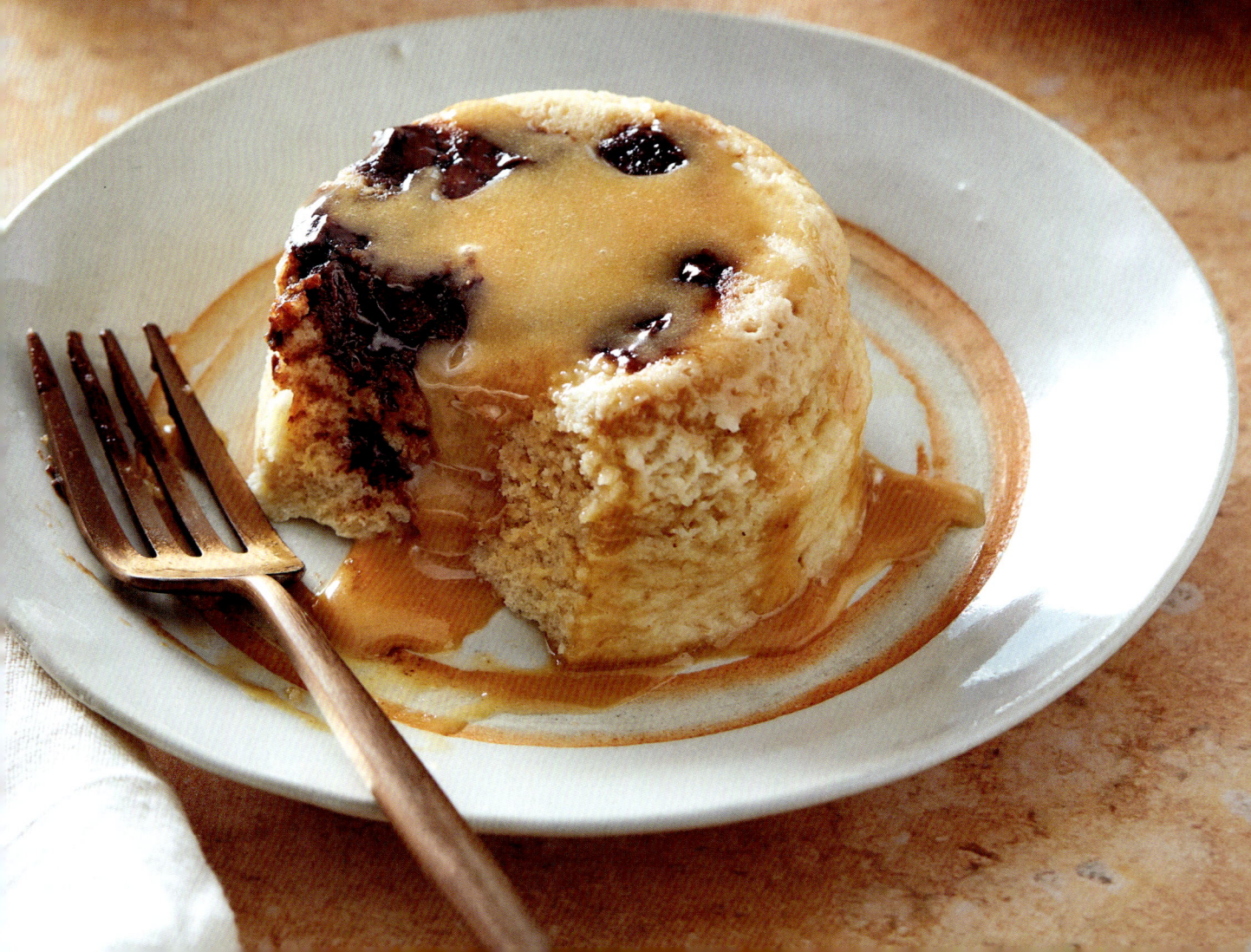

90-Second Peanut Butter Chocolate Mug Cake

This 90-second peanut butter chocolate mug cake is the low-carb-friendly answer to all your sweet cravings. Sour cream is the secret to making the cake deliciously moist. I also add allulose, chocolate chips, and an easy homemade peanut butter glaze to up the indulgence. With just a quick 90-second zap in the microwave, you'll have a warm and super moist single-serving cake that tastes like the real deal.

PREP TIME: 5 MINUTES
COOK TIME: 2 MINUTES
SERVINGS: 1

Neutral oil cooking spray

1 egg white

1½ tablespoons almond flour

½ tablespoon powdered peanut butter

1 tablespoon allulose or sweetener of choice, plus extra for garnish

½ tablespoon baking powder

1 tablespoon sour cream

1½ tablespoons almond milk

15 chocolate chips

FOR THE PEANUT BUTTER GLAZE

½ tablespoon powdered peanut butter

1 tablespoon granulated allulose

2 tablespoons almond milk

½ teaspoon ground cinnamon, for garnish (optional)

1. Spray a large mug with cooking spray.

2. In the mug, combine the egg white (save the yolk for my Smoky Chipotle Aioli [page 208] or an extra-rich omelet), almond flour, powdered peanut butter, allulose, and baking powder.

3. Add the sour cream and almond milk to the dry ingredients.

4. Mix well, then drop in the chocolate chips.

5. Pop the mug into the microwave and microwave for three 30-second increments, 90 seconds in total. With microwaves' intensities varying, this will help control the rise of the mug cake and allow it to cook gradually.

6. **For the peanut butter glaze:** In a small bowl, mix the powdered peanut butter with the allulose and almond milk. Stir well and set aside.

7. Remove the mug cake from the microwave and plate it. (It should slide right out of the mug onto your plate.) Top it with the peanut butter glaze and dust it with some powdered allulose and the cinnamon (if using). You can also enjoy it right out of the mug.

Acknowledgments

I never imagined any of this would happen. I was just a regular guy climbing the corporate ladder in a career that didn't feel right. I lived an unhealthy life and both my physical and mental health suffered. One day in late 2017, I decided to transform my life and begin @shredhappens. At that time, I didn't know how to take photos, make videos, or even how to cook. But as you've learned by now, I did love to eat!

The example my parents set for me growing up undoubtedly gave me the courage and strength to take this big leap in life.

To Maman and Baba: Your sacrifices have instilled in me the confidence and determination to pursue and overcome anything in life. I aspire to be as selfless and generous as you.

To my wife, Madalina: thank you for believing in me when there was nothing. And I really mean nothing. You challenge me to continuously improve, pushing me to levels far beyond what I can grasp in the moment. You're not only an incredible partner but a ferocious coach, motivating me to strive for excellence no matter the task. You never shy away from the tough but necessary conversations. I am the luckiest person in the world.

To Donna Loffredo, Katherine Leak, Theresa Zoro, Odette Fleming, and Abdi Omer, and the rest of the PRH team: Thank you for taking a chance on me as a new author. Donna, I know I can be difficult . . . and . . . persistent. Thank you for advocating for me at every turn.

To Kate Bolen and Zora O'Neill—thank you for your incredible attention to detail and patience with my writing. You've made me so much better.

To Cindy and the CAA team: Thank you for believing in me and seeing the potential in me. I don't take this for granted.

To my incredible cookbook team: Ghazalle Badiozamani, I can't imagine a better photographer to capture the life in each of my recipes. Barrett Washburne, I am forever grateful for your masterful work with each of my dishes. You nailed every single one with such finesse yet so much ease. Paige Hicks, thank you for brilliantly capturing just the right vibe in every shot so perfectly. And of course, Amelia Arend, Paulina Velez, and EJ Muniz—you did all the heavy lifting that made all of this possible.

To Lynne Yeamans, Jenny Davis, and Jan Derevjanik: I couldn't have asked for a more remarkable team for my first cookbook. Thank you for helping bring everything together so beautifully.

To the shredhappens community: Thank you for inviting my recipes and creations into your homes and kitchens. Your stories inspire me to keep going and make my life truly special. Thank you for making this book a reality, because without you, there is no shredhappens.

And finally, to everyone who has supported, encouraged, and believed in me in each stage of my life—thank you from the bottom of my heart. As Steve Jobs once said, "You can't connect the dots looking forward; you can only connect them looking backwards." This book is a result of countless dots somehow being connected over time—each one representing a person, a story, a moment that brought this moment to life. This book is as much yours as it is mine.

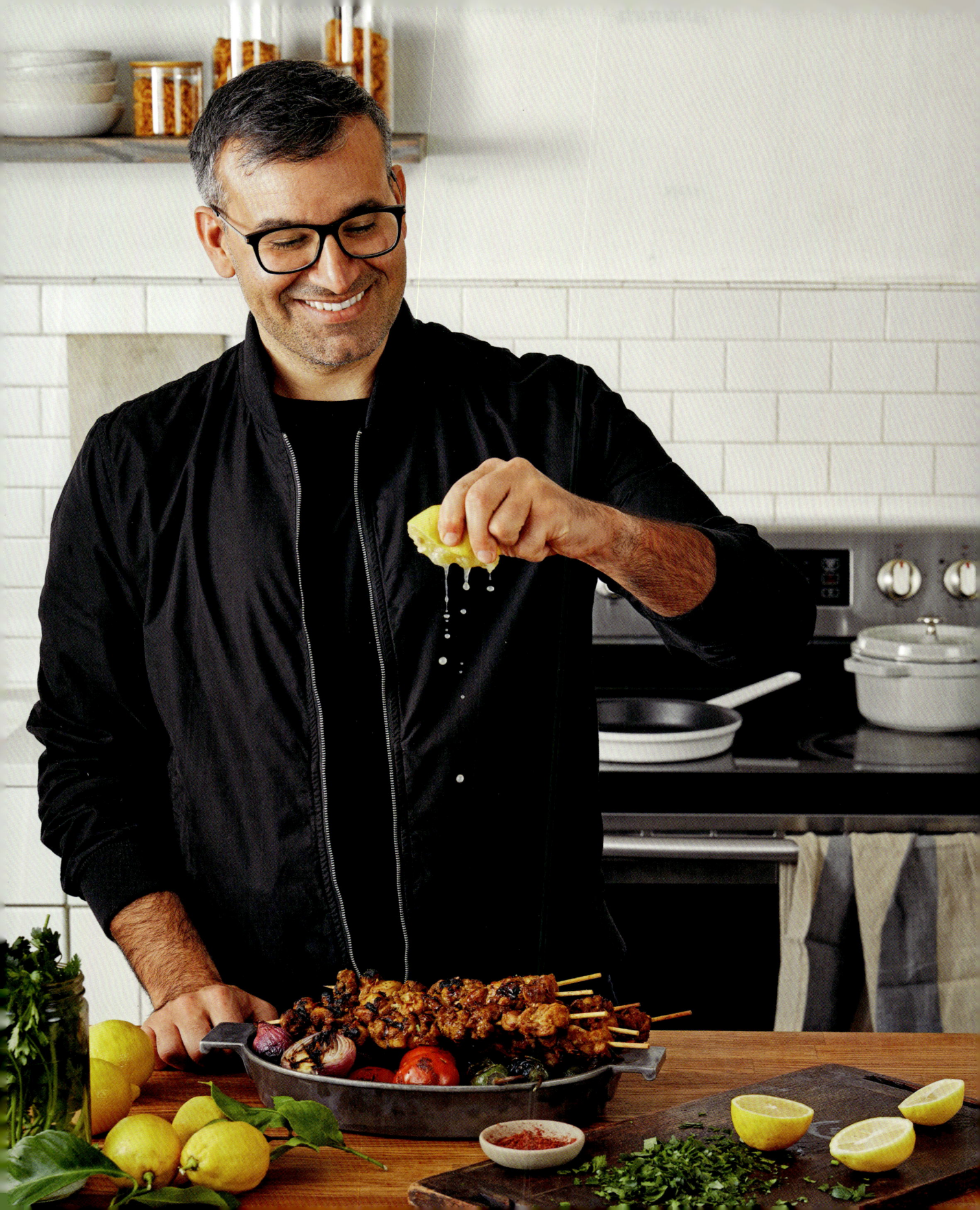

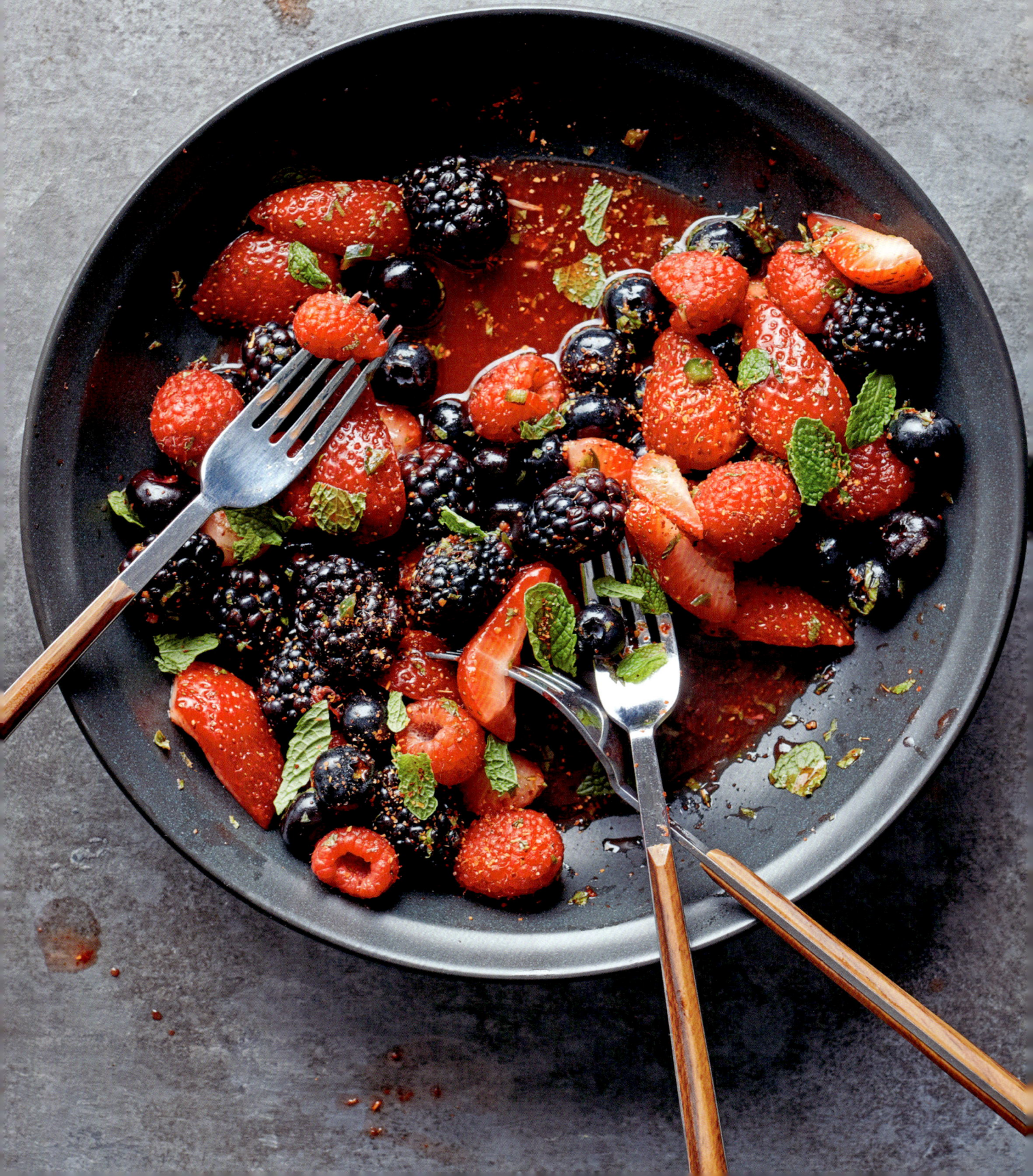

Index

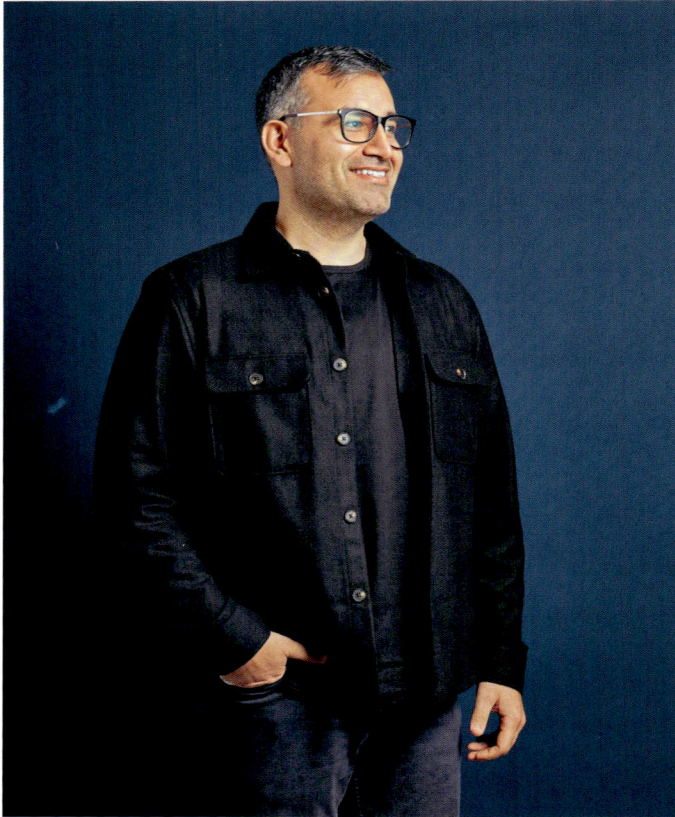

About the Author

ARASH HASHEMI is the creator behind @shredhappens and the co-founder of Kaizen Food Company. Instagram: @ShredHappens